ESSENTIALS

Nursi ship
& Management

EIGHTH EDITION

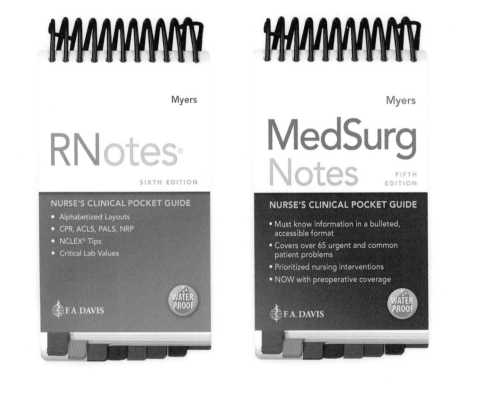

ESSENTIALS OF
Nursing Leadership & Management

EIGHTH EDITION

Sally A. Weiss, EdD, APRN, FNP-C, CNE, ANEF
Faculty
Family Nurse Practitioner Program
Frontier Nursing University
Versailles, Kentucky

Ruth M. Tappen, EdD, RN, FAAN
Christine E. Lynn Eminent Scholar and Professor
Florida Atlantic University College of Nursing
Boca Raton, Florida

Karen A. Grimley, PhD, MBA, RN, NEA-BC, FACHE FAAN
Chief Nursing Executive, UCLA Health
Vice Dean, UCLA School of Nursing
Los Angeles, California

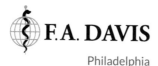

F.A. DAVIS

Philadelphia

F. A. Davis Company
1915 Arch Street
Philadelphia, PA 19103
www.fadavis.com

Printed in the United States of America

Last digit indicates print number: 10 9 8 7 6 5 4 3 2 1

Sponsoring Editor: Haleahy Craven
Content Project Manager: Molly Shaffer
Design and Illustration Manager: Carolyn O'Brien

As new scientific information becomes available through basic and clinical research, recommended treatments and drug therapies undergo changes. The author(s) and publisher have done everything possible to make this book accurate, up to date, and in accord with accepted standards at the time of publication. The author(s), editors, and publisher are not responsible for errors or omissions or for consequences from application of the book, and make no warranty, expressed or implied, in regard to the contents of the book. Any practice described in this book should be applied by the reader in accordance with professional standards of care used in regard to the unique circumstances that may apply in each situation. The reader is advised always to check product information (package inserts) for changes and new information regarding dose and contraindications before administering any drug. Caution is especially urged when using new or infrequently ordered drugs.

Library of Congress Cataloging-in-Publication Data
Names: Weiss, Sally A., 1950- author. | Tappen, Ruth M., author. | Grimley,
    Karen A., author.
Title: Essentials of nursing leadership & management / Sally A. Weiss, Ruth
    M. Tappen, Karen A. Grimley.
Other titles: Essentials of nursing leadership and management
Description: Eighth edition. | Philadelphia, PA : F.A. Davis Company,
    [2024] | Includes bibliographical references and index.
Identifiers: LCCN 2023005799 (print) | LCCN 2023005800 (ebook) | ISBN
    9781719646581 (paperback) | ISBN 9781719649964 (ebook)
Subjects: MESH: Leadership | Nursing, Supervisory | Nursing
    Services--organization & administration | United States
Classification: LCC RT89 (print) | LCC RT89 (ebook) | NLM WY 105 | DDC
    362.17/3068--dc23/eng/20230523
LC record available at https://lccn.loc.gov/2023005799
LC ebook record available at https://lccn.loc.gov/2023005800

Dedication

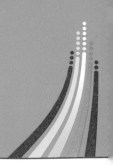

*To my son Stefan and daughter Alyssa,
who understand what it means to continue to grow, strive, and pursue a dream.
To my grandchildren, Sydni, Logan, and Ian,
who taught me that new information and ideas can be learned at any age,
and to my husband, Joel, who has supported me through every edition.*
　　　　—SALLY A. WEISS

*To students, colleagues, family, and friends,
who have taught me so much about leadership.*
　　　　—RUTH M. TAPPEN

*To my kids, Kristina, Kathleen, Meagan, and Ian,
for their love and understanding during this lifelong pursuit of learning.
To my dad for teaching me that the only limits we face are the ones we create,
and to my mom for instilling the value of a good education.*
　　　　—KAREN A. GRIMLEY

Preface

We are pleased to bring our readers this eighth edition of *Essentials of Nursing Leadership & Management*. This new edition has been updated to reflect the dynamic health-care environment, new safety and quality initiatives, diversity, lessons learned during the pandemic, changes in the nursing workforce, and transformations in the nursing practice environment. As in our previous editions, the content, examples, and diagrams were designed with the goal of assisting the new graduate to make the transition to professional nursing practice.

The eighth edition of *Essentials of Nursing Leadership & Management* focuses on essential leadership and management skills and the knowledge needed by the staff nurse as a key member of the interprofessional health-care team and manager of patient care. Issues related to setting priorities, delegation, quality improvement, legal parameters of nursing practice, and ethical issues were also updated for this edition.

This edition discusses current quality and safety issues and the high demands placed on nurses in the current health-care environment. In addition, we continue to bring you comprehensive, practical information on developing a nursing career and addressing the many workplace issues that may arise in practice.

This new edition of *Essentials of Nursing Leadership & Management* will provide a strong foundation for the beginning nurse leader. We want to thank all of the people at F. A. Davis for their continued support and assistance in bringing this edition to fruition. We also want to thank our contributors, reviewers, colleagues, and students for their enthusiastic support. Thank you all.

—SALLY A. WEISS
RUTH M. TAPPEN
KAREN A. GRIMLEY

Reviewers

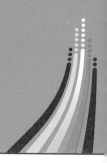

Jenna Boothe, DNP, APRN, FNP-C
Professor
Hazard Community and Technical College
Hazard, Kentucky

Faith Johnson, EdD, MA, BSN, BA,
RN, PHN, CNE
Assistant Faculty
Southwest Minnesota State University
Marshall, Minnesota

Candace Jones, RN, MSN
Professor of Nursing
Greenville Technical College
Greenville, South Carolina

Nancy Mitchell, RN, DNP
Associate Professor
University of South Carolina Aiken
Aiken, South Carolina

Contents

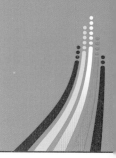

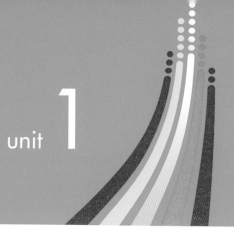

unit 1

Professionalism

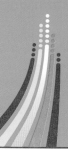

chapter 1

Characteristics of a Profession

OBJECTIVES

After reading this chapter, the student should be able to:

- Explain the qualities associated with a profession.
- Differentiate between a job, a vocation, and a profession.
- Discuss professional behaviors.
- Determine the characteristics associated with nursing as a profession.
- Explain licensure and certification.
- Summarize the relationship between social change and the advancement of nursing as a profession.
- Describe cultural competence and professionalism.
- Discuss some of the issues faced by the nursing profession.
- Explain current changes impacting nursing's future.

Introduction

It is often said that you do not know where you are going until you know where you have been. More than 40 years ago, Beletz (1974) wrote that most people thought of nurses in gender-linked, task-oriented terms: "a female who performs unpleasant technical jobs and functions as an assistant to the physician" (p. 432). Interestingly, physicians in the 1800s viewed nursing as a complement to medicine. According to Warrington (1839), ". . . the prescriptions of the best physician are useless unless they be timely and properly administered and attended to by the nurse" (p. iv).

In its earliest years, most nursing care occurred at home. Even in 1791 when the first hospital opened in Philadelphia, nurses continued to care for patients in their own home settings. It took almost another century before nursing moved into hospitals. These institutions, mostly dominated by male physicians, promoted the idea that nurses acted as "handmaidens" to the better-educated, more capable men in the medical field.

The level of care differed greatly in these early health-care institutions. Those operated by the religious nursing orders gave high-quality care to patients. In others, care varied greatly from good to almost none at all. Although the image of nurses and nursing has advanced considerably since then, some still think of nurses as helpers who carry out the physician's orders.

However, throughout nursing's history, nurses discovered ways to work independently, yet in tandem with the medical profession. The history of public health nursing, the Frontier Nursing Service, and advanced practice nursing provide examples of nursing ingenuity (Breckinridge, 1952; Kub, Kulbok, Miner & Merrill, 2017; Roux & Halstead, 2018). During each of these advances, the country and, at times, the world found themselves immersed in turmoil when struggling to provide health care to individuals. It comes as no surprise that nursing and health care have converged and reached a crossing point. Nurses face a new age for human experience; the very foundations of health practices and therapeutic interventions continue to be dramatically altered by significantly transformed scientific, technological, cultural, political, and social realities (Porter-O'Grady, 2003). The global environment needs nurses more than ever to meet the health-care needs of all. This call to action was seen most recently during the COVID pandemic of 2019 as nurses stepped forward to care for individuals from all walks of life (Luis & Vance, 2020).

Nursing sees itself as a profession rather than a job or vocation and continues with this quest for its place among the health-care disciplines. However, what defines a profession? What behaviors are expected from the members of the profession? Chapter 1 discusses nursing as a profession with its own identity and place within this new and ever-changing health-care system.

Professionalism

Definition of a Profession

A vocation or calling defines "meaningful work" depending on an individual's point of view (Dik & Duffy, 2009). Nursing started as a vocation or "calling." Until Nightingale, most nursing occurred through religious orders. To care for the ill and infirmed was a duty (Kalisch & Kalisch, 2004). In the early years, despite the education required, nursing was considered a job or vocation (Cardillo, 2013).

Professionalism represents a "quality," and providing a definition for a "profession" or "professional" is not as easy as it appears. The term is used all the time; however, what characteristics define a professional? Professionalism is not how you do the job, but how you do the job you do (Feissner, 2015). According to Saks (2012), several theoretical approaches have been applied to creating a definition of a profession, the older of these looking only at knowledge and expertise, whereas later ones include a code of ethics, practice standards, licensure, and certification, as well as expected behaviors (Post, 2014).

Nurses engage in specialized education and training confirmed by successfully passing the National Council Licensure Examination (NCLEX®) and receiving a license to practice in each state. Nurses follow a code of ethics and recognized practice standards and a body of continuous research that forms and directs our practice. Nurses function autonomously within the designated scope of practice, formulating and delivering a plan of care for clients, applying judgments, and utilizing critical thinking skills in decision making (Cardillo, 2013).

Nurses view professionalism as analogous to holding appropriate knowledge about a specific discipline in care delivery accompanied by experience and autonomy (Shohani &

Zamanzadeh, 2017). In today's global health-care environment, nurses experience a new professional independence which requires changing previous definitions for roles and performance (Shohani & Zamanzadeh, 2017).

Present health-care demands have altered nursing's role within the environment. The realization of the impact the nursing profession exerts on health-care and patient outcomes came to the attention of the public during the pandemic as nurses used their knowledge and skills to make judgments that affected patients, families, and local and global communities.

Professional Behaviors

According to Post (2014), professional characteristics or behaviors include:

- Consideration
- Empathy
- Respect
- Ethical and moral values
- Accountability
- Commitment to lifelong learning
- Honesty

In addition, in today's world, professionalism entails having cultural intelligence or the ability to adapt to new cultural environments (Ang, Rockstuhl & Tan, 2015). Workplaces today represent the cultural diversity of the communities nurses service. This welcomed change opens new opportunities but also presents challenges to the "status quo." Incorporating cultural intelligence into professional behaviors is a process and incorporates skills such as cultural competence and cultural humility. It requires a recognition of others' beliefs, values, and practices and a commitment to respect the differences that exist without placing judgment.

Professionalism denotes a commitment to carry out specialized responsibilities and observe ethical principles while remaining responsive to diverse recipients (Al-Rubaish, 2010). Communicating effectively and courteously within the work environment is expected professional behavior. State boards of nursing through the nurse practice acts elaborate expected behaviors in a registered nurse's (RN) professional practice and personal life (National Council of State Boards of Nursing [NCSBN], 2012, 2016). Nurses may lose their licenses for a variety of actions deemed unprofessional or illegal. For example, inappropriate use of social media, posting emotionally charged statements in blogs or forums, driving without a license, and committing felonies outside of professional practice may be cause for suspending or revoking a nursing license.

Commitment to others remains central to a profession. In nursing, this entails commitment to colleagues, lifelong learning, and accountability for one's actions. Professionalism in the workplace means coming to work when scheduled and on time. Coming late to work shows disrespect to your peers and colleagues. It also indicates to your supervisor that this position is not important to you.

Always portray a positive attitude. Although everyone experiences a bad day, projecting personal feelings and issues onto others affects the work environment. Many agencies and institutions have dress codes. Dress appropriately per the employer's expectations. Wearing heavy makeup, colognes, or inappropriate hairstyles demonstrates a lack of professionalism. Finally, always speak professionally to everyone in the work environment. A good rule to follow should be, "If you wouldn't say it in front of your grandmother, do not say it in the workplace" (McKay, 2017).

Work politics often create an unfavorable environment. Stay away from gossip or engaging in negative comments about others in the workplace. Change the topic or indicate a lack of interest in this type of verbal exchange. Negativity is contagious and affects workplace morale. Professionals maintain a positive attitude in the work environment. If the environment affects this attitude, it is time to look for another position (McKay, 2017).

Lastly, professional behavior entails honesty and accountability. If a day off is needed, take a personal or vacation day; save sick days for illness. Own up to errors. In nursing, an error may result in injury or death. The health-care environment should promote a culture of safety, not one of punishment for errors. This is discussed more in later chapters.

Evolution of Nursing as a Profession

Nursing Defined

The changes that have occurred in nursing are reflected in the definitions of nursing that have developed through time. In 1859, Florence Nightingale defined the goal of nursing as putting the client "in the best possible condition for nature to act upon him" (Nightingale, 1992/1859, p. 79).

In 1966, Virginia Henderson focused her definition on the uniqueness of nursing:

> *The unique function of the nurse is to assist the individual, sick or well, in the performance of those activities contributing to health or its recovery (or to peaceful death) that he would perform unaided if he had the necessary strength, will or knowledge. And to do this in such a way as to help him gain independence as rapidly as possible. (Henderson, 1966, p. 21)*

Martha Rogers defined *nursing practice* as "the process by which this body of knowledge, nursing science, is used for the purpose of assisting human beings to achieve maximum health within the potential of each person" (Rogers, 1988, p. 100). Rogers emphasized that nursing is concerned with *all* people, only some of whom are ill.

In the modern nursing era, nurses are viewed as collaborative members of the health-care team. Nursing has emerged as a strong field of its own in which nurses have a wide range of obligations, responsibilities, and accountability. Recent polls show that nurses are considered the most trusted group of professionals because of their knowledge, expertise, and ability to care for diverse populations.

Nightingale's concepts of nursing care became the basis of modern theory development, and in today's language, she used evidence-based practice to promote nursing. Her 1859 book *Notes on Nursing: What It Is and What It Is Not* laid the foundation for modern nursing education and practice. Many nursing theorists have used Nightingale's thoughts as a basis for constructing their view of nursing.

Nightingale believed that schools of nursing must be independent institutions and that women who were selected to attend the schools should be from the higher levels of society. Many of Nightingale's beliefs about nursing education are still applicable, particularly those involved with the progress of students, the use of diaries kept by students, and the need for integrating theory into clinical practice (Roberts, 1937).

The Nightingale school served as a model for nursing education. Its graduates were sought worldwide. Many of them established schools and became matrons (superintendents) in hospitals in other parts of England, the British Commonwealth, and the United States. However, very few schools were able to remain financially independent of the hospitals and thus lost much of their autonomy. This was in contradiction to Nightingale's philosophy that the training schools were educational institutions, not part of any service agency.

The National Council Licensure Examination

Professions require advanced education and an advanced area of knowledge and training. Many are regulated in some way and have a licensure or certification requirement to enter practice. This holds true for teachers, attorneys, physicians, and pilots, just to name a few. The purpose of a professional license is to ensure public safety, by setting a level of standard that indicates an individual has acquired the necessary knowledge and skills to enter into the profession.

Licensure

Licensure for nurses is defined by the NCSBN as the process by which boards of nursing grant permission to an individual to engage in nursing practice after determining that the applicant has attained the competency necessary to perform a unique scope of practice. Licensure is necessary when the regulated activities are complex, require specialized knowledge and skill, and involve independent decision making (NCSBN, 2012). Government agencies grant licenses allowing an individual to engage in a professional practice and use a specific title. State boards of nursing issue nursing licenses. This limits practice to a specific jurisdiction. However, as the NCLEX® is a nationally recognized examination, many states have joined together to form a "compact" where the license in one state is recognized in another. States belonging to the compact passed legislation adopting the terms of the agreement. The state in which the nurse resides is considered the home state, and license renewal occurs in the home state (NCSBN, 2018).

Licensure may be mandatory or permissive. Permissive licensure is a voluntary arrangement whereby an individual chooses to become licensed to demonstrate competence. However, in this situation a mandatory license is not required to practice. Mandatory licensure requires a nurse to be licensed in order to practice. In the United States and Canada, licensure is mandatory.

Licensure by Endorsement

If a state is not a member of the compact, nurses licensed in one state may obtain a license in another state through the process of endorsement. Each application is considered independently and is granted a license based on the rules and regulations of the state.

States differ in the number of continuing education credits required, mandatory courses, and other educational requirements. Some states may require that nurses meet the current criteria for licensure at the time of application, whereas others may grant the license based on the criteria in effect at the time of the original license. When applying for a license through endorsement, a nurse should always contact the board of nursing for the state and ask about the exact requirements for licensure in that state. This information is usually found on the state board of nursing Web site.

NURSYS is a national database that houses information on licensed nurses. Nurses applying for licensure by endorsement may verify their licenses through this database. The nurse's license verification is available immediately to the endorsing board of nursing (NCSBN, 2016). Not all states belong to NURSYS.

Qualifications for Licensure

The basic qualification for licensure requires graduation from an approved nursing program. In the United States, each state may add additional requirements, such as disclosures regarding health or medications that could affect practice. Most states require disclosure of criminal conviction.

Licensure by Examination

A major accomplishment in the history of nursing licensure was the creation of the Bureau of State Boards of Nurse Examiners. The formation of this agency led to the development of an identical examination in all states. The original examination, called the State Board Test Pool Examination, was created by the testing department of the National League for Nursing (NLN). This was completed through a collaborative contract with the state boards. Initially, each state determined its own passing score; however, the states did eventually adopt a common passing score. The examination is called the NCLEX-RN® and is used in all states and territories of the United States. This test is prepared and administered through a professional testing company.

NCLEX-RN®

The NCLEX-RN® is administered through computerized adaptive testing (CAT). Candidates need to register to take the examination at an approved testing center in the state in which they intend to practice. Because of a large test bank, CAT permits a variety of questions to be administered to a group of candidates. Candidates taking the examination at the same time may not necessarily receive the same questions. Once a candidate answers a question, the computer analyzes the response and then chooses an appropriate question to ask next. If the candidate answers the question correctly, the following question may be more difficult; if the candidate answers incorrectly, the next question may be easier.

In April 2016, the NCSBN released the updated test plan. The new test plan redistributed the percentages for each content area and updated the question format with increased use of technology that better simulated patient care situations. More updated information on the NCLEX® test plans may be found on the NCSBN Web site (www.ncsbn.org).

Political Influences and the Advance of Nursing Professionals

Nursing made many advances during the time of social upheaval and change. The passing of the Social Security Act in 1935 strengthened public health services. Public health nursing found itself in an ideal position to step up and assume responsibility for providing care to dependent mothers and children, the blind, and disabled children (Black, 2014). In 1965, under President Lyndon B. Johnson, amendments to the Social Security Act designed to ensure access to health care for the elder adult, the poor, and the disabled resulted in the creation of Medicare and Medicaid (Centers for Medicare and Medicaid Services [CMS], 2017). Health insurance companies emerged and increased in number during this time as well. Hospitals started to rely on Medicare, Medicaid, and insurance reimbursement for services. Care for the sick and new opportunities and roles emerged for nurses within this environment.

Historically, as a profession, nursing has made most of its advances during times of social change. The 1960s through the 1980s brought many changes for both women and nursing. In 1964, President Johnson signed the Civil Rights Act, which guaranteed equal treatment for all individuals and prohibited gender discrimination in the workplace. However, the law lacked enforcement. During this time, the feminist movement gained momentum, and the National Organization for Women was founded to help women achieve equality and give women a voice. Nursing moved forward as well. Specialty care disciplines developed. Advances in technology gave way to the more complex medical–surgical treatments such as cardiothoracic surgery, complex neurosurgical techniques, and the emergence of intensive care environments to care for these patients. These changes fostered the development of specialization for nurses and physicians, creating a shortage of primary care physicians. The public demanded increased access to health care, and nursing again stepped forward by developing an advanced practice role for nurses to meet the primary health-care needs of the public.

Throughout the years, wars created situations that facilitated changes in nursing and its role within society. Wars increased the nation's need for nurses and the public's awareness of nursing's role in society (Kalisch & Kalisch, 2004). Nurses served in the military during both world wars and the Korean conflict and changed nursing practice during the time of war. For the first time, nurses were close to the front and worked in mobile hospital units. Often they lacked necessary supplies and equipment (Kalisch & Kalisch, 2004). They found themselves in situations where they needed to function independently and make immediate decisions, often assuming roles normally associated with the physicians and surgeons.

The Vietnam War afforded nurses opportunities to push beyond the boundaries as they functioned in mobile hospital units in the war theater, often without direct supervision of physicians. These nurses performed emergency procedures such as tracheostomies and chest tube insertions in order to preserve the lives of the wounded soldiers (Texas Tech University, 2017). After functioning independently in the field, many nurses felt restricted by the practice limits placed on them when they returned home.

Challenges for society and nurses continued from the 1980s through 2000. The 1980s were marked by the emergence of HIV and AIDS. Although we know more about HIV and AIDs today than we knew more than 30 years ago, society's fear of the disease stigmatized groups of individuals and created fear among global populations and health-care providers. Nurses became instrumental in educating the public and working directly with infected individuals.

The increase in available technology allowed for the widespread use of life-support systems. Nurses working in critical care areas often faced ethical dilemmas involving the use of these technologies. During this time period, nurses voiced their opinions and concerns and helped in formulating policies addressing these issues within their communities and institutions. The field of hospice nursing received a renewed interest and support (National Hospice and Palliative Care Organization [NHPCO], 2012); therefore, the number of hospice care providers grew and opened new opportunities for nurses.

The first part of the 21st century introduced nurses to situations beyond anyone's imagination. Nursing's response to the terrorist attack on the World Trade Center and during the onset and aftermath of Hurricane Katrina raised multiple questions regarding nurses' abilities to react to major disasters. Nurses, physicians, and other health-care providers attempted to care for and protect patients under horrific conditions. Nurses found themselves trying to function "during unfamiliar and unusual conditions with the health-care environment that may necessitate adaptations to recognized standards of nursing practice" (American Nurses Association [ANA], 2006).

Nursing has recognized the need for the profession to understand and function during human-caused and natural disasters such as 9/11 and hurricanes. The profession has answered the call by increasing disaster preparedness training for nurses.

Nursing and Health-Care Reform

For more than 40 years, Florence Nightingale played an influential part in most of the important health-care reforms of her time. Her accomplishments went beyond the scope of nursing and nursing education, affecting all aspects of health care and social reform.

Nightingale contributed to health-care reform through her work during the Crimean War, where she greatly improved the health and well-being of the British soldiers. She kept accurate records and accountings of her interventions and outcomes, and on her return to England, she continued this work and reformed the conditions in hospitals and health care.

The 21st century brings both challenges and opportunities for nursing. It is estimated that more than 434,000 nurses will be needed by the year 2024

(Bureau of Labor Statistics [BLS], 2017). The severe nursing shortage has increased the demand for more nurses, whereas the passing of the Affordable Care Act (ACA) offers opportunities for nurses to take the lead in providing primary health care to those who need it. More advanced practice nurses (APRNs) will be needed to address the needs of the diverse population in this country. Health-care reform is discussed in more detail in Chapter 16.

Nursing Today

Issues specific to nursing reflect the problems and concerns of the health-care system as a whole. The average age of nurses in the United States is 52 years, with nurses age 65 or older making up 19% of the workforce (Smiley et al., 2020). Because of changes in the economy, many nurses who planned to retire have instead found it necessary to remain in the workforce. However, the recent data collected also noted an increase in men entering the field as well as an increase in younger and more diverse populations seeking nursing careers. As of the 2020 NCSBN statistics, men comprised 9.4% of the RN workforce.

Concerns about the supply of RNs and staffing shortages persist in both the United States and abroad. For the first time, multiple generations of nurses find themselves working together within the health-care environment. The oldest of the generations, the early baby boomers, planned to retire during the last several years; however, economics have forced many to remain in the workplace. They presently work alongside Generation X (born between 1965 and 1979) and the generation known as the millennials (born in 1980 and later). Nurses from the baby boomer generation and Generation X provide the majority of bedside care; whereas the millennials find themselves comfortable with technology, the baby boomers feel the "old ways" worked well.

Generational issues in the nursing workforce present potential conflicts in the work environment as these generations come with differing viewpoints culturally and ethically, as they attempt to work together within the health-care community (Bragg, 2014; Moore, Everly & Bauer, 2016). Each generation brings its own set of core values to the workplace. In order to be successful and work together as cohesive teams, each generation needs to value the others' skills and perspectives. This requires active and assertive communication, recognizing the individual skill sets and cultural perspective of the generations, and placing individuals in positions that fit their specific characteristics.

The related issues of excessive workload, mandatory overtime, scheduling, abuse, workplace violence, and lack of professional autonomy contribute to the concerns regarding the nursing shortage (Clarke, 2015; Spurlock, 2020; Wheatley, 2017).

The coronavirus (COVID-19) pandemic added additional strain to the health-care system globally and nationally. However, the situation proved the professionalism, resiliency, and agility of nurses to assume responsibility and take a leadership role during this uncertain and stressful time. Maintaining a positive professional outlook continues to be critical for an effective response to unexpected and unparalleled disaster situations (Jeong & Kim, 2022). It also brought forward the multitude of issues nurses face in the workplace including staffing issues, increased patient acuity, and lack of recognition for their own self-care and mental health needs. These issues impact the workplace environment and often place patients at risk. Professional behavior requires respect and integrity, as well as safe practice (Spurlock, 2020).

The Future of Professional Nursing

The changes in health care and the increased need for primary care providers have opened the door for nursing. The Institute of Medicine (IOM, 2010) report specifically stated that nurses should be permitted to practice to the full extent of their education. Nurses are educated to care for individuals who have chronic illnesses and need health teaching and monitoring.

APRNs are qualified to diagnose and treat certain conditions. These highly educated nurses are more than physician extenders as they sit for board certification examinations and are licensed by the states in which they practice. Educational requirements for APRNs include a minimum of a master's degree in nursing with a clinical focus and a designated number of clinical hours. Many nurse practitioners are obtaining the doctor of nursing practice (DNP) degree. The American Association of Critical Care Nurses (AACN) and the NLN both promote this as the terminal degree for nurse practitioners. Areas of advanced practice include family nurse practitioner, acute care nurse practitioner, pediatric nurse practitioner, and certified nurse–midwife.

Conclusion

Professional behavior is an important component of nursing practice. It is outlined and guided by state nurse practice acts, the ethical codes, and standards of practice. Acting professionally both while in the workplace and in one's personal life is also an expectation. As nursing moves forward in the 21st century, the need for committed professionals and innovative nurse leaders is greater than ever. Society's demand for high-quality health care at an affordable cost is now law and an impetus for change in how nurses function in the new environment.

Employers, colleagues, and peers depend on new nurses to act professionally and provide safe, quality patient care. Taking advantage of expanding educational opportunities, engaging in lifelong learning, and seeking certification in a specialty demonstrate professional commitment.

Nursing has its roots as a calling and vocation. It originated in the community, moved to hospitals, returned to the community, and is now seen in multiple practice settings. The ACA has opened doors for more opportunities for nurses, and the IOM report on the *Future of Nursing* states that nurses need to be permitted to use their educational skills in the health-care environment.

Often students ask the question: "So what can I do? I am a new graduate." Get involved in your profession by joining organizations and becoming politically active. Continue pursuing excellence and set the stage for those who will come after you.

Study Questions

1. Read *Notes on Nursing: What It Is and What It Is Not* by Florence Nightingale. How much of its content is still true today?

2. What is your definition of nursing? How does it compare or contrast with Virginia Henderson's definition?

3. Review the mission and purpose of the ANA or another national nursing organization online. Do you believe that nurses should belong to these organizations? Explain your answer.

4. Professional behaviors include a commitment to lifelong learning. What does "lifelong learning" mean beyond mandatory continuing education?

5. Formulate your plan to prepare for the NCLEX®.

Case Studies to Promote Clinical Judgment

Case I

Thomas went to nursing school on a U.S. Public Health Service scholarship. He has been directed to go to a rural village in a small Central American country to work in a local health center. Several other nurses have been sent to this village, and the residents forced them to leave.

The village lacks electricity and plumbing; water comes from in-ground wells. The villagers and children suffer from frequent episodes of gastrointestinal disorders.

1. How do you think Florence Nightingale would have approached these issues?

2. What do you think Thomas should do first to gain the trust of the residents of the village?

3. Explain how APRNs would contribute to the health and welfare of the residents of the village.

Case II

The younger nurses in your health-care institution have created a petition to change the dress code policy. They feel it is antiquated and rigid. Rather than wearing uniforms or scrubs on the nursing units, they would prefer to wear more contemporary clothing such as khakis and nice shirts with the agency logo along with laboratory coats. The older-generation nurses feel that this will detract from the nursing image, as patients expect nurses to dress in uniforms or scrubs and this is what defines them as a "profession."

1. What are your thoughts regarding the image of nursing and uniforms?

2. Do you feel that uniforms define nurses? Explain your reasoning.

3. Explain the reasons certain generations may see this as a threat to their professionalism.

4. Which side would you support? Explain your answer with current research.

Case III

Remy is a 40-year-old Vietnamese nurse who was born in this country to first-generation Vietnamese American parents. His grandparents escaped from Saigon in 1974. After completing his master of science degree as an acute care clinical specialist, he was promoted to the role of nurse manager of the emergency department (ED) even though he had only worked in the ED for 2 years. Remy maintains many of his cultural values and beliefs including practicing Buddhism. Since becoming the manager of the ED, Remy has confronted various forms of cultural ignorance and bias. Lately, a small group of nurses has started making comments about the food he brings and his meditation practices, and have begun isolating from him during meals and breaks. These behaviors seem to be instigated by one or two other members of the staff.

1. As a professional within this setting, how might you address this behavior?

2. What importance would cultural intelligence have in this situation?

3. What actions might you take as a leader to indicate that you view this as unprofessional behavior?

NCLEX®-Style Review Questions

1. Nursing has its origins with
   1. Florence Nightingale
   2. The Knights of Columbus
   3. Religious orders
   4. Wars and battles

2. Who stated that the "function of the nurse is to assist the individual, sick or well, in the performance of those activities contributing to health or its recovery (or to peaceful death)"?
   1. Henderson
   2. Rogers
   3. Robb
   4. Nightingale

3. You are participating in a clinical care coordination conference for a patient with terminal cancer. You talk with your colleagues about using the nursing code of ethics for professional RNs to guide care decisions. A non-nursing colleague asks about this code. Which of the following statements best describes this code?
   1. It improves communication between the nurse and the patient.
   2. It protects the patient's right of autonomy.
   3. It ensures identical care to all patients.
   4. It acts as a guide for professional behaviors in giving patient care.

4. The NCLEX® for nurses is exactly the same in every state in the United States. The examination
    1. Guarantees safe nursing care for all patients
    2. Ensures standard nursing care for all patients
    3. Ensures that honest and ethical care is provided
    4. Provides a minimal standard of knowledge for an RN in practice

5. APRNs generally: **Select all that apply.**
    1. Function independently
    2. Function as unit directors
    3. Work in acute care settings
    4. Work in the university setting
    5. Hold advanced degrees

6. Nurses at a community hospital are in an education program to learn how to use a new pressure-relieving device for patients at risk for pressure ulcers. This is which type of education?
    1. Continuing education
    2. Graduate education
    3. In-service education
    4. Professional RN education

7. Which of the following is unique to a professional standard of decision making? **Select all that apply.**
    1. Weighs benefits and risks when making a decision
    2. Analyzes and examines choices more independently
    3. Utilizes concrete thinking
    4. Anticipates when to make choices without others' assistance

8. Nursing practice in the 21st century is an art and science that focuses on
    1. The client
    2. The nursing process
    3. Cultural diversity
    4. The health-care facility

9. Which of the following represent the knowledge and skills expected of the professional nurse? **Select all that apply.**
    1. Accountability
    2. Advocacy
    3. Autonomy
    4. Social networking
    5. Participation in nursing blogs

10. Professional accountability serves the following purpose: **Select all that apply.**
    1. To provide a basis for ethical decision making
    2. To respect the decision of the client
    3. To maintain standards of health
    4. To evaluate new professional practices and reassess existing ones
    5. To belong to a professional organization

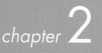
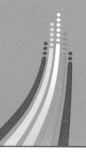

chapter 2

Professional Ethics and Values

OBJECTIVES

After reading this chapter, the student should be able to:

- Discuss ways individuals form values.
- Differentiate between laws and ethics.
- Explain the relationship between personal ethics and professional ethics.
- Examine various ethical theories.
- Explore the concept of virtue ethics.
- Apply ethical principles to an ethical issue.
- Evaluate the influence organizational ethics exerts on nursing practice.
- Identify an ethical dilemma in the clinical setting.
- Discuss current ethical issues in health care and possible solutions.

Doctors at the Massachusetts General Hospital for Children faced an ethical challenge when a pair of conjoined twins born in Africa arrived several years ago seeking surgery that could save only one of them. The twins were connected at the abdomen and pelvis, sharing a liver and bladder, and had three legs. An examination by doctors at the hospital determined that only one of the girls was likely to survive the surgery, but that if doctors did not act, both would die. The case had posed the hospital with the challenge both of ensuring that the parents understood the risks of the procedure and that the hundreds of medical professionals needed to perform the complex series of operations to separate the children were comfortable with the ethics of the situation (Malone, 2017). Which child should live, and which child should die?

This is only one of many modern ethical dilemmas faced by health-care personnel. If you were a member of the ethics committee, what decision might you make? How would you come to that decision? Which twin would live and which would die?

In previous centuries, health-care practitioners had neither the knowledge nor the technology to make determinations regarding prolonging life, sustaining life, or even creating life. The main function of nurses and physicians was to support patients and families through times of illness, help them toward recovery, or provide comfort until death. There were very few complicated decisions such as, "Who shall live and who shall die?" During the latter part of the 20th century and through the first part of the 21st century, technological advances such as multiple-organ transplantation, use of stem cells, new biologically based pharmaceuticals, artificial intelligence (AI) and robotics, and sophisticated life-support systems created unique situations stimulating serious conversations and debates. The costs of these life-saving treatments and technologies presented new dilemmas as to who should provide and pay for them, as well as who should receive them.

Health care saw its first technological advances in 1943 when Willem Kolff, a Dutch physician, built the first dialysis machine (Henderson, 2009). The next major advancement occurred during 1947 and 1948 as the polio epidemic raged through Europe and the United States. This devastating disease initiated the development of units for patients who required manual ventilation (the "iron lung"). During this period, Danish physicians invented a method of manual ventilation by placing a tube into the trachea of polio patients. This initiated the creation of mechanical ventilation as we know it today. The development of mechanical ventilation required more intensive nursing care and patient observation. The care and monitoring of patients proved to be more efficient when nurses kept patients in a single care area, hence the term *intensive care.*

In 1954, Dr. Richard Lawler performed the first kidney transplant in the United States. However, due to the lack of immunosuppressive therapies, the patient rejected the kidney. This sparked an interest in organ transplantation, but the ethics of obtaining organs for transplant emerged as an issue (Barker & Markmann, 2013). The late 1960s brought greater technological advances. Open heart surgery, in its infancy at the time, became available for patients who were seriously ill with cardiovascular disease. These patients required specialized nursing care and nurses specifically educated in the use of advancing technologies. These new therapies and monitoring methods provided the impetus for the creation of intensive care units and the critical care nursing specialty (Vincent, 2013).

In the past, the vast majority of individuals receiving critical care services would have died. However, the development of new drugs and advances in biomechanical technology permit health-care personnel to challenge nature. These advances have enabled providers to offer patients treatments that in many cases increase their life expectancy and enhance their quality of life. However, this progress is not without its shortcomings as it also presents new perplexing questions.

The ability to prolong life has created some heart-wrenching situations for families and complex ethical dilemmas for health-care professionals. Decisions regarding terminating life support on an adolescent involved in a motor vehicle accident, instituting life support on a 65-year-old productive father, or sanctioning a mother's pregnancy in order to provide stem cells for her older child who has a terminally ill disease are just a few examples. At what point do parents say good-bye to their neonate who was born far too early to survive outside the womb? Families and professionals face some of the most difficult ethical decisions at times such as these. How is death defined? When does it occur? Perhaps these questions need to be asked: "What is life? Is there a difference between life and living?"

More recently, the pandemic brought forward ethical issues for providers, patients, and families. The safety of nurses and other providers who worked on the front lines also presented ethical issues for the health-care community (Morley et al., 2020). Initially, the scarcity of appropriate medications and technological resources along with the lack of personal protective equipment (PPE) triggered more questions than answers. Which patients should receive monoclonal antibodies and/or other medications? Who should be placed on a ventilator? Should PPE be reused or recycled?

To find answers to these questions, health-care professionals look to philosophy, especially the branch that deals with human behavior. Through time, to assist in dealing with these issues, the field of biomedical ethics (or simply bioethics) evolved. This subdiscipline of ethics, the philosophical study of morality, is the study of medical morality, which concerns the moral and social implications of health care and science in human life (Numminen et al., 2017). The rapid developments in technology make this subdiscipline more important as health-care professionals and scientists face greater challenges such as questions regarding who owns medical and genetic data. How do we set boundaries on our capabilities of significantly improving physical or cognitive human skills and aptitudes? These continuous advancements bring forward unique moral, ethical, and legal issues (Piergentili et al., 2021).

In order to understand biomedical ethics, it is important to appreciate the basic concepts of values, belief systems, ethical theories, and morality. The following sections will define these concepts and then discuss ways nurses can help the interprofessional team and families resolve ethical dilemmas.

Values

Individuals talk about value and values all the time. The term *value* refers to the worth of an object or thing. However, the term *values* refers to how individuals feel about ideas, situations, and concepts. *Merriam-Webster's Collegiate Dictionary* defines *value* as the "estimated or appraised worth of something, or that quality of a thing that makes it more or less desirable, useful" (Merriam-Webster Dictionary, 2017). Values, then, are judgments about

the importance or unimportance of objects, ideas, attitudes, and attributes. Individuals incorporate values as part of their conscience and worldview. Values provide a frame of reference and act as pilots to guide behaviors and assist people in making choices.

Morals

Morals arise from an individual's conscience. They act as a guide for individual behavior and are learned through family systems, instruction, and socialization. Morals find their basis within individual values and have a larger social component than values (Ma, 2013). They focus more on "good" versus "bad" behaviors. For example, if you value fairness and integrity, then your morals include those values, and you judge others based on your concept of morality (Maxwell & Narvaez, 2013).

Values and Moral Reasoning

Reasoning is the process of making inferences from a body of information and entails forming conclusions, making judgments, or making inferences from knowledge for the purpose of answering questions, solving problems, and formulating a plan that determines actions (McHugh & Way, 2018). Reasoning allows individuals to think for themselves and not to take the beliefs and judgments of others at face value. Moral reasoning relates to the process of forming conclusions and creating action plans centered on moral or ethical issues.

Values, viewpoints, and methods of moral reasoning have developed through time. Older worldviews have now emerged in modern history, such as the emphasis on virtue ethics or a focus on what type of person one would prefer to become (McLeod-Sordjan, 2014). Virtue ethics are discussed later in this chapter.

Value Systems

A value system is a set of related values. For example, one person may value (believe to be important) societal aspects of life, such as money, objects, and status. Another person may value more abstract concepts such as kindness, charity, and caring. Values may vary significantly, based on an individual's culture, family teachings, and religious upbringing. An individual's system of values frequently affects how that person makes decisions. For example, one person may base a decision on cost, whereas another person placed in the same situation may base the decision on a more abstract quality, such as kindness. Values fall into different categories:

- Intrinsic values are those related to sustaining life, such as food and water (Zimmerman & Zalta, 2014).
- Extrinsic values are not essential to life. They include the value of objects, both physical and abstract. Extrinsic values are not an end in themselves but offer a means of achieving something else. Things, people, and material items are extrinsically valuable (Zimmerman & Zalta, 2014).
- Personal values are qualities that people consider important in their private lives. Concepts such as strong family ties and acceptance by others are personal values.
- Professional values are qualities considered important by a professional group. Autonomy, integrity, and commitment are examples of professional values.

People's behaviors are motivated by values. Individuals take risks, relinquish their own comfort and security, and generate extraordinary efforts because of their values (Zimmerman & Zalta, 2014). Patients who have traumatic brain injuries may overcome tremendous barriers because they value independence. Race car drivers may risk death or other serious injury because they value competition and winning.

- Cultural values are a specific society's or group's core principles that are demonstrated in the attitudes and behaviors of the group. An entire community follows these rules or principles (Hanel et al., 2018).

Values also generate the standards by which people judge others. For example, someone who values work more than leisure activities will look unfavorably on a coworker who refuses to work throughout the weekend. A person who believes that health is more important than wealth would approve of spending money on a relaxing vacation or perhaps joining a health club rather than investing the money. An individual from a culture that values family may forego a long-awaited vacation or trip with friends to attend a family gathering.

Often people adopt the values of individuals they admire. For example, a nursing student may begin to value humor after observing it used effectively with patients. Values provide a guide for decision making and give additional meaning to

life. Individuals develop a sense of satisfaction when they work toward achieving values they believe are important (Tuckett, 2015).

How Values Are Developed

Values are learned (Taylor, 2012). Ethicists attribute the basic question of whether values are taught, inherited, or passed on by some other mechanism to Plato, who lived more than 2,000 years ago. A recent theory suggests that values and moral knowledge are acquired much in the same manner as other forms of knowledge, through real-world experience. Moral knowledge may change over time based on experiences and society's progress (Severini, 2021).

Values can be taught directly, incorporated through societal norms, and modeled through behavior. Children learn by watching their parents, friends, teachers, and religious leaders. Through continuous reinforcement, children eventually learn about and then adopt values as their own. Because of the values they hold dear, people often make great demands on themselves and others, ignoring the personal cost. For example:

> Niesa grew up in a family where educational achievement was highly valued. Not surprisingly, she adopted this as one of her own values. Niesa became a physician, married, and had a son, Dino. She placed a great deal of effort on teaching her son the necessary educational skills in order to get him into the "best private school" in the area. As he moved through the program, his grades did not reflect his mother's great effort, and he felt that he had disappointed his mother as well as himself. By the time Dino reached 9 years of age, he had developed a variety of somatic complaints such as stomach ailments and headaches.
>
> Culture plays a major role in value development. Cultural influences determine what an individual from a specific culture considers important. Cultural values often come into conflict when a situation arises and one individual's cultural background comes into conflict with that of the majority culture (Bian et al., 2019).

Values change with experience and maturity. For example, young children often value objects, such as a favorite blanket or toy. Older children are more likely to value a specific event, such as a family vacation. As children enter adolescence, they place more value on peer opinions than those of their parents. Young adults often place value on certain ideals such as heroism. The values of adults are formed from all these experiences as well as from learning and thought.

The number of values that people hold is not as important as what values they consider important. Choices are influenced by values. The way people use their own time and money, choose friends, link to family, and pursue a career are all influenced by values.

Values Clarification

Values clarification is deciding what one believes is important. It is the process that helps people become aware of their values. Values play an important role in everyday decision making. For this reason, nurses need to be aware of what they do and do not value. This process helps them to behave in a manner that is consistent with their values.

Both personal and professional values influence nurses' decisions (McLeod-Sordjan, 2014). Understanding one's own values simplifies solving problems, making decisions, and developing better relationships with others when one begins to realize how others develop their values. Kirschenbaum (2011) suggested using a three-step model of choosing, prizing, and acting with seven substeps to identify one's own values (Box 2-1).

You may have used this method when making the decision to go to nursing school. For some people, nursing is a first career; for others, a second career. Using the model in Box 2-1, the valuing process is analyzed:

1. **Choosing** After researching alternative career options, you freely choose nursing school. This choice was most likely influenced by such factors as educational achievement and abilities, finances, support and encouragement from others, time, and feelings about people.
2. **Prizing** Once the choice was made, you were satisfied with it and told your friends about it.
3. **Acting** You entered school and started the journey toward your new career. Later in your career, you may decide to return to school for a bachelor's or master's degree in nursing.

As you progressed through school, you probably started to develop a new set of values—your professional values. Professional values are those

---

box 2-1

Values Clarification

Choosing
1. Choosing freely
2. Choosing from alternatives
3. Deciding after giving consideration to the consequences of each alternative

Prizing
4. Being satisfied about the choice
5. Being willing to declare the choice to others

Acting
6. Making the choice a part of one's worldview and incorporating it into behavior
7. Repeating the choice

Source: Adapted from Raths, L. E., Harmon, M., & Simmons, S. B. (1979). Values and teaching. Charles E. Merrill.

---

established as being important in your practice. The values include caring, quality of care, and ethical behaviors (McLeod-Sordjan, 2014).

Belief Systems

Belief systems are an organized way of thinking about why people exist in the universe. The purpose of belief systems is to explain issues such as life and death, good and evil, and health and illness. Usually these systems include an ethical code that specifies appropriate behaviors. People may have a personal belief system, participate in a religion that provides such a system, or follow a combination of the two.

Members of primitive societies worshiped events in nature. Unable to understand the science of weather, for example, early civilizations believed these events to be under the control of someone or something that needed to be appeased. Therefore, they developed rituals and ceremonies to pacify these unknown entities. They called these entities "gods" and believed that certain behaviors either pleased or angered the gods. Because these societies associated certain behaviors with specific outcomes, they created a belief system that enabled them to function as a group.

As higher civilizations evolved, belief systems became more complex. Archaeology has provided evidence of the religious practices of ancient civilizations that support the evolution of belief systems (Ball, 2015). The Aztec, Mayan, Incan, and Polynesian cultures had a religious belief system composed of many gods and goddesses for the same functions. The Greek, Roman, Egyptian, and Scandinavian societies believed in a hierarchal system of gods and goddesses. Although given various names by the different cultures, it is very interesting that most of the deities had similar purposes. For example, the Greeks looked at Zeus as the king of the Greek gods, whereas Jupiter was his Roman counterpart. Thor was the king of the Norse gods. All three used a thunderbolt as their symbol. Sociologists believe that these religions developed to explain what was then unexplainable. Human beings have a deep need to create order from chaos and to have logical explanations for events. Religion offers theological explanations to answer questions that cannot be explained by "pure science."

Along with the creation of rites and rituals, religions also developed codes of behaviors or ethical codes. These codes contribute to the social order and provide rules regarding how to treat family members, neighbors, and the young and the old. Many religions also developed rules regarding marriage, sexual practices, business practices, property ownership, and inheritance.

For some individuals, the advancement of science has minimized their need for belief systems, as science can now provide explanations for many previously unexplainable phenomena. In fact, the technology explosion has created an even greater need for belief systems. Technological advances often place people in situations where they may welcome rather than oppose religious convictions to guide difficult decisions. Many religions, particularly Christianity, focus on the will of a supreme being; technology, for example, is considered a gift that allows health-care personnel to maintain the life of a loved one. Other religions, such as certain branches of Judaism, focus on free choice or free will, leaving such decisions in the hands of humankind. For example, many Jewish leaders believe that if genetic testing indicates that an infant will be born with a disease such as Tay-Sachs that causes severe suffering and ultimately death, terminating the pregnancy may be an acceptable option.

Belief systems often help survivors in making decisions and living with them afterward. So far, technological advances have created more questions than answers. As science explains more and more previously unexplainable phenomena, people need beliefs and values to guide their use of this new knowledge.

Ethics and Morals

Although the terms *morals* and *ethics* are often used interchangeably, *ethics* usually refers to a standardized code as a guide to behaviors, whereas *morals* usually refers to an individual's personal code for acceptable behavior. Moral orientation is a concept associated with the values that guide a person's behavior, often making decisions based on reward and punishment (i.e., reward good behaviors and punish bad ones) (Bian et al., 2019).

Ethics

Ethics is the part of philosophy that deals with the rightness or wrongness of human behavior. It is also concerned with the motives behind that behavior. *Bioethics,* specifically, is the application of ethics to issues that pertain to life and death. The implication is that judgments can be made about the rightness or goodness of health-care practices.

Ethical Theories

Several ethical theories have emerged to justify moral principles (Baumane-Vitolina et al., 2016). *Deontological theories* take their norms and rules from the duties that individuals owe each other by the goodness of the commitments they make and the roles they take upon themselves. The term *deontological* comes from the Greek word *deon* (duty). This theory is attributed to the 18th-century philosopher Immanuel Kant (Kant, 1949). Deontological ethics considers the intention of the action. In other words, it is the individual's good intentions or goodwill (Kant, 1949) that determines the worthiness or goodness of the action.

Teleological theories take their norms or rules for behaviors from the consequences of the action. This theory is also called utilitarianism. According to this concept, what makes an action right or wrong is its utility or usefulness. Usefulness is considered to be the right amount of "happiness" the action carries. "Right" encompasses actions that result in good outcomes, whereas "wrong" actions end in bad outcomes. This theory originated with David Hume, a Scottish philosopher. According to Hume, "Reason is and ought to be the slave of passions" (Hume, 1978, p. 212). Based on this idea, ethics depends on what people want and desire. The passions determine what is right or wrong.

However, individuals who follow teleological theory disagree on how to decide on the "rightness" or "wrongness" of an action because individual passions differ.

Principalism is an arising theory receiving a great deal of attention in the biomedical ethics community. This theory integrates existing ethical principles and tries to resolve conflicts by relating one or more of these principles to a given situation (Hine, 2011; Varelius, 2013). Ethical principles actually influence professional decision making more than ethical theories.

Ethical Principles

Ethical codes are based on principles that can be used to judge behavior. Ethical principles assist decision making because they are a standard for measuring actions. They may be the basis for laws, but they themselves are not laws. Laws are rules created by governing bodies. Laws operate because the government holds the power to enforce them. They are usually quite specific, as are the consequences for disobeying them. Ethical principles are not confined to specific behaviors. They act as guides for appropriate behaviors. They also consider the situation in which a decision must be made. Ethical principles speak to the essence of the law rather than to the exactness of the law. Here is an example:

> Mrs. Gustav, 88 years old, was admitted to the hospital in acute respiratory distress. She was diagnosed with aspiration pneumonia and soon became septic, developing acute hypoxemic respiratory failure (AHRF). She had a living will, and her attorney was her designated health-care surrogate. Her competence to make decisions remained uncertain because of her illness. The physician presented the situation to the attorney, indicating that without a feeding tube and tracheostomy, Mrs. Gustav would die. According to the laws governing living wills and health-care surrogates, the attorney could have made the decision to withhold all treatments. However, he believed he had an ethical obligation to discuss the situation with his client. The client requested the tracheostomy be performed and the feeding tube inserted, which was done.

The ethical principles most important to nursing practice include autonomy, nonmaleficence, beneficence, justice, fidelity, confidentiality, veracity, and accountability. In some situations, two or more ethical principles may conflict with each other, leading to an ethical dilemma. Making a decision under these circumstances causes difficulty and often results in extreme stress for those who need to make the decision.

Autonomy

Autonomy is the freedom to make decisions for oneself. This ethical principle requires that nurses respect patients' rights to make their own choices about treatments. Informed consent before treatment, surgery, or participation in research provides an example of autonomy. To be able to make an autonomous choice, individuals need to be informed of the purpose, benefits, and risks of the procedures. Nurses accomplish this by assessing the individuals' understanding of the information provided to them and supporting their choices.

Closely linked to the ethical principle of autonomy is the legal issue of competence (Varkey, 2021). A patient needs to be deemed competent in order to make a decision regarding treatment options. When patients refuse treatment, health-care personnel and family members who think differently often question the patient's "competence" to make a decision. Of note is the fact that when patients agree with health providers' treatment decisions, rarely is their competence questioned (Shahriari et al., 2013).

Nurses often find themselves in a position to protect a patient's autonomy. They do this by preventing others from interfering with the patient's right to proceed with a decision. If a nurse observes that a patient received insufficient information to make an appropriate choice, is being coerced into a decision, or lacks an understanding of the consequences of the choice, then the nurse may act as a patient advocate to ensure the principle of autonomy (Rahmani et al., 2010; Varkey, 2021).

Closely tied to autonomy is beneficence. Historically, beneficence took precedence over other principles. However, allowing beneficence to supercede autonomy relates to "paternalism," such as a parent making a decision for a child, because they know what is best (Varkey, 2021). Sometimes nurses fall into this domain and have difficulty with the principle of autonomy because it also requires respecting another person's choice, even when the nurse disagrees. According to the principle of autonomy, nurses may not replace a patient's decision with their own, even when the nurses deeply believe that the patient made the wrong choice. Nurses may, however, discuss concerns with patients and ensure that patients considered the consequences of the decision before making it (Rahmani et al., 2010).

Nonmaleficence

The ethical principle of nonmaleficence requires that no harm be done, either deliberately or unintentionally. This rather complicated word comes from Latin roots, *non,* which means not; *male* (pronounced mah-leh), which means bad; and *facere,* which means to do.

The principle of nonmaleficence also requires nurses to protect individuals who lack the ability to protect themselves because of their physical or mental condition. An infant, a person under anesthesia, and a person suffering from dementia are examples of individuals with limited ability to protect themselves from danger or those who may cause them harm. Nurses are ethically obligated to protect their patients when the patients are unable to protect themselves.

Often, treatments meant to improve patient health lead to harm. This is not the intention of the nurse or of other health-care personnel, but it is a direct result of treatment. Nosocomial infections because of hospitalization are harmful to patients. The nurses, however, did not deliberately cause the infection. The side effects of chemotherapy or radiation may also result in harm. Chemotherapeutic agents cause a decrease in immunity that may result in a severe infection, and radiation may burn or damage the skin. For this reason, many choose not to pursue treatments.

The obligation to do no harm extends to the nurse who for some reason is not functioning at an optimal level. For example, a nurse who is impaired by alcohol or drugs knowingly places patients at risk. According to the principle of nonmaleficence, other nurses who observe such behavior have an ethical obligation to protect patients. More recently, such as during the COVID-19 pandemic causing times when providers are in high demand, nonmaleficence needs to be considered. What happens when a nurse has a highly infectious disease (Ayanian, 2020)? Consider the following:

Mori wakes up with a fever, sore throat, and respiratory symptoms. He has been caring for COVID-19 patients and he is scheduled to report to work in 2 hours. He has been fully vaccinated and followed all the safety protocols. He knows that the unit is short-staffed. Should Mori tell the nurse manager about his symptoms and remain at home and face the discontent of his colleagues or remain quiet, take extra precautions, and go to work, risking the health of his fellow workers and patients? How does he balance his own health and welfare, duty to others, and "do no harm?"

Beneficence

The word *beneficence* also comes from Latin: *bene,* which means well, and *facere,* which means to do.

The principle of beneficence demands that good be done for the benefit of others and also supports the variety of moral guidelines to protect, support, and prevent harm (Varkey, 2021). For nurses, this means more than delivering competent physical or technical care. It requires helping patients meet all their needs, whether physical, social, or emotional. Beneficence is caring in the truest sense, and caring fuses thought, feeling, and action. It requires knowing and being truly understanding of the situation and the thoughts and ideas of the individual (Benner & Wruble, 1989).

Sometimes physicians, nurses, and families withhold information from patients for the sake of beneficence. This behavior represents paternalism, and it does not allow competent individuals to make their own decisions based on all available information. In an attempt to be beneficent, the principle of autonomy is violated. It may also violate the informed consent (Varkey, 2021). This is just one example of the ethical dilemmas encountered in nursing practice. In today's environment focused on patient-centered care and the inclusion of the patient and their families and/or significant others in the decision-making process, the balance between autonomy and beneficence holds great importance (Picker Institute, 2020). For instance:

Mrs. Liu was admitted to the oncology unit with ovarian cancer. She is scheduled to begin chemotherapy treatments. Her two children and her husband have requested that the physician ensure that Mrs. Liu not be told her diagnosis because they believe she would not be able to cope with it. The physician communicated this information to the nursing staff and placed an order in the patient's electronic medical record (EMR). After the first treatment, Mrs. Liu became very ill. She refused the next treatment, stating she did not feel sick until she came to the hospital. She asked the nurse what could possibly be wrong with her that she needed a medicine that made her sick when she did not feel sick before. She then said, "Only people who get cancer medicine get this sick! Do I have cancer?"

As the nurse, you understand the order that the patient not be told her diagnosis. You also understand your role as a patient advocate. Consider the following questions:

1. To whom do you owe your duty: to the patient or the family?
2. How do you think you may be able to be a patient advocate in this situation?
3. What information would you communicate to the family members, and how could you assist them in dealing with their mother's concerns?

Justice

The principle of justice obliges nurses and other health-care professionals to treat every person equally regardless of gender, sexual orientation, religion, ethnicity, disease, or social standing (Johnstone, 2011). This principle also applies in the work and educational settings. Based on this principle, all individuals should be treated and judged by the same criteria. The following example illustrates this:

Mr. Laury was found on the street by the police, who brought him to the emergency department. He was assessed and admitted to a medical unit. Mr. Laury was in deplorable condition: His clothes were dirty and ragged, he was unshaven, and he was covered with blood. His diagnosis was chronic alcoholism, complicated by esophageal varices and end-stage liver disease. Several nursing students overheard the staff discussing Mr. Laury. The essence of the conversation was that no one wanted to care for him because he was "dirty and smelly," and he brought this

condition on himself. The students, upset by what they heard, went to the clinical faculty to discuss the situation. The clinical faculty explained that based on the ethical principle of justice, all individuals have a right to good care despite their economic or social position.

The concept of distributive justice necessitates the fair allocation of responsibilities and advantages, especially in a society where resources may be limited. Considered an ethical principle, distributive justice refers to what society, or a larger group, feels is indebted to its individual members regarding: (a) individual needs, contributions, and responsibilities; (b) the resources available to the society or organization; and (c) the society's or organization's responsibility to the common good (Capp et al., 2001). Increased health-care costs through the years and access to care have become social and political issues. In order to understand distributive justice, we must address the concepts of need, individual effort, ability to pay, contribution to society, and age (Zahedi et al., 2013). This principle came to the forefront during the pandemic as resources quickly diminished and the need for care, hospital beds, and access to care accelerated. Within the health-care setting, this necessitates that patients who present with comparable cases be treated in a similar manner, and for there to be predominant equality of access to limited health resources (Fisher et al., 2020).

Age has become a controversial issue as it leads to questions pertaining to quality of life (Skedgel et al., 2015). The other issue regarding age revolves around technology in neonatal care. How do health-care providers place a value on one person's life being higher than that of another? Should millions of dollars be spent preserving the life of an 80-year-old man who volunteers in his community, plays golf twice a week, and teaches reading to underprivileged children, or should money be spent on a 26-week-old fetus who will most likely require intensive therapies and treatments for a lifetime, adding up to millions of health-care dollars? In the social and business world, welfare payments are based on need, and jobs and promotions are usually distributed on the basis of an individual's contributions and achievements. Is it possible to apply these measures to health-care allocations?

Philosopher John Rawls addressed the issues of fairness and justice as the foundation of social structures (Ekmekci & Arda, 2015). Rawls addresses the issue of fair distribution of social goods using the idea of the original position to negotiate the principles of justice. The original position based on Kant's (1949) social contract theory presents a hypothetical situation where individuals, known as negotiators, act as trustees for the interests of all individuals. These individuals are knowledgeable in the areas of sociology, political science, and economics. However, this position places certain limitations on them known as the *veil of ignorance*, which eliminates information about age, gender, socioeconomic status, and religious convictions. With the absence of this information, the vested interests of all parties disappear. According to Rawls, in a just society the rights protected by justice are not political bargaining issues or subject to the calculations of social interests. Simply put, everyone has the same rights and liberties (Ekmekci & Arda, 2015).

Fidelity

The principle of fidelity requires loyalty. It is a promise that all individuals will fulfill all commitments made to themselves and to others. For nurses, fidelity includes the professional's loyalty to fulfill all responsibilities and agreements expected as part of professional practice. Fidelity is the basis for the concept of accountability—taking responsibility for one's own actions (Ostlund et al., 2015).

Confidentiality

The principle of confidentiality states that anything patients say to nurses and other health-care providers must be held in the strictest confidence. Confidentiality presents both an ethical and legal issue. Exceptions only exist when patients give permission for the sharing of information or when the law requires the release of specific information. Sometimes simply sharing information without revealing an individual's name can be a breach of confidentiality if the situation and the individual are identifiable.

Nurses come into contact with people from all walks of life. Within communities, individuals know other individuals who know others, creating "micro-communities" of information. Individuals have lost families, employment, and insurance coverage because nurses shared confidential information and others acted on that knowledge (Beltran-Aroca et al., 2016).

In today's electronic environment, the principle of confidentiality has become a major concern, especially in light of the security breaches that have occurred throughout the last several years. There is a difference between confidentiality and security. Confidentiality means privacy, whereas security refers to keeping information safe and inaccessible by those who are not authorized to view it (Keshta & Odeh, 2020). Many health-care institutions, insurance companies, and businesses use electronic media to transfer sensitive and confidential information, allowing more opportunities for a breakdown in confidentiality. Health-care institutions and providers have attempted to address the situation through the use of passwords, limited access, and cybersecurity. However, it has become more apparent that the securest of systems remains vulnerable to hacking and illegal access.

Veracity

Veracity requires nurses to be truthful. Truth is fundamental to building a trusting relationship. Intentionally deceiving or misleading a patient is a violation of this principle. Deliberately omitting a part of the truth is deception and violates the principle of veracity. This principle often creates ethical dilemmas. When is it permissible to lie? Some ethicists believe it is never appropriate to deceive another individual. Others think that if another ethical principle overrides veracity, then lying is acceptable (Sokol, 2007). Lying or omitting information violates the patient's autonomy (Varkey, 2021). Consider this situation:

Ms. Allen has been told that her father suffers from Alzheimer's disease. The nurse practitioner wants to come into the home to discuss treatment options. Ms. Allen refuses, explaining that under no circumstances should the nurse practitioner tell her father the diagnosis. Ms. Allen bases her concern on past statements made by her father. She explains to the nurse practitioner that if her father finds out his diagnosis, he will take his own life. The nurse practitioner provides information on the newest treatments and available medications that might help. However, these treatments and medications are only available through a research study. To participate in the study, the patient needs to be aware of the benefits and the risks. Ms. Allen continues refusing to allow anyone to tell her father his diagnosis because of her certainty that he will commit suicide.

The nurse practitioner faces a dilemma: Does he abide by Ms. Allen's wishes based on the principle of beneficence, or does he abide by the principle of veracity and inform his patient of the diagnosis? If he goes against Ms. Allen's wishes and tells the patient his diagnosis, and he commits suicide, has nonmaleficence been violated? Did the practitioner's action cause harm? What would you do in this situation?

Accountability

Accountability is linked to fidelity and means accepting responsibility for one's own actions. Nurses are accountable to their patients and to their colleagues. When providing care to patients, nurses are responsible for their actions, good and poor. If something was not done, do not chart it and then tell a colleague that it was completed. An example of violating accountability is the story of Anna:

Anna was a registered nurse who worked nights on an acute care medical unit. She was an excellent nurse; however, as the acuity of the patients' conditions increased, she was unable to keep up with both patients' needs and the technology, particularly intravenous fluids and lines. The pumps confused her, so often she would take the fluids off the pump and "monitor her IVs" the way she did in the past. She started to document that all the IVs were infusing as they should, even when they were not. Each morning the day shift would find that the actual infused amount did not agree with the documentation, even though "pumps" were found for each patient. One night, Anna allowed an entire liter of intravenous fluids to be infused in 2 hours into a patient who had heart failure. When the day staff came on duty, they found the patient expired, the bag empty, and the tubing filled with blood. The IV was attached to the pump. Anna's documentation showed 800 mL left in the bag. It was not until after a lawsuit was filed that Anna assumed responsibility for her behavior.

The idea of a standard of care evolves from the principle of accountability. Standards of care provide a rule for measuring nursing actions and safety issues. According to the Institute of Medicine (IOM), organizations also hold accountability for patient care and the actions of personnel. Based on the Institute for Healthcare Improvement (IHI), health-care organizations have a duty to ensure a safe environment and that all personnel receive appropriate training and education (IHI, 2018).

Ethical Codes

A code of ethics is a formal statement of the rules of ethical behavior for a particular group of individuals. A code of ethics is one of the hallmarks of a profession. This code makes clear the behavior expected of its members.

The American Nurses Association (ANA) *Code of Ethics for Nurses With Interpretive Statements* (Olsen & Stokes, 2016) provides values, standards, and principles to help nursing function as a profession. The ANA developed the original code in 1985; it has gone through several revisions during the years since its development and may be viewed online at www.nursingworld.org. In 2020, based on Provision 2 and Provision 5 of the *Code*, the ANA added information pertaining to the ethical issues nurses confronted during the COVID-19 pandemic. These provisions refer to nurses' obligations to care for their patients and for themselves. These two provisions came into conflict during the pandemic as nurses found themselves placed in high-risk situations while providing for their patients (ANA, 2020).

Ethical codes remain subject to change. They reflect the values of the profession and the society for which they were developed. Changes occur as society and technology evolve. For example, years ago no thought was given to do not resuscitate (DNR) orders or withholding food or fluids. Technological advances have since made it possible to keep people in a type of twilight life, comatose and unable to participate in living in any way, thus making DNR and withholding very important issues in health care. Technology and scientific advancements increased knowledge and skills, but the ability to make decisions regarding care continues to be guided by ethical principles.

Virtue Ethics

Virtue ethics focuses on virtues or moral character, rather than on duties or rules that emphasize consequences of actions. Consider the following:

Carlos is driving along the highway and discovers a crying child sitting by a fallen bicycle. It is obvious that the child needs assistance. From one ethical standpoint (utilitarianism), helping the child will increase Carlos's feelings of "doing good." The deontological stance states that by helping, Carlos is behaving in accordance with a moral rule such as "Do unto others. . . ." Virtue ethics looks at the fact that, by helping, Carlos would be acting charitable or benevolent.

Plato and Aristotle are considered the founders of virtue ethics. Its roots can be found in Chinese philosophy. During the 1800s, virtue ethics disappeared, but in the late 1950s it re-emerged as an Anglo-American philosophy. Neither deontology nor utilitarianism considered the virtues of moral character and education and the question: "What type of person should I be, and how should I live?" (Sakellariouv, 2015). Virtues include qualities such as honesty, generosity, altruism, and reliability. They are concerned with many other elements as well, such as emotions and emotional reactions, choices, values, needs, insights, attitudes, interests, and expectations. Nursing has practiced virtue ethics for many years.

Nursing Ethics

Up to this point, the ethical principles discussed apply to ethics for nurses; however, nurses do not customarily find themselves enmeshed in the biomedical ethical decision-making processes that gain attention. The ethical principles that guide nursing practice are rooted in the philosophy and science of health care.

Relationships are the center of nursing ethics. Nursing ethics, viewed from the perspective of nursing theory and practice, deals with the experiences and needs of nurses and their perceptions of these experiences (Johnstone, 2011).

Organizational Ethics

Organizational ethics focus on the workplace at the organizational level. Every organization, even one with hundreds of thousands of employees, consists of individuals. Each individual makes personal decisions about how to behave in the workplace (Carucci, 2016), and every person has the opportunity to make an organization a more or less ethical place. These individual decisions exert a powerful effect on the lives of many others in the organization as well as the surrounding community.

Most organizations create a set of values that guide the organizational ideals, practices, and expectations (Leonard, 2018). Although given varying "names," such as core values, practice values, and so on, they lay the groundwork for expectations for employees. What is most important is that employees see that the organization practices what it states. Leadership, especially senior leadership, is the most critical factor in promoting an ethical culture. During the pandemic, health-care organizations had a moral and ethical obligation to support their nurses and other providers. Much of this revolved around physical and psychological support. This unprecedented event raised many questions regarding the role of organizations and the ethics revolving around balancing physical resources, human resources, and patient care (Sahebi et al., 2020). Because of this situation, an ethical concern developed surrounding the extent that providers had a professional patient-care duty as the pandemic disturbed routine duties and increased workload. Additionally, a clash between civil duty and the organization's self-interest made nurses more vulnerable (Sahebi et al., 2020).

When looking for a professional position, it is important to consider the organizational culture and ethical guides. What are the values and beliefs of the organization? Do they blend with yours, or are they in conflict with your value system? To discover this information, look at the organization's mission, vision, and value statements. Speak with other nurses who work in the organization. Do they see consistency between what the organization states and what it actually expects from employees? For example, if an organization states that it collaborates with the nurses in decision making, do nurses sit on committees that provide input toward the decision-making process (Choi et al., 2014)? Conflicts between a nurse's professional values and those of the organization result in moral distress for the nurse.

Ethical Issues on the Nursing Unit

Organizational ethics refer to the values and expected behaviors entrenched within the organizational culture. The nursing unit represents a subculture within a health-care organization. Ideally, the nursing unit should mirror the ethical atmosphere and culture of the organization. This requires the individuals who staff the unit to embrace the same values and model the expected behaviors (Choi et al., 2014).

Conflicts with the values and ethics among individuals who work together on a unit often create issues that result in moral suffering for some nurses. Moral suffering occurs when nurses experience a feeling of uneasiness or concern regarding behaviors or circumstances that challenge their own morals and beliefs (Epstein & Hamric, 2009; Morley, 2016). These situations may be the result of unit policies, physician's orders that the nurse believes may not be beneficial for the patient, professional behaviors of colleagues, or family attitudes about the patient (Morley, 2016).

Perhaps one of the most disconcerting ethical issues nurses on the patient care unit face is the one that challenges their professional values and ethics. Friendships often emerge from work relationships, and these friendships may interfere with judgments. Similarly, strong negative feelings may cloud a nurse's ability to view a situation fairly and without prejudice. Consider the following:

> Anela and Oskar attended nursing school together and developed a strong friendship. They work together in the neonatal unit of a large teaching hospital. The hospital provides full tuition reimbursement for graduate education, so both decided to return to graduate school together and enrolled in a nurse practitioner program. Anela made a medication error that she decided not to report, an error that resulted in a neonate going into respiratory arrest; the baby subsequently developed an anoxic brain injury. Oskar realized what happened and confronted Anela, who begged him not to say anything. Oskar knew the error needed to be reported, but how would this affect his friendship with Anela? Taking this situation to the other extreme, if a friendship had not been involved, would Oskar react the same way? What would you do in this situation?

When working with others, it is important to hold true to your personal values and moral standards. Practicing virtue ethics, that is, "doing the right thing," may cause difficulty because of the possible consequences of the action. Nurses should support each other, but not at the expense of patients or each other's professional duties. There are times when not acting virtuously may cause a colleague more harm.

Moral Distress in Nursing Practice

Moral distress occurs when nurses know the action they need to take, but for some reason find themselves unable to act (Fourie, 2015; Silverman et al., 2021). This is usually the result of external forces or loyalties (Hamric, 2014). Therefore, the action or actions they take create conflict as the decision goes against their personal and professional values, morals, and beliefs (Morley, 2016; Silverman et al., 2021). These situations challenge nurses' integrity and authenticity.

Studies have shown that nurses exposed to moral distress suffer from emotional and physical problems and eventually leave the bedside and the profession. Sources of moral distress vary; however, contributing factors include end-of-life challenges, nurse–physician conflicts, workplace bullying or violence, disrespectful interactions, and fear for their own safety and well-being (Oh & Gastmans, 2015; Silverman et al., 2021). Nursing organizations such as the American Association of Critical Care Nurses (AACN, 2018) have developed guidelines addressing the issue of moral distress.

Ethical Dilemmas

What is a dilemma? The word *dilemma* is of Greek derivation. A lemma was an animal resembling a ram and having two horns. Thus came the saying, "stuck on the horns of a dilemma." The story of Hugo illustrates a hypothetical dilemma with a touch of humor:

> One day Hugo, dressed in a bright red cape, walked through his village into the countryside. The wind caught the corners of his cape, and it was whipped in all directions. As he continued down the dusty road, Hugo happened to pass by a lemma. Hugo's bright red cape caught the lemma's attention. Lowering its head, with its two horns posed in attack position, the animal started chasing Hugo down the road. Panting and exhausted, Hugo reached the end of the road only to find himself blocked by a huge stone wall. He turned to face the lemma, which was ready to charge. A decision needed to be made, and Hugo's life depended on this decision. If he moved to the left, the lemma would gore his heart. If he moved to the right, the lemma would gore his liver. No matter what his decision, Hugo would be "stuck on the horns of the lemma."

Similar to Hugo, nurses are often faced with difficult dilemmas. Also, as Hugo found, a dilemma can be a choice between two serious alternatives. An ethical dilemma occurs when a problem exists that forces a choice between two or more ethical principles. Deciding in favor of one principle will violate the other. Both sides have goodness and badness to them; however, neither decision satisfies all the criteria that apply (Jie, 2015).

Ethical dilemmas also carry the added burden of emotions. Feelings of anger, frustration, and fear often override rational decision making. Consider the case of Mr. Rodney:

Mr. Rodney, 85 years old, was admitted to the neuroscience unit after suffering a left hemispheric bleed while playing golf with his friends. He had a total right hemiplegia and a Glasgow Coma Scale (GCS) score of 8. He had been receiving intravenous fluids for four days, and the neurologist raised the question of placing a jejunostomy tube for enteral feedings. The older of his two children asked what the chances of his recovery were. The neurologist explained that Mr. Rodney's current state was probably the best he could attain but that "miracles happen every day," and that some diagnostic tests might help in determining the prognosis. The family requested the tests. After the results were available, the neurologist explained that the prognosis remained grave and that the intravenous fluids were insufficient to sustain life. The jejunostomy tube would be a necessity if the family wished to continue with food and fluids. After the neurologist left, the family asked the nurse, Gloria, who had been caring for Mr. Rodney during the previous 3 days, "If this was your father, what would you do?" Once the family asked Gloria this question, the situation became an ethical dilemma for her as well.

If you were Gloria, how might you respond? Depending on your answer, what ethical principles would be in conflict here?

Resolving Ethical Dilemmas Faced by Nurses

Ethical dilemmas can occur in any aspect of life, personal or professional. This section focuses on the resolution of professional dilemmas. The various

box 2-2

Questions to Help Resolve Ethical Dilemmas

- What are the medical facts?
- What are the psychosocial facts?
- What are the patient's wishes?
- What values are in conflict?

models for resolving ethical dilemmas consist of 5 to 14 sequential steps. Each step begins with a complete understanding of the dilemma and concludes with the evaluation of the implemented decision.

The nursing process provides a helpful mechanism for finding solutions to ethical dilemmas. The first step is assessment, including identification of the problem. The simplest way to do this is to create a statement that summarizes the issue. The remainder of the process evolves from this statement (Box 2-2).

Assessment

Ask yourself, "Am I directly involved in this dilemma?" An issue is not an ethical dilemma for nurses unless they find themselves directly involved in the situation or have been asked for their opinion. Some nurses involve themselves in situations even when no one solicited their opinion. This is generally unwarranted unless the issue involves a violation of the professional code of ethics.

Nurses are frequently in the position of hearing both sides of an ethical dilemma. Often individuals only want an empathetic listener. At other times, when guidance is requested, nurses can help people work through the decision-making process (remember the principle of autonomy) (Barlow et al., 2018).

Collecting data from all the decision makers helps identify the reasoning process used by the individuals as they struggle with the issue. The following questions assist in the information-gathering process:

- **What are the medical facts?** Find out how the physicians, nurse practitioners, and all members of the interprofessional health-care team view the patient's condition and treatment options. Speak with the patient if possible, and determine the patient's understanding of the situation.
- **What are the psychosocial facts?** What is the emotional state of the patient right now? The patient's family? What kind of relationship exists between the patient and the patient's family? What are the patient's living conditions?

Who are the individuals who form the patient's support system? How are they involved in the patient's care? What is the patient's ability to make medical decisions about personal care? Do financial considerations need to be taken into account? What does the patient value? What does the patient's family value? The answers to these questions will provide a better understanding of the situation. Ask more questions, if necessary, to complete the picture. The social facts of a situation also include the institutional policies, legal aspects, and economic factors. The personal belief systems of the providers may also influence this aspect.

- **What are the cultural beliefs?** Cultural beliefs play a major role in ethical decisions. Some cultures do not allow surgical interventions as they fear that the "life force" may escape. Many cultures forbid organ donation. Other cultures focus on the sanctity of life, thereby requesting that providers use all available methods for sustaining life.

- **What are the patient's wishes?** Remember the ethical principle of autonomy? With very few exceptions, if the patient is competent, then decisions the patient makes take precedence. Too often, the family's or provider's worldview and belief system overshadow those of the patient. Nurses can assist by maintaining the focus on the patient. If the patient is unable to communicate, try to discover if the individual discussed the issue in the past. If the patient completed a living will or advance directives and designated a health-care surrogate, this helps determine the patient's wishes. By interviewing family members, the nurse can often learn about conversations where the patient voiced personal feelings about treatment decisions. Using guided interviewing, the nurse can encourage the family to share anecdotes that provide relevant insights into the patient's values and beliefs.

- **What values are in conflict?** To assess values, begin by listing each person involved in the situation. Then identify values represented by each person. Ask such questions as, "What do you feel is the most pressing issue here?" and "Tell me more about your feelings regarding this situation." In some cases, there may be little disagreement among the people involved, just a different way of expressing individual beliefs. However, in others, a serious value conflict may exist.

Planning

For planning to be successful, everyone involved in the decision must be included in the process. Thompson and Thompson (1992) listed three specific and integrated phases of this planning:

1. **Determine the goals of treatment.** Is cure a goal, or is the goal a peaceful death at home? These goals need to be patient-focused, reality-centered, and attainable. They should be consistent with current medical treatment and, if possible, measurable according to an established period.

2. **Identify the decision makers.** As mentioned earlier, nurses may not be decision makers in these health-related ethical dilemmas. It is important to know who the decision makers are and their belief systems. A patient who has the capability to participate makes the task less complicated. However, critically ill or terminally ill patients may be too exhausted to speak for themselves or ensure their voices are heard. When this happens, the patient needs an advocate, which might be family members, friends, spiritual advisors, or nurses. A family member may need to be designated as a primary decision maker or *health-care surrogate*. The creation of living wills, advance directives, and the appointment of a health-care surrogate while a person is healthy often eases the burden for the decision makers during a later crisis. These are discussed in more detail in Chapter 3.

3. **List and rank all the options.** Performing this task involves all decision makers. It is sometimes helpful to begin with the least desired choice and methodically work toward the preferred treatment choice that will most likely produce the desired outcome. Engaging all participating parties in a discussion identifying each one's beliefs regarding attaining a reasonable outcome using available medical expertise often helps. Often sharing ideas in a controlled situation allows everyone involved to realize that everyone wants the same goal but perhaps has varying opinions on how to reach it.

Implementation

During the implementation phase, the patient or surrogate (substitute) decision maker(s) and members of the health-care team reach a mutually acceptable decision. This occurs through open discussion and negotiation. An example of negotiation follows:

Olivia's mother, Angela, has Stage IV ovarian cancer. She and Olivia have discussed treatment options. Angela's physician suggested the use of a new chemotherapeutic agent that has demonstrated success in many cases. Angela states emphatically that she has "had enough" and prefers to spend her remaining time doing whatever she chooses. Olivia wants her mother to try the medication. To resolve the dilemma, the oncology nurse practitioner and physician speak with Olivia and her mother. Everyone reviews the facts and expresses their feelings. Seeing Olivia's distress, Angela says, "OK, I will try the drug for a month. If there is no improvement after this time, I want to stop all treatment and live out the time I have with my daughter and her family." All agreed that this was a reasonable decision.

The role of the nurse during the implementation phase is to ensure the communication remains open. Ethical dilemmas are emotional issues, filled with guilt, sorrow, anger, and other strong emotions. These strong feelings create communication failures among decision makers. Remind yourself of the three ethical principles: autonomy, beneficence, and nonmaleficence, and think, "I am here to do what is best for this patient."

Keep in mind that an ethical dilemma is not always a choice between two attractive alternatives. Many dilemmas revolve around two unattractive, even unpleasant choices. In the previous scenario, Angela's choices did not include what she truly wants: good health and a long life.

Once an agreement is reached, the decision makers must accept it. Sometimes an agreement cannot be reached because the parties are unable to reconcile their conflicting belief patterns or values. At other times, caregivers are unable to recognize the worth of the patient's point of view. Occasionally, the patient or surrogate may make a request that is not institutionally or legally possible. When this occurs, a different institution or physician may be able to honor the request. In some instances, a patient or surrogate may ask for information that reflects illegal acts.

When this happens, the nurse needs to explore whether the patient and the family considered the consequences of their proposed actions. This now presents a dilemma for the nurse as, depending on the request, the nurse may need to notify upper-level administration or the authorities. This conflicts with the principle of confidentiality. It may be necessary to bring other counselors into the discussion (with the patient's permission) to negotiate the agreement.

Evaluation

As in the nursing process, the purpose of evaluation in resolving ethical dilemmas is to determine whether the desired outcomes have occurred. In the case of Mr. Rodney, some of the questions that could be posed by Gloria to the family are as follows:

- "I have noticed the amount of time you have been spending with your father. Have you observed any changes in his condition?"
- "I see the neurologist spoke to you about the test results and your father's prognosis. How do you feel about the situation?"
- "Now that the neurologist spoke to you about your father's condition, have you considered future alternatives?"

Changes in patient status, availability of medical treatment, and social factors may call for reevaluation of a situation. The course of treatment may need to be altered. Continued communication and cooperation among the decision makers are essential.

Another model, the MORAL model created by Thiroux in 1977 and refined for nursing by Halloran in 1992, has gained popularity and is considered a standard for dealing with ethical dilemmas (Toren & Wagner, 2010). This ethical decision-making model is easily implemented in all patient care settings (Box 2-3).

---

box 2-3

The MORAL Model

M: Massage the dilemma.
O: Outline the option.
R: Resolve the dilemma.
A: Act by applying the chosen option.
L: Look back and evaluate the complete process, including actions taken.

Current Ethical Issues

Probably one of the most well-known events that brought attention to some of the ethical dilemmas regarding end-of-life issues occurred in 1988 when Dr. Jack Kevorkian (sometimes called Dr. Death by the media) openly admitted to giving some patients, at their request, a lethal dose of medication, resulting in the patients' deaths. His statement raised the consciousness of the American people and the health-care system about the issues of euthanasia and assisted suicide. Do individuals have the right to consciously end their own lives when they are suffering from a terminal condition? If they are unable to perform the act themselves, should others assist them in ending their lives? Should assisted suicide be legalized? Physician-assisted suicide is currently legal in 11 jurisdictions, including the District of Columbia. Oregon was one of the first states to pass legislation, and in 2018 Hawaii recognized this legal right with the passage of the *Our Choice Act* (ProCon.org, 2018, 2021).

The Terri Schiavo case gained tremendous media attention, probably becoming the most important case of clinical ethics as it brought forward the deep divisions and fears that reside in society regarding life and death, as well as the role of the government and courts in these decisions (Quill, 2005). Many aspects of the case may never be completely clarified; however, it raised many questions that laid the groundwork for present ethical decisions in similar situations and beyond.

The primary goal of nursing and health-care professions is to keep people alive and well or, if this cannot be done, to help them live as comfortably as possible and achieve a peaceful death. To accomplish this end, health-care professionals struggle to improve their knowledge and skills so they can care for their patients and provide the best quality of life possible. The costs involved in achieving this goal can be astronomical.

Questions are being raised more and more about who should receive the benefits of technology. The competition for resources also creates ethical dilemmas. Other difficult questions, such as who should pay for care when the illness may have been caused by poor health practices such as smoking and substance abuse, are now under consideration. Many employers and health insurance companies evaluate the health status of individuals before determining the cost of their health-care premiums. For example, individuals who smoke or are overweight are considered to have a higher risk for chronic disease. Individuals with less risky behaviors and better health indicators may pay less for coverage (Centers for Disease Control and Prevention [CDC], 2015).

Practice Issues Related to Technology

Technology and Treatment

In issues of technology, the principles of beneficence and nonmaleficence may be in conflict. For example, a specific advancement in medical technology administered with the intention of "doing good" may cause harm. At times, this is an accepted consequence and the patient is aware of the risk. However, in situations where little or no improvement is expected, the issue becomes whether the benefit outweighs the risk. Suffering from induced technology may include multiple components for the patient and family.

Today, many infants born prematurely or with extremely low birthweights who long ago would have been considered unable to survive are maintained on mechanical devices in highly sophisticated neonatal units. This process may keep the infants alive only to die later or live with chronic, and often severe, disabilities. These children require highly technological treatments and specialized medical, educational, and supportive services.

The use of ultrasound throughout a pregnancy is supported by evidence-based practice and is a standard of care. In the past, these pictures were mostly two-dimensional and used to determine fetal weight and size in relation to the mother's pelvic anatomy. Today, this technology has evolved to where the fetus's internal organ structure is visualized, and defects not known before are detectable. This presents parents with additional options, leading to other decisions.

Technology and Genetics

The Human Genome Project (HGP) allowed mapping and sequencing of human genes (NIH, 2021). This knowledge permitted scientists and medical researchers the ability to explore, identify, and manipulate genetic causes and predispositions to diseases and other conditions. *Genetic diagnosis* is a process that involves analyzing the parents or an embryo for a genetic disorder. This is done before in vitro fertilization. Once the egg is fertilized, the embryos are tested, and only those without genetic flaws are implanted. *Genetic screening* of parents has also entered the standard of care, particularly in the presence of a family history. Parents are offered this option when seeking prenatal care. Some parents refuse to have genetic testing as their value and belief systems preclude them from making a decision that may lead to terminating the pregnancy.

Genetic screening leads to issues pertaining to reproductive rights and also opens new issues. What is a disability versus a disorder, and who decides? Is a disability a disease, and does it need to be prevented? The technology is also used to determine whether individuals are predisposed to certain diseases such as Alzheimer's or Huntington's chorea. This has created additional ethical issues regarding genetic screening. For example:

> Christy, who is 32 years old, is diagnosed with a nonhormonally dependent breast cancer. She has two daughters, ages 6 and 4 years old, respectively. Christy's mother and maternal grandmother had breast cancer, and her maternal grandfather died from prostate cancer. Neither her mother nor grandmother survived more than 5 years posttreatment. Christy's physician suggested she obtain genetic testing for the *BRCA1* and *BRCA2* genes before deciding on a treatment plan. Christy meets with the nurse geneticist and asks the following questions: "If I am positive for the genes, what are my options? Should I have a bilateral mastectomy with reconstruction? Will I be able to get health insurance coverage, or will the company charge me a higher premium? What are the future implications for my daughters?"

As the nurse, how might you address these concerns?

Genetic engineering is the ability to change the genetic nature of an organism. Researchers have created disease-resistant fruits and vegetables as well as certain medications using this process. Theoretically, genetic engineering allows for the genetic alteration of an embryo, eliminating genetic flaws and creating healthier babies. Envision being able to "engineer your child." Imagine, as Aldous Huxley did in *Brave New World* (1932), being able to create a society of perfect individuals: "We also predestine and condition. We decant our babies as socialized human beings, as Alphas or Epsilons as future sewer workers or future . . . he was going to say future World controllers but correcting himself said

future directors of Hatcheries instead" (p. 12). The ethical implications pertaining to genetic technology are profound. For example, some of the questions raised by the HGP related to:

- Fairness in the use of genetic information
- Privacy and confidentiality of obtained genetic information
- Genetic testing of an individual because of a family history

However, genetics has also allowed health-care providers to identify individuals who may have a greater risk for heart disease and diabetes and begin early treatment and lifestyle changes to minimize or prevent the onset or complications of these disorders.

Pharmacogenetics presently incorporates pharmacology and genetics and allows more targeted treatments for individuals by addressing their genetic makeup.

Testing allows physicians and other providers to determine if a particular medication is appropriate for a specific patient (Luzum et al., 2021). Resources are limited in this area and the testing expensive. What are the ethical implications of genetic testing to determine if a medication is appropriate for an individual based on their genetic make-up?

DNA Use and Protection

In 2015, Butler approached the subject of DNA use and protection. Presently, DNA is mostly used in forensic science for the identification of individuals, military personnel, or possible criminal evidence. However, questions remain as to the protection of this information and what is considered legal usage. The birth of companies that offer individuals the ability to discover their DNA and ancestral origins presents a greater level of concern both legally and ethically. This technology allowed law enforcement agencies to identify suspects involved in violent crimes through accessing relatives' DNA housed within these company databases (Rainey, 2018). Within the last few years, 3% to 5% of the funding available for the HGP has been set aside to study the many social, ethical, and legal implications that will result from better understanding of human heredity and its impact on disease (Feeney et al., 2021).

Stem Cell Use and Research

Stem cell use and research issues have emerged during this decade. Stem cell transplants for the treatment of certain cancers are considered an acceptable treatment option when others have failed. They are usually harvested from a matching donor. The ethics of stem cell use focuses on how to access them. Should fetal tissue be used to harvest stem cells? Companies now offer prospective parents the option of obtaining and storing fetal cord blood and tissue for future use should the need arise. Although this is costly and not covered by insurance, many parents opt to do this.

When faced with the prospect of a child who is dying from a terminal illness, some parents have resorted to conceiving a sibling for the purpose of harvesting stem cells from the sibling to save the life of the ill child. Nurses who work in pediatrics and pediatric oncology units may find themselves dealing with this situation. It is important for nurses to examine their own feelings regarding these issues and understand that, regardless of their personal beliefs, the family is in need of sensitivity and the best nursing care. Other issues emerging in stem cell research revolve around "curing" debilitating diseases such as Parkinson's disease and spinal cord injury (Sivandzade & Cucullo, 2021).

Artificial Intelligence

AI is a branch of computer sciences and technology that focuses on the creation of intelligent machines that possess the capability to think and function similar to humans. They problem-solve, learn from experience, and are capable of speech recognition and voice modulation. Siri™ and Alexa are two examples of AI.

These "machines" form neural networks similar to brain function learning from previous introductions and immersement in an experience. The advances in research, construction, and application of AI to real-world scenarios created a need to look at the ethical issues associated with this technology (Hagendorff, 2020). Industries such as the military, business, and science and technology hold a vested interest in AI applications stimulating fierce global competition to maintain the lead in this area (Greene et al., 2019). New to the health-care arena is the concept of AI and its role in determining and guiding health-care decision making. However, what are the ethics of using AI in ethical decision making? As machines do not "feel" in the sense of humans, are they capable of making better or fairer decisions? Can machines be taught moral behaviors (Haggendorff, 2020)?

This futuristic approach to health-care decision making leads to more questions than answers. Ethicists and scientists will need to construct a connective pathway between the AI technology and ethical principles.

Professional Dilemmas

Most of this chapter dealt with patient issues; however, ethical problems may involve leadership and management issues as well. What should you do about an impaired coworker? Personal loyalties may cause conflict with professional ethics, creating an ethical dilemma. For this reason, most nurse practice acts address this concern and require the reporting of impaired professionals while also providing rehabilitation for those who need it.

Other professional dilemmas revolve around competence. How do you deal with incompetent health-care personnel? This situation frustrates both staff and management. Regulations created to protect individuals from unjustified loss of position and the magnitude of paperwork, remediation, and the time it takes to terminate an incompetent health-care worker often compel management to tolerate the situation.

Employing institutions that provide nursing services have an obligation to establish a process for reporting and handling practices that jeopardize patient safety (Gong et al., 2015). The behaviors of incompetent staff place patients and other staff members in jeopardy. Eventually, the incompetency may lead to legal action that could have been avoided if appropriate leadership pursued a different approach.

Ethical Issues Raised by the COVID-19 Pandemic

Several ethical issues emerged during the pandemic. Some occurred more globally within the public health domain while others transpired at the direct point of care. Issues such as limited resources and ill health-care providers were addressed earlier in the chapter. However, ethical dilemmas such as falsifying COVID testing for financial gain, refusal to treat COVID patients in private offices and clinics because of possible exposure, and delaying surgeries that may have ultimately had fatal outcomes (Al-Jabir et al., 2020). Other issues revolved around mandating vaccinations, delaying procedures other than surgeries, and the closing of emergency services in some areas (Kooli, 2021).

Conclusion

Nurses and other health-care personnel find themselves confronting more ethical dilemmas in this ever-changing health-care environment. More questions are being raised with fewer answers available. New guidelines need to be developed to assist in finding viable solutions to these challenging questions. Technology wields enormous power to alter the human organism, the promise to eradicate diseases that plague humankind, and the ability for health-care professionals to prolong human life. However, fiscal resources and economics may force the health-care profession to rethink answers to questions such as, "What is life versus living?" and "When is it okay to terminate a human life?" Will society become the brave new world of Aldous Huxley? Again and again the question is raised, "Who shall live and who shall die?" How will you answer?

Study Questions

1. What is the difference between intrinsic and extrinsic values? Make a list of your intrinsic values.

2. Consider a decision you recently made that you based on your values. How did you make your choice?

3. Describe how you could use the valuing process of choosing, prizing, and acting in making the decision considered in Question 2.

4. Which of your personal values would be primary if you were assigned to care for an anencephalic infant whose parents have decided to donate the baby's organs?

5. The parents of the anencephalic infant in Question 4 confront you and ask, "What would you do if this were your baby?" What do you think would be most important for you to consider in responding to them?

6. Your friend is single and feels that her "biological clock is ticking." She decides to undergo in vitro fertilization using donor sperm. She tells you that she has researched the donor's background extensively and wants to show you the "template" for her child. She asks for your professional opinion about this situation. How would you respond? Identify the ethical principles involved.

7. During the past several weeks, you have noticed that your closest friend, Jamie, has been erratic and making poor patient care decisions. On two separate occasions you quietly intervened and "fixed" his errors. You have also noticed that he volunteers to give pain medications to other nurses' patients, and you see him standing very close to other nurses when they remove controlled substances from the medication distribution system. Today, you watched him go to the center immediately after another colleague and then saw him go into the men's room. Within about 20 minutes his behavior changed completely. You suspect that he is taking controlled substances. You and Jamie have been friends for more than 20 years. You grew up together and went to nursing school together. You realize that if you approach him, you may jeopardize this close friendship that means a great deal to you. Using the MORAL ethical decision-making model, devise a plan to resolve this dilemma.

Case Study to Promote Clinical Judgment

Andy is assigned to care for a 14-year-old girl, Amanda, admitted with a large tumor located in the left groin area. During an assessment, Amanda shares her personal feelings with Andy. She tells him that she "feels different" from her friends. She is ashamed of her physical development because all her girlfriends have "breasts" and boyfriends. She is very flat-chested and embarrassed. Andy listens attentively to Amanda and helps her focus on some of her positive attributes and talents.

A computed tomography (CT) scan is ordered and reveals that the tumor extends to what appears to be the ovary. A gynecological surgeon is called in to evaluate the situation. An ultrasonic-guided biopsy is performed. It is discovered that the tumor is actually an enlarged lymph node, and the "ovary" is actually a testis. Amanda has both male and female gonads.

When the information is given to Amanda's parents, they do not want her to know. They feel that she was raised as "their daughter." They ask the surgeon to remove the male gonads and leave only the female gonads. That way, "Amanda will never need to know." The surgeon refuses to do this. Andy believes the parents should discuss the situation with Amanda as they are denying her choices. The parents are adamant about Amanda not knowing anything. Andy returns to Amanda's room, and Amanda begins asking all types of questions regarding the tests and the treatments. Andy hesitates before answering, and Amanda picks up on this, demanding he tell her the truth.

1. How should Andy respond?

2. What ethical principles are in conflict?

3. What are the long-term effects of Andy's decision?

NCLEX®-Style Review Questions

1. Several studies have shown that although care planning and advance directives are available to clients, only a minority actually complete them. Which of the following has been shown to be related to completing an advance directive? **Select all that apply.**
   1. African American race
   2. Younger age
   3. History of chronic illness
   4. Lower socioeconomic status
   5. Higher education

2. *The ANA Code of Ethics With Interpretive Statements* guides nurses in ethical behaviors. Provision 3 of the *ANA Code of Ethics* says: "The nurse promotes, advocates for, and strives to protect the health, safety, and rights of the patient." Which of the following best describes an example of this provision?
   1. Respecting the patient's privacy and confidentiality when caring for him
   2. Serving on a committee that will improve the environment of patient care
   3. Maintaining professional boundaries when working with a patient
   4. Caring for oneself before trying to care for another person

3. Health Insurance Portability and Accountability Act (HIPAA) regulations guard confidentiality. In several situations, confidentiality can be breached and information can be reported to other entities. Which of the following meet these criteria? **Select all that apply.**
   1. The patient is from a correctional institution.
   2. The situation involves child abuse.
   3. An injury occurred from a firearm.
   4. The patient is a physician.
   5. The breach of information was unintentional.

4. A patient asks a nurse if he has to agree to the health provider's treatment plan. The nurse asks the patient about his concerns. Which ethical principle is the nurse applying in this situation? **Select all that apply.**
   1. Beneficence
   2. Autonomy
   3. Veracity
   4. Justice

5. Which best describes the difference between patient privacy and patient confidentiality?
    1. Confidentiality occurs between persons who are close, whereas privacy can affect anyone.
    2. Privacy is the right to be free from intrusion into personal matters, whereas confidentiality is protection from sharing a person's information.
    3. Confidentiality involves the use of technology for protection, whereas privacy uses physical components of protection.
    4. Privacy involves protection from being watched, whereas confidentiality involves protection from verbal exchanges.

6. A nurse is working on an ethics committee to determine the best course of action for a patient who is dying. The nurse considers the positive and negative outcomes of the decision to assist with choices. Which best describes the distinction of using a list when making an ethical decision?
    1. The nurse can back up her reasons for why she has decided to provide a certain type of care.
    2. The nurse can compare the benefits of one choice over another.
    3. The nurse can communicate the best choice of action to the interdisciplinary team.
    4. The nurse can provide care based on developed policies and standards.

7. A nurse is caring for a patient who feels that life should not be prolonged when hope is gone. She has decided that she does not want extraordinary measures taken when her life is at its end. She has discussed her feelings with her family and health-care provider. The nurse realizes that this is an example of
    1. Affirming a value
    2. Choosing a value
    3. Prizing a value
    4. Reflecting a value

8. Which of the following demonstrates a nurse as advocating for a patient? The nurse
    1. Calls a nursing supervisor in conflicting situations
    2. Reviews and understands the law as it applies to the client's clinical condition
    3. Documents all clinical changes in the medical record in a timely manner
    4. Assesses the client's point of view and prepares to articulate this point of view

9. A nurse's significant other undergoes exploratory surgery at the hospital where the nurse is an employee. Which practice is most appropriate?
    1. The nurse is an employee; therefore, access to the chart is permissible.
    2. Access to the chart requires a signed release form.
    3. The relationship with the client provides the nurse special access to the chart.
    4. The nurse can ask the surgeon to discuss the outcome of the surgery.

10. A nurse is providing care to a patient whose family has previously brought suit against another hospital and two physicians. Under which ethical principle should the nurse practice?
    1. Justice
    2. Veracity
    3. Autonomy
    4. Nonmaleficence

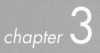

chapter 3

Nursing Practice and the Law

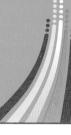

OBJECTIVES

After reading this chapter, the student should be able to:

- Describe three major forms of laws.
- Identify the differences among the various types of laws.
- Clarify the criteria that determine negligence from malpractice.
- Differentiate between an intentional and an unintentional tort.
- Support the use of standards of care in determining negligence and malpractice.
- Explain how nurse practice acts protect the public.
- Differentiate between internal standards and external standards.
- Examine the role advance directives play in protecting client rights.
- Discuss the legal implications of the Health Insurance Portability and Accountability Act (HIPAA).
- Identify legal issues surrounding the use of electronic medical records (EMRs).

OUTLINE

The courtroom seemed cold and sterile. Scanning her surroundings with nervous eyes, Naomi knew how Alice must have felt when the Queen of Hearts screamed for her head. The image of the White Rabbit running through the woods, looking at his watch, yelling, "I'm late! I'm late!" flashed before her eyes. For a few moments, she indulged herself in thoughts of being able to turn back the clock and rewrite the past. The future certainly looked grim at that moment. The calling of her name broke her reverie. Ms. Cornish, the attorney for the plaintiff, wanted her undivided attention regarding the inauspicious day when she committed a fatal medication error. That day, the client died following a cardiac arrest because Naomi failed to follow the standard of practice for administering a chemotherapy medication. She removed the appropriate medication from the automated system; however, she made a calculation error and did not check this against the order. Her 15 years of nursing experience meant little to the court. She stood alone. She was being sued for malpractice, with the possibility of criminal charges should she be found guilty of contributing to the client's death.

As client advocates, nurses have a responsibility to deliver safe and effective care to their clients. This expectation requires nurses to have professional knowledge at their expected level of practice and be proficient in technical skills. A working knowledge of the legal system, client rights, and behaviors that may result in lawsuits helps nurses to act as client advocates. As long as nurses practice according to the established standards of care, they may be able to avoid the kind of day in court Naomi experienced.

General Principles

Meaning of Law

The word *law* holds several meanings. For the purposes of this chapter, law refers to any system of regulation that governs the conduct of individuals within a community or society, in response to the need for regularity, consistency, and justice (Riches & Allen, 2013). In other words, law means those rules that prescribe and control social conduct in

a formal and legally binding manner. Laws are created in one of three ways:

1. *Statutory laws* are created by various legislative bodies, such as state legislatures or Congress. Some examples of federal statutes include the Patient Self-Determination Act of 1990 (PSDA), the Americans with Disabilities Act, and, more recently, the Affordable Care Act. State statutes include the state nurse practice acts and the Good Samaritan Act. Laws that govern nursing practice fall under the category of statutory law.
2. *Common law* is the traditional unwritten law of England, based on custom and use. It dates back to 1066 A.D. when William of Normandy won the Battle of Hastings (Riches & Allen, 2013). This law develops within the court system as the judicial system makes decisions in various cases and sets precedents for future cases. A decision rendered in one case may affect decisions made in later cases of a similar nature. For this reason, one case sets a precedent for another.
3. *Administrative law* includes the procedures created by administrative agencies (governmental bodies of the city, county, state, or federal government) involving rules, regulations, applications, licenses, permits, hearings, appeals, and decision making. These governing boards have the duty to meet the intent of laws or statutes.

Sources of Law

The Constitution

The U.S. Constitution is the foundation of American law. The Bill of Rights, composed of the first 10 amendments to the Constitution, laid the foundation for the protection of individual rights. These laws define and limit the power of government and protect citizens' rights, such as freedom of speech, assembly, religion, and the press. They also prevent the government from intruding into personal choices. State constitutions may expand individual rights but cannot limit nor deprive people of rights guaranteed by the U.S. Constitution.

Constitutional law evolves. As individuals or groups bring suits that challenge interpretations of the Constitution, decisions are made concerning the application of the law to that particular event. An example of this is the protection of "freedom of speech." Is the use of obscenities protected? Can one person threaten or criticize another? The freedom to criticize is protected; however, threats are not. The definition of obscenity has been clarified by the U.S. Supreme Court based on three separate cases. The decisions made in these cases evolved into what is referred to as the *Miller test* (Department of Justice, 2015).

Statutes

Statutes are written laws created by a government or accepted governing body. Localities, state legislatures, and the U.S. Congress generate statutes. Local statutes are usually referred to as ordinances. Requiring all residents to use a specific city garbage bag is an example of a local ordinance.

At the federal level, conference committees comprising representatives of both houses of Congress negotiate the resolution of differences on the working of a bill before it is voted upon by both houses of Congress and sent to the president to be signed into law. If the bill does not meet with the approval of the executive branch of government, the president holds the right to veto it. If that occurs, the legislative branch needs enough votes to override the veto, or the bill will not become law.

Administrative Law

Federal agencies concerned with health-care–related laws include the Department of Health and Human Services (DHHS), the Department of Labor, and the Department of Education. Agencies that focus on health-care law at the state level involve state health departments and licensing boards.

Administrative agencies are staffed with professionals who develop the specific rules and regulations that direct the implementation of statutory laws. These rules need to be reasonable and consistent with existing statutory law and the intent of the legislature. The targeted individuals and groups review and comment before these rules go into effect. For example, specific statutory laws give the state boards of nursing (SBONs) the authority to issue and revoke licenses. This means that each SBON holds the responsibility to oversee the professional nurse's competence.

Types of Laws

Another way to view the legal system is to divide laws into categories, such as public law and private law. Public law encompasses state, constitutional, administrative, and criminal law, whereas private law (civil law) covers contracts, torts, and property.

Criminal Law

Criminal or penal law focuses on crime and punishment. Societies created these laws to protect citizens from threatening actions. Criminal acts, although directed toward individuals, are considered offenses against the state. The perpetrator of the act is punished, and the victim receives no compensation for injury or damages. Criminal law subdivides into three categories:

1. **Felony** the most serious category, including such acts as homicide, grand larceny, and nurse practice act violations.
2. **Misdemeanor** includes lesser offenses such as traffic violations or shoplifting of a small dollar amount.
3. **Juvenile** crimes carried out by individuals younger than 18 years of age; specific ages vary by state and crimes.

There are occasions when a nurse breaks a law and is tried in criminal court. A nurse who obtains or distributes controlled substances illegally, either for personal use or for the use of others, is violating the law. Falsification of records of controlled substances is also a criminal action. In some states, altering a patient record may lead to both civil and criminal action depending on the treatment outcome (Zhong et al., 2016). Although the following is an older case, it provides an excellent example of negligence resulting in criminal charges brought against a nurse:

In *New Jersey State v. Winter*, Nurse V needed to administer a blood transfusion. Because she was in a rush, she neglected to check the paperwork properly and therefore failed to follow the established standard of practice for blood administration. The client was transfused with incompatible blood, suffered a transfusion reaction, and died. Nurse V then intentionally attempted to conceal her conduct. She falsified the records, disposed of the blood and administration equipment, and did not notify the client's health-care provider of the error. The jury found Nurse V guilty of simple manslaughter and sentenced her to 5 years in prison (Sanbar, 2007).

In the March 2022 case of *Tennessee v. Vaught*, a jury convicted a registered nurse (RN), RaDonda Vaught, of "reckless homicide and impaired adult abuse after she was accused of inadvertently injecting a patient with a deadly dose of a paralyzing drug" (Timms, 2022). Ms. Vaught mistakenly removed the drug vecuronium instead of the ordered Versed from the electronic dispensing system and gave the vecuronium to the patient. Ms. Vaught self-reported the error. According to the trial records, Ms. Vaught initially typed "VE" into the dispenser's search system "without realizing that she should have been looking for its generic name, midazolam" (Kelman, 2022a). When the system failed to produce Versed, Ms. Vaught initiated an override and this provided a larger selection of medications. When she entered for "VE" again, the drug dispenser provided the vecuronium. During her testimony before the Tennessee Board of Nursing (TBN), Vaught discussed the use of the override function and that it had become common practice due to a glitch in the upgraded electronic health records (EHR) system. The hospital was not brought into the suit although the Tennessee Bureau of Investigation supported the argument that systemic errors within the Vanderbilt system led to the error (Kelman, 2022a). The case presented by the prosecution focused on Vaught ignoring the warnings built into the electronic dispensing system. She was convicted of two felonies for a fatal drug error. Nurses across the country organized sending letters and signing petitions to the judge who resided over the case. At the sentencing hearing, the judge decided to give Vaught three years probation and granted her a judicial diversion. Once Vaught completes the three years probation, her record will be expunged (Kelman, 2022b).

The American Nurses Association (ANA) has voiced concern regarding this conviction. First, in the realm of a *just culture* and a *culture of safety*, when "criminalizing the honest reporting of mistakes" (ANA, 2022), will nurses and other providers feel safe reporting errors? Second, most inadvertent errors are system errors; in this case, an issue from an upgrade in the EHR caused delays in medication dispensing and the hospital system instructed the nursing staff to override the system to prevent late administration of medications (Kelman, 2022a). Lastly, there are more "effective and just mechanisms to examine errors, establish system improvements and take corrective action" (ANA).

Civil Law

Civil laws usually involve the violation of one person's rights by another person. Areas of civil law that particularly affect nurses are tort law, contract law, antitrust law, employment discrimination, and labor laws.

Tort

The remainder of this chapter focuses primarily on tort law. By definition, tort law consists of a body of rights, obligations, and remedies that courts apply during civil proceedings for the purpose of providing relief for individuals who suffered harm from the wrongful acts of others. Tort laws serve two basic functions: (1) to compensate a victim for any damages or losses incurred by the defendant's actions (or inaction) and (2) to discourage the defendant from repeating the behavior in the future (LaMance, 2018). The individual who incurs the injury or damage is known as the plaintiff, whereas the person who caused the injury or damage is referred to as the defendant. Tort law recognizes that individuals, in their relationships to one another, have a general duty to avoid harm. For example, automobile drivers have a duty to drive safely so that others will not be harmed. A construction company has a duty to build a structure that meets building codes and will not collapse, resulting in harm to the individuals using it (Viglucci & Staletovich, 2017). Nurses have a duty to deliver care in such a manner that the consumers of care are not harmed. These legal duties of care may be violated intentionally or unintentionally.

Quasi-Intentional Tort

A quasi-intentional tort includes voluntary wrongful acts based on speech. These are committed by a person or entity against another person or entity that inflicts economic harm or damage to reputation. For example, a defamation of character through slander or libel or an invasion of privacy is considered a quasi-intentional tort (Garner, 2014).

Negligence

Negligence is an unintentional tort of acting or failing to act as an ordinary, reasonable, prudent person, resulting in harm to the person to whom the duty of care is owed (Garner, 2014). For negligence to occur, the following elements must be present: duty, breach of duty, causation, and harm or injury (Jacoby & Scruth, 2017). All four elements need to be present in the determination of negligence.

Nurses find themselves in these situations when they fail to meet a specified standard of practice or standard of care. The duty of care is the standard (Wade, 2015). For example, if a nurse administers the incorrect medication to a client, but the client does not suffer any injury, the element of harm is not met. However, if a nurse administers the appropriate pain medication to a client and fails to raise the side rails and the client falls and breaks a hip, all four elements of negligence have been satisfied. The law defines the standard of care as that which any reasonable, prudent practitioner with similar education and experience would do or not do in a similar circumstance (Jacoby & Scruth, 2017; Sanbar, 2007).

Malpractice

Malpractice is the term applied to professional negligence (Sohn, 2013). This term is used when the fulfillment of duties requires specialized education. In most malpractice suits, the facilities employing the nurses who cared for a client are named as the defendants in the suit. These types of cases fall under the legal principle known as *vicarious liability* (West, 2016).

Three doctrines come under the principle of vicarious liability: *respondeat superior,* the borrowed servant doctrine, and the "captain of the ship" doctrine. The captain of the ship doctrine, an adaptation of the borrowed servant rules, emerged from the case of *McConnell v. Williams* and refers to medical malpractice (*McConnell v. Williams,* 1949). The ruling declared that the person in charge is held accountable for all those falling under the leader's supervision, regardless of whether the "captain" is directly responsible for the alleged error or act of alleged negligence, and despite the others' positions as hospital employees (Stern, 1949).

An important principle in understanding negligence is *respondeat superior* ("let the master answer") (Thornton, 2010). This doctrine holds employers liable for any negligence by their employees when the employees were acting under the scope of employment. The "borrowed servant" rules come into play when an employee may be subject to the control and direction of an entity other than the primary employer. In this particular situation, someone other than an individual's primary employer is held accountable for that individual's actions. This was the basis for the ruling in *McConnell v. Williams* and its application to the captain of the ship doctrine. Consider the following scenario:

> A nursing clinical faculty member instructed students not to administer any medication without the faculty member's direct supervision. Marcos, a second-level student, was unable to find the faculty member, so Marcos decided to administer digoxin to his client without faculty supervision. The ordered dose was 0.125 milligrams. Marcos requested that one of the nurses access the automated medication dispensing system for him. The unit dose came as 0.5 milligrams/milliliter. Marcos administered the entire amount of medication without checking the dose, the client's digoxin level, and the potassium levels. The client became toxic, developed a dysrhythmia, and was transferred to the intensive care unit. The family sued the hospital and the nursing school for malpractice. The clinical faculty was also sued under the principle of *respondeat superior,* even though specific instructions were given to students regarding administering medications without direct faculty supervision.

Other Laws Relevant to Nursing Practice

Good Samaritan Laws

Fear of being sued often prevents trained professionals from providing assistance in emergency situations. To encourage physicians and nurses to respond to emergencies, many states developed what are now known as Good Samaritan laws. These laws protect health-care professionals from civil liability as long as they behave in the same manner as an ordinary reasonable and prudent professional in the same or similar circumstances. In other words, the professional standards of care still apply. However, if the provider receives a payment for the care given, the Good Samaritan laws do not hold.

Confidentiality

It is possible for nurses to find themselves involved in lawsuits other than those involving negligence. For example, clients have the right to confidentiality, and it is the duty of the professional nurse to ensure this right (Guglielmo, 2013). This assures the client that information obtained by a nurse while providing care will not be communicated to anyone who does not have a need to know. This includes giving information without a client's signed release or removing documents from a health-care provider with a client's name or other information.

The Health Insurance Portability and Accountability Act (HIPAA) of 1996 was passed as an effort to preserve confidentiality, protect the privacy of health information, and improve the portability and continuation of health-care coverage. The HIPAA gave Congress until August 1999 to pass this legislation. Congress failed to act, and the DHHS took over developing the appropriate regulations (Charters, 2003). The latest version of HIPAA can be found on the Department of Health and Human Services (DHHS) website at www.hhs.gov.

The increased use of electronic medical records (EMRs) and transfer of client information presents many confidentiality issues. It is important for nurses to be aware of the guidelines protecting the sharing and transfer of information through electronic sources. Although most health-care institutions have internal procedures to protect client confidentiality, several major health-care organizations recently found themselves victims of hacking and were held accountable for the dissemination of private information. However, it is exceptionally difficult to file lawsuits for these types of breaches (Worth, 2017).

Consider the following example:

> Evan was admitted to the hospital for pneumonia. With Evan's permission, an HIV test was performed, and the result was positive. This information was available on the computerized laboratory printout. A nurse inadvertently left the laboratory results up on the computer screen, which partially faced the hallway. One of Evan's coworkers, who had come to visit him, saw the report on the screen and reported the test results to Evan's supervisor. When Evan returned to work, he was terminated for "poor job performance," although he had superior evaluations. In the process of filing a discrimination suit against his employer, Evan discovered that the information about his health status had come from this source. A lawsuit was filed against the hospital and the nurse involved based on a breach of confidentiality.

Telehealth

Telehealth, sometimes referred to as telemedicine, refers to using "electronic information and telecommunications technologies to support and promote long-distance clinical healthcare, patient and professional health-related education, public health and health administration" (Balestra, 2018, p. 33). Originally providers established this method of providing care to extend access to patients living in rural areas. During the pandemic, health-care practices and institutions imposed restrictions on the number of patients and significant others allowed in these settings. To try and ensure care and maintain communication, many providers and health-care agencies resorted to telehealth to interface with patients and their families.

Several issues arose surrounding the implementation of telehealth visits and communication including confidentiality, health equity, and access to resources. Nurses found themselves involved in telehealth delivery systems in several ways: (a) assisting providers in connecting with patients in the office setting, (b) meeting with patients to review information from a previous visit or obtain pre-visit information, and (c) speaking with hospitalized patients' families to provide updates on their loved one's condition or connect patients with their families. The potential for violating patient confidentiality exists in any one of these situations. Therefore, systems used to interface with patients need to be HIPAA compliant. However, for the most part, the communication methods used in the acute care setting relied on external applications such as FaceTime or Zoom technologies. Neither of these can be considered HIPAA compliant. For this reason, appropriate identification of the patient and family remains imperative to ensure confidentiality to the best of the nurse's knowledge (Balestra, 2018; Rose et al., 2021).

Social Networking

Another issue affecting confidentiality involves social networking. The definition of *social media* is extensive and consistently changing. The term usually refers to Internet-based tools that permit individuals and groups to meet and communicate; to share information, ideas, personal messages, images, and other content; and to collaborate with other users in real time (Geraghty et al., 2021; Ventola, 2014). Social media use is widespread across all ages and professions and is universal throughout the world.

Social media modalities provide health-care professionals with Internet-based methods that assist them in sharing information; engaging in discussions on health-care policy and practice issues; encouraging healthy behaviors; connecting with the public; and educating and interacting with patients, caregivers, students, and colleagues (Geraghty et al., 2021; Ventola, 2014). These modalities convey information about a person's personality, values, and priorities, and the first impression generated by this content can be lasting (Bernhardt et al., 2014).

Employers, academic institutions, and other organizations often view social media content and develop perceptions about prospective employees, students, and possible clientele based on this content (Denecke et al., 2015). A person who consciously posts personal information on social media sites has willingly given access to anyone to view it for any purpose. Therefore, it is only logical that those who do not use discretion in deciding what content to post online may also be unable to exercise sensible professional judgment.

Several years ago Microsoft conducted a survey revealing that 79% of employers accessed online information regarding potential employees, and only 7% of job candidates knew of this possibility (MacMillan, 2013).

However, the increased use of social networking comes with a downside. A major threat centers on issues such as breaches of confidentiality and defamation of character. The posting of unprofessional content has the potential to damage the reputations of health-care professionals, students, and affiliated institutions. Recently, a surgeon posted videos of herself dancing in the operating room while engaged in performing surgery on patients. A mishap occurred during one of the surgeries, and the patient suffered a respiratory arrest. Patients and the public saw the videos, and therefore several malpractice suits have been filed against the physician (Hartung, 2018).

Behaviors associated with unprofessional actions include violations of patient privacy; the use of profanity or biased language; images of sexual impropriety or drunkenness; and inappropriate comments about patients, an employer, or a school (Peck, 2014). Nursing boards have also disciplined nurses for violations involving online disclosure of patients' personal health information and have imposed sanctions ranging from letters of concern to license suspensions (MacMillan, 2013). In 2009, a U.S. District Court upheld the expulsion of a nursing student for violating the school's honor code because the student made offensive comments regarding the race, sex, and religion of patients (Peck, 2014).

The increased use of smartphones has led to increased violations of confidentiality (Ventola, 2014). These infractions often occur without intent yet pose a risk to both clients and health-care personnel. Posting pictures and information on social networking sites that involve clinical experiences or work experiences can present a risk to patient confidentiality and violate HIPAA regulations. To comply with the HIPAA Privacy Rule, clinical information or stories posted on social media that deal with clients or patients must have all personal identifying information removed. The HIPAA Privacy Rule places heavy financial penalties and possible criminal charges on the unauthorized release of *individually identifiable* health information by health-care providers, institutions, and other entities that provide confidential physical or psychological care. For this reason, many institutions have implemented policies that affect employees and student affiliations. These policies may result in employee termination or cancellation of agreements with outside agencies using the health-care institution.

Take the following example:

Several nursing students who received scholarships from an affiliated health-care organization, composed of multiple hospitals, were working their required shift in the emergency department (ED). The staff brought in a birthday cake for one of the ED physicians. One of the students snapped a "selfie" with the staff and the physician and posted it on her social network page. The computer screen with the names and information of the clients in the ED at the time was clearly visible behind the group. Another staff member noticed this and immediately notified the chief nursing officer of the hospital. The nursing student lost her scholarship, was terminated from her job, was required to return all monies to the organization, and was identified as a "do not hire" within the organization. Disciplinary actions were instituted against the staff involved in the incident. Because this organization owned all the hospitals, clinics, and physician practices within the geographic area, the student needed to attempt to gain employment in an area 50 miles from her home.

Patients and their families often develop feelings of gratitude toward the nurses who cared for them. Sometimes patients may think they built a friendship with their caregivers and reach out to "friend them" via social media. Nurses need to ensure that they keep the lines clear between friendship and professionalism. Blurring these may cause legal issues for the nurse at a later time.

At all times, remember that nurses represent their employing organization. Although staff may feel that what they post online is their own personal choice, often their institutions and licensing organizations view the posts in a different light resulting in legal issues.

Slander and Libel

Slander and libel are categorized as quasi-intentional torts. The term *slander* refers to the spoken word, whereas *libel* refers to the written word. Nurses rarely think of themselves as being guilty of slander or libel, but making a false verbal statement about a client's condition that may result in an injury is considered slander. Making a false written statement is libel. For example, verbally stating that a client who had blood drawn for drug testing has a substance abuse problem, when in fact the client does not carry that diagnosis, could be considered a slanderous statement.

Slander and libel also refer to statements made about coworkers or other individuals whom you may encounter in both your professional and educational life. Think before you speak and write. Sometimes what may appear to be harmless to you, such as a complaint, may contain statements that damage another person's credibility personally and professionally. Consider this example:

> Several nurses on a unit were having difficulty with a nurse manager. Rather than approach the manager or follow the chain of command, they decided to send a written statement to the chief executive officer (CEO) of the hospital. In this letter, they embellished some of the incidents that occurred and took statements that the nurse manager made out of context, changing the meaning of the remarks. The CEO called the nurse manager to the office and reprimanded her for these events and statements that had in fact not occurred, documented the meeting, and developed an action plan that was placed in her personnel file. The nurse manager sued the

nurses for slander and libel based on the premise that her personal and professional reputation had been tainted. She also filed a complaint against the hospital CEO for failure to appropriately investigate the situation, demanding a verbal and written apology.

False Imprisonment

False imprisonment is confining individuals against their will by either physical (restraining) or verbal (detaining) means. The following represent examples of false imprisonment:

- Using restraints on individuals without the appropriate written consent or following protocols
- Restraining mentally challenged individuals who do not represent a threat to themselves or others
- Detaining unwilling clients in an institution when they desire to leave
- Keeping persons who are medically cleared for discharge for an unreasonable amount of time
- Removing clients' clothing to prevent them from leaving the institution
- Threatening clients with some form of physical, emotional, or legal action if they insist on leaving

Sometimes clients are a danger to themselves and to others. Nurses need to decide on the appropriateness of restraints as a protective measure. Nurses should always try to obtain the cooperation of the client before applying any type of restraint and follow the institutional protocols and standards for restraint use (Springer, 2015). The first step is to attempt to identify a reason for the risky or threatening behavior and resolve the problem. If this fails, document the need for restraints, consult with the health-care provider, and conduct a complete assessment of the patient's physical and mental status. Systematic documentation and continuous assessment are of highest importance when caring for clients who have restraints. Any changes in client status must be reported and documented. Failure to follow these guidelines may result in greater harm to the client and possibly a lawsuit for the staff. Consider the following example:

> Mr. Harvey, an 87-year-old man, was admitted from home to the ED with severe lower abdominal pain and vomiting of three days' duration. Before admission, he and his wife lived alone,

remained active in the community, and cared for themselves without difficulty. Physical assessment revealed severe dehydration and acute distress. Physical examination revealed a ruptured appendix. A surgeon was called, and after a successful surgery, Mr. Harvey was sent to the intensive care unit for 24 hours. He was transferred to the surgical floor awake, alert, oriented, and in stable condition. Later that night he became confused, irritable, and anxious. He attempted to climb out of bed and pulled out his indwelling urinary catheter. The nurse restrained him. The next day his irritability and confusion continued. Mr. Harvey's nurse placed him in a chair, tying and restraining his hands. When his wife came to the hospital three hours later, she found him in the chair, completely unresponsive. He had died of cardiopulmonary arrest. A lawsuit of wrongful death and false imprisonment was brought against the nurse manager, the nurses caring for Mr. Harvey, and the institution. It was determined that the primary cause of Mr. Harvey's behavior was hypoxemia. A violation of law occurred with the failure of the nursing staff to notify the physician of the client's condition and to follow the institution's standard of practice on the use of restraints.

To protect themselves against charges of negligence and false imprisonment in cases similar to this one, nurses should discuss safety needs with clients, their families, or other members of the health-care team. Careful assessment and documentation of client status remain imperative and are also components of good nursing practice. Confusion, irritability, and anxiety often result from metabolic causes that need correction, not restraint.

There are statutes and case laws specific to the admission of clients to psychiatric institutions. Most states have guidelines for emergency involuntary hospitalization for a specific period of time. Involuntary admission is considered necessary when clients demonstrate a danger to themselves or others. Specific procedures and legal guidelines must be followed. A determination by a judge or administrative agency or certification by a specified number of health-care providers that a person's mental health justifies detention and treatment may be required. Once admitted, these clients may not be restrained unless the guidelines established by state law and the institution's policies provide for this possibility. Clients who voluntarily admit themselves to psychiatric institutions are also protected against false imprisonment. Nurses working in areas such as the ED, mental health facilities, and so forth, need to be cognizant of these issues and find out the policies of their state and employing institution.

Assault and Battery

Assault is threatening to do harm. Battery is touching another person without that person's consent. The significance of an assault lies in the threat: "If you don't stop pushing that call bell, I'll sedate you" is considered an assaultive statement. Battery would occur if the sedation was given when it was refused, even if the medical personnel deemed it necessary for the "client's good." With few exceptions, clients have the right to refuse treatment. Holding down a violent client against that client's will and injecting medication is considered battery. Most medical treatments, particularly surgery, would be considered battery if clients failed to provide informed consent.

Standards of Practice

Avedis Donabedian, credited as the "Father of Quality Assurance," said, "Standards are professionally developed expressions of the range of acceptable variations from a norm or criterion" (Best & Neuhauser, 2004, p. 472). Concern for the quality of care is a major part of nursing's responsibility to the public. Therefore, the nursing profession is accountable to the consumer for the quality of its services.

One defining characteristic of a profession is the ability to set its own standards. Nursing standards were established as guidelines for the profession to ensure acceptable quality of care. Clear statements of the scope of practice including specialty nursing practice and standards of specialty practice and professional performance assist and promote continued awareness and recognition of nurses' varied professional contributions (Finnel et al., 2015).

State Boards of Nursing (SBONs) and professional organizations develop standards and delineate responsibilities (Finnel et al., 2015). Statutes written by the government, professional organizations, and health-care institutions establish standards of practice. The nurse practice acts of each state define the boundaries of practice within those states. Nurses are bound to follow these rules and standards as outlined by the state boards.

Standards of practice are also used as criteria to determine whether appropriate care has been delivered. In practice, they represent the minimum acceptable level of care. They take many forms. Some are written and appear as criteria of professional organizations, job descriptions, and agency policies and procedures. Many may be found in textbooks and find their basis in evidence-based practice (Moffett & Moore, 2011). Nurses are judged on generally accepted standards of practice for their level of education, experience, position, and specialty area (Finnel et al., 2015).

The role of the SBONs is to protect the public. The courts have upheld the authority of boards of nursing to regulate standards of practice. The boards accomplish this through direct or delegated statutory language (Maloney & Harper, 2016). The ANA developed specific standards of practice for general practice areas and in several clinical areas (ANA, 2015, 2021; see Appendix 1). "Specialty organizations align with those broad parameters by developing and revising their own specific scope and standards of practice. Standards of professional practice include a description of the standard followed by multiple competency statements that serve as evidence for compliance with the standard" (Maloney & Harper, 2016, p. 327).

Institutions develop internal standards of practice. The standards are usually explained as a specific institutional policy (for example, guidelines for the appropriate administration of a specific chemotherapeutic agent), and the institution includes these standards in its policy and procedure manuals. The guidelines are based on current literature and research (evidence-based practice). It is the nurse's responsibility to meet the institution's standards of practice, whereas it is the institution's responsibility to notify the health-care personnel of any changes and instruct the personnel about the changes. Institutions may accomplish this task through written memos or meetings and in-service education.

With the expansion of advanced nursing practice, the need to clarify the legal distinctions and scope of practice among the varied levels of education and certification has become increasingly important (Feringa et al., 2018). Patient care has become more complex and nursing skills more technologically advanced, causing some blurring of boundaries. In certain high-acuity areas, nurses make independent decisions based on protocols and standards developed by the institution. However, these practices remain institution-specific with the expectation that the nurse has received the appropriate education to implement the protocols (Feringa et al., 2018). Nurses need to realize that the same practices may be unacceptable in another setting.

These changes in practice require nurses to familiarize themselves with the boundaries among the professional demands and the scope and standards of practice within the discipline and various specialties. The nurse practice acts help nurses clarify their roles at the varied practice levels (Altman et al., 2016).

Use of Standards in Nursing Negligence and Malpractice Actions

When omission of prudent care or acts committed by a nurse or those under the nurse's supervision cause harm to a client, standards of nursing practice are among the elements used to determine whether malpractice or negligence exists. Other criteria may include but are not limited to:

- National, state, or local (community—those used universally within the community) standards
- Institutional policies that alter or adhere to the nursing standards of care
- Expert opinions on the appropriate standard of care at the time
- Available literature and research that substantiates a standard of care or changes in the standard

Patient's Bill of Rights

In 1973 the American Hospital Association (AHA) approved a statement called the Patient's Bill of Rights, which was revised in October 1992. Patient rights were developed with the belief that hospitals and other health-care institutions and providers would support them with the goal of delivering effective client care. In 2003 the Patient's Bill of Rights was replaced by the Patient Care Partnership. These standards were derived from the ethical principle of autonomy.

In 2010, President Obama announced new regulations that included a set of protections that applied to health coverage that started in September, 6 months after the Congress enacted the Affordable Care Act. This addition was designed to protect children and eventually all Americans who have preexisting conditions and help them obtain and keep coverage, offer a choice of health-care providers, and end the lifetime limits on the ability to receive care (Centers for Medicare and Medicaid Services [CMS], 2010).

Informed Consent

Informed consent is a legal document in all 50 states and is critical to both ethical and legal principles considering a patient's understanding of a procedure or treatment, and respect for their autonomy (Grant, 2021). It requires health-care providers to divulge the benefits, risks, and alternatives to a suggested treatment, nontreatment, or procedure. It allows for fully informed, rational persons to maintain involvement in their health and health-care decisions (Grant, 2021; Hall et al., 2012). "While the concept of informed consent evolved under the theory of legal battery, it is now considered under the legal domain of negligence" (Moore et al., 2014, p. 923).

Although the concept of consent goes as far back as ancient legal and philosophical principles, the modern legal model for "simple" consent was based on the case of *Schloendorff v. Society of New York Hospital* in 1914. In this case, a young woman agreed to an examination of her uterus while under anesthesia, but she had not consented to surgery. Her surgeon discovered a tumor and removed her uterus. Although the New York court dismissed the patient's claim for reasons that were not related to providing consent, the case gave the judge a chance to discuss and contribute to the development of the legal concept of informed consent. The judge noted that it was the patient's "understanding" that there was only to be an examination, and that the patient's understanding was crucial to determining consent. The New York Court of Appeals issued a decision that laid the groundwork for informed consent and instituted a patient's "right to determine what shall be done with his body" (Moore et al., 2014).

Without informed consent, many of the procedures performed on clients in a health-care setting may be considered battery or unwarranted touching. When clients consent to treatment, they give health-care personnel the right to deliver care and perform specific treatments without fear of prosecution. Although physicians and other practitioners performing procedures or care are responsible for obtaining informed consent, nurses often find themselves involved in the process.

It is the responsibility of the practitioner who is performing the procedure or treatment to give information to a client about the benefits and risks of treatment and outcomes (The Joint Commission [TJC], 2016). Although the nurse may witness the signature of a patient or client for a procedure or surgery, the nurse should not be providing details such as the benefits, risks, or possible outcomes. The individual institution is not responsible for obtaining the informed consent unless (a) the physician or practitioner is employed by the institutions or (b) the institution was aware or should have been aware of the lack of informed consent and failed to act on this fact (Hall et al., 2012). Some institutions require the physician or independent practitioner to obtain informed consent by getting the patient's signature at the time the provider offers the explanation for treatment.

Although some nurses believe that they only need to obtain the client's signature on the informed consent document, nursing professionals have a larger responsibility in evaluating a client's ability to give informed consent. The nurse's role is to (a) act as the patient's advocate, (b) protect the patient's dignity, (c) identify fears or concerns, and (d) determine the patient's level of understanding and approval of the proposed care.

Every client brings a different and unique response depending on the patient's personality, level of education, emotions, and cognitive status. A good practice is to ask the client to restate the information offered. This helps confirm that the client has received an appropriate amount of information and understands it. The nurse remains obliged to report any concerns about the client's understanding regarding what the nurse said or any concerns about the client's ability to make decisions.

The defining opinion on the requirements of informed consent emerged from the case of *Canterbury v. Spence*. In this situation, a young patient developed paralysis after spinal surgery (Moore et al., 2014). The patient and the family asked the surgeon if the operation was serious, and he responded, "Not any more than any other operation." The suit was litigated as a "failure to obtain informed consent due to battery" (p. 923); however, the court determined that this constituted an issue of negligence. Besides putting informed consent completely within the concept of negligence, this landmark case put forth many of the elements of informed consent we recognize today. The informed consent form should contain all the possible negative outcomes as well as the positive ones. The following are some criteria to help ensure that a client has given an informed consent (Bal & Choma, 2012; Gupta, 2013):

- A mentally competent adult has voluntarily given the consent.
- The client understands exactly as to what the client is consenting.
- The consent includes the risks involved in the procedure, alternative treatments that may be available, and the possible result if the treatment is refused.
- The consent is written.
- A minor's parent or guardian needs to give consent for treatment.

Ideally, a nurse should be present when the health-care provider who is performing the treatment, surgery, or procedure is explaining benefits and risks to the client.

To give informed consent, the client must receive complete information and understand the risks and benefits. Clients have the right to refuse treatment, and nurses must respect that right. If a client refuses the recommended treatment plan, then that individual needs to be fully informed of the possible consequences of the decision in a nonforceful, noncoercive manner. This caveat remains exceptionally important; if clients consent because they feel coerced and the outcome is less than favorable, all parties involved in obtaining the consent may find themselves at risk (Hall et al., 2012).

Implied consent occurs when consent is assumed (Moore et al., 2014). This often occurs in emergency situations when an individual is unable to give consent. State laws support the right of health-care providers to act in an emergency without the expressed consent of the patient. It is also important to note that complications of that procedure may be legally defensible if the providers acted in a reasonable, prudent manner. A recent civil case, *Futral v. Webb*, supported this. In this lawsuit, a patient presented in shock and with altered mental status. The ED provider placed a subclavian line for fluids and caused a hemothorax. A chest tube was then inserted; however, the patient became bradycardic, arrested, and died. The patient's family sued the provider; however, the jury ruled in favor of the provider and the hospital based on the fact that the complication was a known and accepted risk of the procedure. They also asserted that the provider acted in the best interests of the patient

when unable to receive expressed consent (Moore et al., 2014).

Nurses may find themselves involved in emergent situations where consent may be implied. Trauma centers often have protocols in place that address provider roles and actions in order to avoid legal actions. In these cases, follow the health-care institution policies, carefully document the client's status, attempt to reach significant others, and identify pertinent assessment data.

Staying Out of Court

Prevention

Unfortunately, the public's trust in the health-care industry and the medical profession has declined during recent years. Consumers are better informed and more assertive in their approach regarding care. They demand safe and effective care that promotes positive outcomes. If clients and their families perceive that the provider exhibits an impersonal attitude and uncaring behaviors, they are more likely to sue for what they believe are errors in treatment.

The same applies to nurses. If nurses demonstrate a caring attitude and interest toward their clients and families, a relationship develops. Individuals rarely initiate lawsuits against those they view as "caring friends." Demonstrating care and concern and making clients and families aware of choices and explaining situations helps decrease liability. Nurses who involve clients and families in care and decisions about care reduce the likelihood of a lawsuit. Tips to prevent legal problems are listed in Box 3-1.

---

box 3-1

Tips for Avoiding Legal Problems

- Keep yourself informed regarding new research related to your area of practice.
- Insist that the health-care institution keep personnel apprised of all changes in policies and procedures and in the management of new technological equipment.
- Always follow the standards of care or practice for the institution.
- Delegate tasks and procedures only to appropriate personnel.
- Identify clients at risk for problems, such as falls or the development of decubiti.
- Establish and maintain a safe environment.
- Document precisely and carefully.
- Write detailed incident reports and file them with the appropriate personnel or department.
- Recognize certain client behaviors that may indicate the possibility of a lawsuit.

table 3-1

Common Causes of Negligence

Problem	Prevention
Client falls	Identify clients at risk.
	Place notices about fall precautions.
	Follow institutional policies on the use of restraints.
	Always be sure beds are in their lowest positions.
	Use side rails appropriately.
Equipment injuries	Check thermostats and temperature in equipment used for heat or cold application.
	Check wiring on all electrical equipment.
Failure to monitor	Observe IV infusion sites as directed by institutional policy.
	Obtain and record vital signs, urinary output, cardiac status, and so on, as directed by institutional policy and more often if client condition dictates.
	Check pertinent laboratory values.
Failure to communicate	Report pertinent changes in client status.
	Document changes accurately.
	Document communication with appropriate source.
Medication errors	Follow the Seven Rights.
	Monitor client responses.
	Check client medications for multiple drugs for the same actions.

All health-care personnel remain accountable for their own actions and adherence to accepted standards of care. Most negligence and malpractice suits arise from the violation of the accepted standards of practice and the policies of the employing institution. Common causes of negligence are listed in Table 3-1. Expert witnesses are called to cite the accepted standards and assist attorneys on both sides in formulating legal strategies pertaining to those standards.

Appropriate Documentation

The adage "not documented, not done" holds true in nursing. According to the law, if something is not documented, then the responsible party did not do whatever needed to be done. If a nurse did not "do" something, then the nurse will be left open to negligence or malpractice charges.

Nursing documentation needs to be legally credible. The move to computerized charting, known by various names, has decreased some concerns but added others. Catalano (2014) provided several tips regarding electronic documentation. Nurses need to be cognizant that in the electronic record, everything documented exists and does not disappear. In other words, nurses cannot simply rip up the paper and start a new sheet or new form. Many systems require wrong information to be deleted, and this leaves an "electronic footprint." It also requires a valid explanation for the deletion and insertion. All applicable spaces and areas need to be completed, and nurses must avoid copying and pasting at all costs. Although some nurses seem to feel this saves time, it also opens up a new area for documentation errors if a piece of information is incorrect or deleted.

Even when nurses are using an electronic method for documentation, some of the "old rules" still apply:

- Remember to only use approved abbreviations.
- Document at the time care was provided.
- Keep documentation objective.
- Ensure appropriateness (document only what could be discussed comfortably in a public setting).
- Always use the barcodes on both clients and medications.
- Avoid shortcuts on documentation.

Common Actions Leading to Malpractice Suits

- Failure to assess a client appropriately
- Failure to report changes in client status to the appropriate personnel
- Failure to document in the patient record
- Falsifying documentation or attempting to alter the patient record
- Failure to report a coworker's negligence or poor practice
- Failure to provide appropriate education to patients and families
- Violation of an internal or external standard of practice

In the case of *Tovar v. Methodist Healthcare* (2005), a 75-year-old female came to the ED reporting a headache and weakness in her right arm. Although the physician wrote an order for admission to the neurological care unit, three hours passed before the patient was transferred. After the patient was admitted to the unit, nurses called a physician regarding the client's status; however, it took

90 minutes for another physician to return the call. Three hours later, the nurses called to report a change in the patient's neurological status. A STAT computerized tomography scan was ordered, which revealed a massive brain hemorrhage. The courts established the following based on the standard of care:

> *Nursing personnel provided poor documentation of the clinical status of Ms. Rodriguez between 5 p.m. and 9 p.m. Despite the patient's obvious deterioration at that time, they meekly accepted inadequate responses of Dr. Garrison and Dr. Osonma with no further calls to physicians until 12:30 a.m. when the patient was in extremis. The appropriate standard of care for nursing personnel treating a patient with acute neurological process is to promptly and expeditiously transfer the patient to the appropriate setting and carefully inform the treating physicians of changes in the patient's clinical status so that appropriate care can be rendered. The nursing personnel failed to perform these critical functions in their management of Ms. Rodriguez, thereby breaching the standard of care. (Tovar v. Methodist Healthcare, 2005)*

The nurses were also cited for:

1. Delay in transferring the patient to the neurological care unit
2. Failure to advocate for the patient

If a Problem Arises

When served with a summons or complaint, people often panic, allowing fear to overcome reason. First, simply answer the complaint. Failure to do this may result in a default judgment, causing greater distress and difficulties.

Second, individuals may take steps to protect themselves if named in a lawsuit. If a nurse carries malpractice, notify the carrier immediately. Legal representation can be obtained to protect personal property. Never sign any documents without consulting the malpractice insurance carrier or legal representative.

Institutions usually have lawyers to defend themselves and their employees. Whether or not you are personally insured, contact the legal department of the institution where the act occurred. Maintain a file of all papers, proceedings, meetings, e-mails, texts, and phone conversations about the case. Do not discuss the case with anyone outside of the appropriate individuals, and do not withhold any information from your attorneys, even if the information may be harmful to you. Concealing information usually causes more damage. Let the attorneys and the insurance company help decide how to handle the difficult situation. They are in charge of damage control.

Sometimes, nurses believe they are not being adequately protected or represented by the attorneys from their employing institution. If this happens, consider hiring a personal attorney who is experienced in malpractice law. This information can be obtained through either the state bar association or the local trial lawyers association.

Anyone has a right to sue; however, that does not always mean a case exists. Many negligence and malpractice cases find in favor of the health-care providers, not the client nor the client's family. Consider the case of *Grant v. Pacific Medical Center, Inc.* (2014). In this case, the plaintiff failed to prove negligence and malpractice and then filed an appeal of the dismissal of the original verdict in the malpractice case. The Supreme Court of the State of Washington upheld the original verdict established by the Court of Appeals. See the following for the summary of this case:

> Patricia A. Grant, a veteran with multiple health concerns, received health care through the Department of Defense Health Care Program, delivered by the Family Health Plan at Pacific Medical Centers, Inc. The allegations in the petitioner's complaint selectively refer to care received in 2009 by Linda Oswald, MD, a board-certified family practice physician. Ms. Grant's medical history includes morbid obesity, mental illness, hypertension, plantar fasciitis, and diabetes. Ms. Grant also underwent multiple prior surgeries, including a Roux Y gastric bypass procedure performed at Valley Medical Center in June 2009. Three months later Ms. Grant was referred to a board-certified gastroenterologist for a complaint of nausea, vomiting, and other gastrointestinal system issues. Ms. Grant's providers at the health-care institution referred her to multiple, board-certified specialists for her continuing medical issues of nausea and vomiting.
>
> At both the trial court level and in her ensuing appeal, Ms. Grant failed to make a "showing sufficient to establish the existence of the key

element of her case—the applicable standard of care in Washington and that a breach of this standard occurred causing her injury. She bore the burden of proof and her failure to produce medical evidence in support of her allegations was fatal to her case and summary judgment was appropriate" (p. 7).

In this case, the Court of Appeals based its decision on existing well-established law and stated the following:

Ms. Grant failed to produce any expert medical testimony to the trial court to establish the standard of care, a violation of the standard of care or proximate causation; and equally failed to raise any legitimate issues in this regard to the Court of Appeals. (p. 8)

Professional Liability Insurance

We live in a litigious society. Although a variety of opinions exist on this issue, in today's world nurses need to consider obtaining personal liability insurance (Pohlman, 2015). Although physicians get sued more than nurses, health-care institutions realize the contributions of all members of the health-care team. A nurse can be found liable under the specific circumstances mentioned in this chapter. Even in a case of a frivolous lawsuit, where the patient fails to incur damages but hopes to collect on a settlement, the nurse faces expenses (Pohlman, 2015).

If a nurse is charged with malpractice and found guilty, the employing institution holds the right to sue the nurse to reclaim damages. When a nurse has personal liability insurance, the company provides legal counsel. The company may also negotiate with another company on the nurse's behalf. Many liability policies also cover assault, violations of HIPAA, libel, slander, and property damage.

End-of-Life Decisions and the Law

When a heart ceases to beat, a client is in a state of cardiac arrest. In health-care institutions and in the community, it is common to initiate cardiopulmonary resuscitation (CPR) when this occurs. In health-care institutions, an elaborate mechanism is put into action when a patient "codes." Much controversy exists concerning when these mechanisms should be used and whether individuals who have no chance of regaining full viability should be resuscitated.

Do Not Resuscitate Orders

A do not resuscitate order (DNR) is a specific directive to health-care personnel not to initiate CPR measures. In the past, only physicians could write DNR orders; however, in many states, nurse practitioners and physician assistants may also write a DNR order (Hayes et al., 2017). Therefore, it is imperative that a nurse check with the institutional policy to ensure that this is an acceptable practice. These types of orders are only written after the provider has consulted with the client or the client's family. Clients have the right to request a DNR order; however, they may not fully understand the ramifications of their request.

Although New York State has one of the most complete laws regarding DNR orders for acute and long-term care facilities, all states have legislation regarding this request. In 2007, the American Bar Association (ABA), in collaboration with the DHHS, developed a document addressing the overall legal and policy issues regarding DNR requests and orders (Sabatino, 2007). This document outlined the overall existence of common law cases and policies that support a patient's right to self-determination. This action has been supported by the ANA (1992, 2005). It is important for nurses to familiarize themselves with the policies and procedures of the employing institution. The nurse's roles in DNR orders are listed in Box 3-2.

Advance Directives

The legal dilemmas that may arise in relation to DNR orders often require court decisions. For this reason, in 1990, Senator John Danforth of Missouri and Senator Daniel Moynihan of New York introduced the PSDA to address questions regarding life-sustaining treatment. The act was created to allow people the opportunity to make decisions about treatment in advance of a time when they might become unable to participate in the decision-making process. Through this mechanism, families can be spared the burden of having to decide what the family member would have wanted.

Federal law mandates that health-care institutions that receive federal monies (from Medicare or Medicaid) inform clients of their right to create advance directives (H.R. 5067, 1995). The PSDA

---

box 3-2

The Nurse's Role in DNR Orders

The ANA recommends that:

- Clinical nurses actively participate in timely and frequent discussions on changing goals of care and initiate DNR or allow natural death (AND) discussions with patients and their families and significant others.

ANA Position Statement 10 Nursing Care and Do Not Resuscitate (DNR) and Allow Natural Death (AND) Decisions

- Clinical nurses ensure that DNR orders are clearly documented, reviewed, and updated periodically to reflect changes in the patient's condition.
- Nurse administrators ensure support for the clinical nurse to initiate DNR discussions.
- Nursing home directors and hospital nursing executives develop mechanisms whereby the AND form accompanies all interorganizational transfers.
- Nurse administrators have an obligation to assure palliative care support for all patients.
- Nurse educators teach that there should be no implied or actual withdrawal of other types of care for patients with DNR orders. DNR does not mean "do not treat." Attention to language is paramount, and euphemisms such as "doing everything," "doing nothing," or "withdrawing care or treatment" to indicate the absence or presence of a DNR order should be strictly avoided.
- Nurse educators develop and provide specialized education for nurses, physicians, and other members of the interdisciplinary health-care team related to DNR, including conversations on moving away from DNR and toward AND language.

- Nurse researchers explore all facets of the DNR process to build a foundation for evidence-based practice.
- All nurses ensure that, whenever possible, the DNR decision is a subject of explicit discussion between the health-care team, patient, and family (or designated surrogate), and that actions taken are in accordance with the patient's wishes.
- All nurses facilitate and participate in interdisciplinary mechanisms for the resolution of disputes between patients, families, and clinicians' DNR orders (Cantor et al., 2003).
- All nurses actively participate in developing DNR policies within the institutions where they work. Specifically, policies should address, consider, or clarify the following:
  - Guidance to health-care professionals who have evidence that a patient does not want CPR attempted but for whom a DNR order has not been written
  - Required documentation to accompany the DNR order, such as a progress note in the medical record indicating how the decision was made
  - The role of various health-care practitioners in communicating with patients and families about DNR orders
  - Effective communication of DNR orders when transferring patients within or between facilities
  - Effective communication of DNR orders among staff that protects against patient stigmatization or confidentiality breaches
  - Guidance to practitioners on specific circumstances that may require reconsideration of the DNR order (e.g., patients undergoing surgery or invasive procedures)
  - The needs of special populations (e.g., pediatrics and geriatrics)

Source: American Nurses Association. (2012). Position statement on nursing care and do not resuscitate decisions. American Nurses Association.

(S.R. 13566) provides guidelines for developing advance directives concerning what will be done for individuals if they are no longer able to participate actively in making decisions about care options. More information regarding the PSDA may be found at www.congress.gov.

Living Will and Durable Power of Attorney for Health Care (Health-Care Surrogate)

The two most common forms of advance directives are living wills and durable power of attorney. Living wills and other advance directives describe individual preferences regarding treatment in the event of a serious accident or illness. These legal documents indicate an individual's wishes regarding care decisions (Sabatino, 2010). A living will is a legally executed document that states an individual's wishes regarding the use of life-prolonging medical treatment in the event that the individual is no longer competent to make informed treatment decisions (Sabatino, 2010). A condition is considered

terminal when, to a reasonable degree of medical certainty, there is little likelihood of recovery or the condition is expected to cause death. A terminal condition may also refer to a severe neurological entity, a persistent vegetative state characterized by a permanent and irreversible condition of unconsciousness in which there is (a) absence of voluntary action or cognitive behavior of any kind and (b) an inability to communicate or interact purposefully with the environment (Shea & Bayne, 2010).

Another function of the advance directive is to designate a health-care surrogate. The role of the health-care surrogate is to make the client's wishes known to medical and nursing personnel. Chosen by the client, the health-care surrogate is usually a family member or close friend. Imperative in the designation of a health-care surrogate is a clear understanding of the client's wishes should the need arise.

In some situations, clients are unable to express themselves adequately or competently, although they may not be considered "terminally ill." For example, clients who have been diagnosed with a cognitive impairment such as Alzheimer's disease or other forms of dementia cannot communicate their wishes, clients under anesthesia are temporarily unable to communicate, and the condition of a comatose client fails to allow for expression of health-care wishes. In these situations, the designated health-care surrogate can make treatment decisions on behalf of the client. However, when a client regains the ability to make personal decisions and is capable of expressing them effectively, the client resumes control of all decision making pertaining to medical treatment. Nurses and other providers may be held accountable when they go against a client's wishes regarding DNR orders.

In the case of *Wendland v. Sparks* (Reagan, 1998), the physician and nurses were sued for not "initiating CPR." In this case, the client had been hospitalized for more than 2 months for a lung disease and multiple myeloma. Although improving at the time, during the hospitalization the client experienced three cardiac arrests. Even after this, she had not requested a DNR order, nor had her family. After one of the arrests, the client's husband stated to the physician that he wanted his wife to be placed on life support if necessary. The client suffered a fourth cardiac arrest. One nurse went to obtain the crash cart while another contacted the physician who happened to be in the area. The physician checked the client's heart rate, respirations, and pupillary reaction and stated, "I just cannot do this to her." She ordered the nurses to stop resuscitation, and the physician pronounced the client. The nurses stated if they had not been given a direct order by the physician, they would have continued their attempts at resuscitation. The court ruled in favor of the family, indicating that the physician exercised faulty judgment. The nurses were cleared as they followed a physician order.

Nursing Implications

The PSDA does not specify who should discuss treatment decisions or advance directives with clients. Because directives are often implemented on care units, nurses must be knowledgeable regarding living wills, advance directives, and health-care surrogates. They need to be prepared to answer questions that clients may ask about the directives and forms used by the health-care institution.

The responsibility for creating an awareness of individual rights often falls on nurses because they act as client advocates. The responsibility for educating the professional staff about policies resides with the health-care institution. Nurses who are unsure of the existing policies and procedures of the institution should contact the appropriate department for clarification.

Conclusion

Nurses need to understand the legalities involved in the delivery of safe and effective health care that promotes positive outcomes. It is important to be familiar with the standards of care established within your institution and the rules and regulations that govern nursing practice within your state because these are the standards to which you will be held accountable. Health-care consumers have a right to expect quality care and that their health information will remain confidential. Caring for clients safely and avoiding legal difficulties requires nurses to adhere to standards of care and their scope of practice and carefully document changes in client conditions.

Study Questions

1. How do federal laws, court decisions, and SBONs affect nursing practice? Give an example of each.

2. Obtain a copy of the nurse practice act in your state. What are some of the penalties for violation of the rules and regulations?

3. Review the minutes or documents of a state board meeting. What were the most common issues for nurses to be called before the board of nursing? What were the resulting disciplinary actions?

4. The next time you are on your clinical unit, look at the nursing documentation done by several different staff members. Do you believe it is adequate? Explain your rationale.

5. How does your clinical institution handle medication errors?

6. If a nurse is found to be less than proficient in the delivery of safe care, how should the nurse manager remedy the situation?

7. Discuss where appropriate standards of care may be found. Explain whether each is an example of an internal or external standard of care.

8. Explain the importance of federal agencies in setting standards of care in health-care institutions.

9. What is the difference between consent and informed consent?

10. Look at the forms for advance directives and DNR policies in your institution. Do they follow the guidelines of the PSDA?

11. What are the most common errors nurses commit that lead to negligence or malpractice?

12. What impact would a law that prevents mandatory overtime have on nurses, nursing care, and the health-care industry? Find out if your state has mandatory overtime legislation.

Case Study to Promote Clinical Judgment

Mr. Evans, 40 years old, was admitted to the hospital's medical–surgical unit from the ED with a diagnosis of acute abdomen. He had a 20-year history of Crohn's disease and had been on prednisone, 20 mg, every day for the past year. Three months ago, he was started on the new biological agent etanercept, 50 mg, subcutaneously every week. His last dose was 4 days ago. Because he was allowed nothing by mouth (NPO), total parenteral nutrition was started through a triple-lumen central venous catheter line, and his steroids were changed to Solu-Medrol, 60 mg, by intravenous (IV) push every 6 hours. He was also receiving several IV antibiotics and medication for pain and nausea.

During the next 3 days, his condition worsened. He was in severe pain and needed more analgesics. One evening at 9 p.m., it was discovered that his central venous catheter line was out. The RN notified the physician, who stated that a surgeon would come in the morning to replace it. The nurse failed to ask the physician what to do about the IV steroids, antibiotics, and fluid replacement; the client was still NPO. She also failed to ask about the etanercept. At 7 a.m., the night nurse noticed that the client had had no urinary output since 11 p.m. the night before. She documented that the client had no urinary output but forgot to report this information to the nurse assuming care responsibilities on the day shift.

The client's physician made rounds at 9 a.m. The nurse for Mr. Evans did not discuss the fact that the client had not voided since 11 p.m., did not request orders for alternative delivery of the steroids and antibiotics, and did not ask about administering the etanercept. At 5 p.m. that evening, while Mr. Evans was having a computed tomography (CT) scan, his blood pressure dropped to 70 mm Hg, and because no one was in the scan room with him, he coded. He was transported to the intensive care unit and intubated. He developed severe sepsis and acute respiratory distress syndrome.

1. List all the problems you can find with the nursing care in this case.

2. What were the nursing responsibilities in reporting information?

3. What do you think was the possible cause of the drop in Mr. Evans's blood pressure and his subsequent code?

4. If you worked in risk management, how would you discuss this situation with the nurse manager and the staff?

NCLEX®-Style Review Questions

1. Which common practice puts the nurse at liability for invasion of patient privacy?
   1. During care, the nurse reveals information about the patient to those in the room.
   2. The nurse releases information about the patient to nursing students who will be caring for the patient the next day.
   3. The nurse conducts a patient care session about a patient whose care is difficult and challenging.
   4. Confidential information regarding an admitted patient is released to third-party payers.

2. The health-care facility has sponsored a continuing education offering on emergency management of pandemic influenza. At lunch, a nurse is overheard saying, "I'm not going to take care of anyone who might have that flu. I have kids to think about." What is true of this statement? **Select all that apply**.
   1. The nurse has a greater obligation than a layperson to care for the sick or injured in an emergency.
   2. This statement reflects defamation and may result in legal action against the nurse.
   3. This statement is a breach of the Code of Ethics for Nurses.
   4. The nurse has this right as no nurse–patient contract has been established.

3. After 3 years of uneventful employment, the nurse made a medication error that resulted in patient injury. What hospital response to this event is ethical?
   1. The hospital was supportive and assistive as the nurse coped with this event.
   2. The nurse was dismissed for incompetence.
   3. The hospital quality department advised the nurse not to tell the patient about the error.
   4. The nurse was reassigned to an area in which there is no direct patient care responsibility.

4. An RN new to the ED documented that "the patient was intoxicated and acted in a crazy manner." The team leader told the RN that this type of documentation can lead to
   1. Assault
   2. Wrongful publication
   3. Defamation of character
   4. Slander

5. An RN sees an older woman fall in the mall. The RN helps the woman. The woman later complains that she twisted and sprained her ankle. The RN is protected from litigation under
   1. Hospital malpractice insurance
   2. Good faith agreement
   3. Good Samaritan law
   4. Personal professional insurance

6. An RN has asked a licensed practical nurse (LPN) to trim the toenails of a diabetic patient. The LPN trims them too short, which results in a toe amputation from infection. The patient files a lawsuit against the hospital, the RN, and the LPN. What might all three be found guilty of?
   1. Unintentional tort
   2. Intentional tort
   3. Negligence
   4. Malpractice

7. An RN is obtaining a signature on a surgical informed consent document. Before obtaining the signature, the RN must ensure which of the following? **Select all that apply**.
   1. The client is not sedated.
   2. The doctor is present.
   3. A family member is a witness.
   4. The signature is in ink.
   5. The patient understands the procedure.

8. A patient is transported to the ED by rescue after being involved in a motor vehicle accident. The patient is alert and oriented but keeps stating he is having trouble breathing. Oxygen is started, but the patient is still showing signs of dyspnea. The patient suddenly develops respiratory arrest and dies. During the resuscitation process, it is discovered that the nurse failed to open the correct oxygen valve. The family sues the hospital and the nurse for
   1. Malpractice
   2. Negligence
   3. Nonmaleficence
   4. Equipment failure

9. A patient tells a nurse that he has an advance directive from 6 years ago. The nurse looks at the medical record for the advance directive. What content should the nurse expect to find in the advance directive? **Select all that apply**.
   1. Decisions regarding treatments
   2. When to take the patient to the hospital
   3. Do not resuscitate orders
   4. Who should be notified in the case of illness, injury, or death
   5. Durable power of attorney for health care
   6. HIPAA protocols

10. An RN calls a health-care provider to report that a patient's condition is deteriorating. The physician gives orders on the telephone to draw arterial blood gases. What should the nurse do next when receiving telephone orders from a health-care provider?
    1. Call the respiratory therapist to obtain the blood gases.
    2. Give the order to the unit secretary to ensure it is entered quickly.
    3. Enter the order directly into the system as it was given to the RN.
    4. Write the order down and read it back to the provider.

Leading and Managing

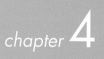
Leadership and Followership

Nurses study leadership to learn how to work effectively with other people. Nurses work with an extraordinary variety of people: technicians, aides, unit managers, housekeepers, patients, patients' families, physicians, respiratory therapists, physical therapists, epidemiologists, social workers, psychologists, information technology staff, and more. In this chapter, the most prominent leadership theories are introduced. Then, the characteristics and behaviors that can make you, a new nurse, an effective leader and follower as well are discussed.

Leadership

Are You Ready to Be a Leader?

You may be thinking, "I'm just beginning my career in nursing. How can I be expected to be a leader now?" This is an important question. You will need time to refine your clinical skills and learn how to function in a new environment. However, you can begin to assume some leadership functions within your new nursing roles right away. Leadership is a function of your actions, that is, what you do. It is not dependent on having a high-level position within your organization (Blanchard & Miller, 2014). In fact, leadership should be seen as a dimension of nursing practice (Scott & Miles, 2013). Consider the following example:

Billie Thomas was a new staff nurse at Green Valley Nursing Care Center. After orientation, she was assigned to a rehabilitation unit with high admission and discharge rates. Billie noticed that admissions and discharges were assigned rather haphazardly. Anyone who was "free" at the moment was directed to handle them. Sometimes, unlicensed assistive personnel (UAP) were directed to admit or discharge residents. Billie believed this was inappropriate because the unlicensed staff were not prepared to do assessments and had no preparation to do discharge planning.

Billie had an idea how the admission and discharge processes could be improved but was not sure that she should bring it up because she was so new. "Maybe they've already thought of this," she said to a former classmate. They began to talk about what they had learned in their leadership course before graduation. "I just keep hearing our instructor saying, 'There's only one manager, but anyone can be a leader.'"

"If you want to be a leader, you have to act on your idea. Why don't you talk with your nurse manager?" her friend asked.

"Maybe I will," Billie replied.

Billie decided to speak with her nurse manager, an experienced rehabilitation nurse who seemed not only approachable but also open to new ideas. "I have been so busy getting our new electronic health record (EHR) system online before the surveyors come that I wasn't paying attention to that," the nurse manager told her. "I'm glad you brought it to my attention."

Billie's nurse manager raised the issue at the next executive meeting, giving credit to Billie for having brought it to her attention. The other nurse managers had the same response. "We were so focused on the new EHR system that we overlooked that. We need to take care of this situation as soon as possible. Billie Thomas is a leader!"

Leadership Defined

Successful nurse leaders are those who engage others to work together effectively in pursuit of a shared goal. Examples of shared goals in nursing would be providing excellent care, reducing infection rates, designing cost-saving procedures, and improving end-of-life care.

Leadership is a much broader concept than management. Although managers need to be leaders, management itself is focused specifically on achievement of organizational goals. Leadership, on the other hand:

> . . . occurs whenever one person attempts to influence the behavior of an individual or group—up, down, or sideways in the organization—regardless of the reason. It may be for personal goals or for the goals of others, and these goals may or may not be congruent with organizational goals. Leadership is influence (Hersey & Campbell, 2004, p. 12).

In order to lead, say Hersey and Campbell, one must develop three important competencies: (1) Diagnose: ability to understand the situation you want to influence, (2) Adapt: make changes that will close the gap between the current situation and what you are hoping to achieve, and (3) Communicate. No matter how much you diagnose or adapt, if you cannot communicate effectively, you will probably not meet your goal (Hersey & Campbell, 2004). Some call people who are leaders but not managers "informal leaders" (Lawson & Fleshman 2020).

What Makes a Person a Leader?

Leadership Theories

There are many different ideas about how a person becomes a good leader. Despite years of research and discussion of this subject, no one idea has emerged as the clear winner. The reason for this may be that different qualities and behaviors are most important in different situations. In nursing, for example, some situations require quick thinking and fast action. Others require time to figure out the best solution to a complicated problem. Different leadership qualities and behaviors are needed in these two instances. The result is that there is not yet a single best answer to the question, "What makes a person a leader?"

Consider some of the best-known leadership theories and the many qualities and behaviors that have been identified as those of the effective nurse leader, which are discussed next.

Trait Theories

At one time or another, you have probably heard someone say, "She's a born leader." Many believe that some people are natural leaders, whereas others are not. It is true that leadership may come more easily to some than to others, but everyone can be a leader, given the necessary knowledge and opportunity to develop one's personal leadership skills. In other words, you can learn how to be a leader, building on your strengths and improving or working around areas of weakness (Owen, 2015).

An important 5-year study of 90 outstanding leaders by Warren Bennis published in 1984 identified four common traits of leaders. These traits hold true today:

1. **Management of attention** These leaders communicated a sense of goal direction that attracted followers.
2. **Management of meaning** These leaders created and communicated meaning and purpose.
3. **Management of trust** These leaders demonstrated reliability and consistency.
4. **Management of self** These leaders knew themselves well and worked within their strengths and weaknesses (Bennis, 1984).

Behavioral Theories

The behavioral theories focus on what the leader does. One of the most influential behavioral theories is concerned with leadership style (White & Lippitt, 1960) (Table 4-1). The ideas behind these three styles are reflected in many of the newer theories as well.

The three styles are:

1. **Autocratic leadership (also called directive, controlling, or authoritarian)** The autocratic leader gives orders and makes decisions for the group. For example, when a decision needs to be made, an autocratic leader says, "I've decided that this is the way we're going to solve our problem." Although this is an efficient way to

---

table 4-1

Comparison of Autocratic, Democratic, and Laissez-Faire Leadership Styles

	Autocratic	Democratic	Laissez-Faire
Amount of freedom	Little freedom	Moderate freedom	Much freedom
Amount of control	High control	Moderate control	Little control
Decision making	By the leader	Leader and group together	By the group or by no one
Leader activity level	High	High	Minimal
Assumption of responsibility	Leader	Shared	Abdicated
Output of the group	High quantity, good quality	Creative, high quality	Variable, may be poor quality
Efficiency	Very efficient	Less efficient than autocratic style	Inefficient

Source: Adapted from White, R. K., & Lippitt, R. (1960). Autocracy and democracy: An experimental inquiry. Harper & Row.

run things, it discourages creativity and may reduce team member motivation. More control communicates less trust and may lower morale within the team (Owen, 2015).

2. **Democratic leadership (also called participative)** Democratic leaders share leadership. Important plans and decisions are made with the team (Chrispeels, 2004). Although this appears to be a less efficient way to run things, it is more flexible and usually increases motivation and creativity. In fact, involving team members, giving them "permission to think, speak and act," brings out the best in them and makes them more productive, not less (Wiseman & McKeown, 2010, p. 3). Decisions may take longer to make, but once made, everyone supports them (Buchanan, 2011).

3. **Laissez-faire leadership (also called permissive or nondirective)** The laissez-faire ("let someone do") leader takes very little initiative and fails to encourage others to do it. It is really a lack of leadership. For example, when a decision needs to be made, a laissez-faire leader may postpone making the decision or never make the decision at all. In most instances, the laissez-faire leader leaves people feeling confused and frustrated because there are no goals, no guidance, and no direction. Some mature, self-motivated individuals thrive under laissez-faire leadership because they need little direction; however, most people flounder under this minimal leadership.

Pavitt summed up the differences among these three styles: a democratic leader tries to move the group toward its goals, an autocratic leader tries to move the group toward the leader's goals, and a laissez-faire leader makes no attempt to move the group (1999, p. 330ff).

Task Versus Relationship

Another important distinction is between a task focus and a relationship focus (Blake et al., 1981) on the part of the leader. Some nurse leaders emphasize the tasks to be done (e.g., administering medication, completing patient records) and fail to recognize that interpersonal relationships (e.g., attitude of physicians toward nursing staff, treatment of housekeeping staff by nurses) affect both the morale and productivity of employees. Others focus on the interpersonal aspects and ignore the quality of the job being done as long as people get along with each other. The most effective leader is able to balance the two, attending to both the task and the relationship aspects of working together.

Motivation Theories

The concept of motivation seems simple: We will act to get what we want but avoid doing whatever we don't want to do. However, what generates motivation is still enveloped in mystery. The study of motivation as a focus of leadership began in the 1920s with the historic Hawthorne studies. Several experiments were conducted to see if increasing light and, later, improving other working conditions would increase the productivity of workers in the Hawthorne, Illinois, electrical plant. This proved to be true, but then something curious happened: When the improvements were taken away, the workers continued to show increased productivity. The researchers concluded that the explanation was found not in the *conditions* of the experiments but in the *attention* given to the workers by the experimenters.

Frederick Herzberg and David McClelland also studied the factors that motivated workers in the workplace. Their findings are similar to the elements in Maslow's hierarchy of needs. Table 4-2 summarizes these three historical motivation theories that continue to be used by leaders today (Herzberg, 1966; Herzberg et al., 1959; Maslow, 1970; McClelland, 1961).

Situational Theories

People and leadership are far more complex than the early theories recognized. Situations can change rapidly, requiring more complex theories to explain leadership of them (Bennis et al., 2001).

Instead of assuming that one particular approach works in all situations, situational theories recognize the complexity of work situations and encourage the leader to consider many factors when deciding what action to take. Adaptability is the key to the situational approach (McNichol, 2000).

Situational theories emphasize the importance of understanding all the factors that affect a particular group of people in a particular environment. The most well-known is Hersey and Campbell's situational leadership model. The appeal of this model is that it focuses on both the task and the follower: The key is to marry the readiness of the follower with the tasks at hand. "Readiness is defined as the extent to which a follower demonstrates

table 4-2

Leading Motivation Theories

Theory	Summary of Motivation Requirements
Maslow, 1970	Categories of need: Lower needs (listed first in the following list) must be fulfilled before others are activated. Physiological Safety Belongingness Esteem Self-actualization
Herzberg et al., 1959	Two factors that influence motivation. The absence of hygiene factors can create job dissatisfaction, but their presence does not motivate or increase satisfaction. 1. *Hygiene factors:* company policy, supervision, interpersonal relations, working conditions, salary 2. *Motivators:* achievement, recognition, the work itself, responsibility, advancement
McClelland, 1961	Motivation results from three dominant needs. Usually all three needs are present in each individual but vary in importance depending on the position a person has in the workplace. Needs are also shaped through time by culture and experience. 1. *Need for achievement:* performing tasks on a challenging and high level 2. *Need for affiliation:* good relationships with others 3. *Need for power:* being in charge

Source: Adapted from Hersey, P., & Campbell, R. (2004). Leadership: A behavioral science approach. Leadership Studies Publishing.

the ability and willingness to accomplish a specific task" (Hersey & Campbell, 2004, p. 114). "The leader needs to spell out the duties and responsibilities of the individual and the group" (Hersey & Campbell, 2004, p. 114).

Followers' readiness levels can range from unable, unwilling, and uncertain to able, willing, and confident. The leader's behavior will focus on appropriately fulfilling the followers' needs, which are identified by their readiness level and the task. Leader behaviors will range from telling, guiding, and directing to delegating, observing, and monitoring.

For example, think about where you fell in this model during your first clinical rotation. Compare that time with where you are now. In the beginning, your clinical instructor gave you clear instructions, closely guiding and directing you. Now, your instructor is most likely delegating, observing, and monitoring. As you move into your first nursing position, you may return to the needing, guiding, and directing stage. However, you may soon become a leader or instructor for new nursing students, guiding and directing them.

Transformational Leadership

Although the situational theories were an improvement over earlier, more simplistic theories, there was still something missing. Meaning, inspiration, and vision were not given enough attention (Tappen, 2001). These are the distinguishing features of transformational leadership.

The transformational theory of leadership emphasizes that people need a sense of mission that goes beyond good interpersonal relationships or an appropriate reward for a job well done (Bass & Avolio, 1993). This is especially true in nursing. Caring for people, sick or well, is the goal of the profession. Most people chose nursing in order to do something for the good of humankind; this is their vision. One responsibility of nursing leadership is to help nurses see how their work helps them achieve this vision.

Transformational leaders can communicate their vision in a manner that is so meaningful and exciting that it can reduce negativity (Leach, 2005), increase staff nurse engagement (Manning, 2016), and inspire commitment in the people with whom they work (Trofino, 1995). Dr. Martin Luther King Jr. had a vision for America: "I have a dream that one day my children will be judged by the content of their character, not the color of their skin" (quoted by Blanchard & Miller, 2007, p. 1). Great leaders share their vision with their followers. You can do the same with your colleagues and team. If successful, the goals of the leader and staff will "become fused, creating unity, wholeness, and a collective purpose" (Barker, 1992, p. 42). See Box 4-1 for an example of a leader with visionary goals.

box 4-1

BHAGs, Anyone?

This is leadership on the very grandest scale. BHAGs are Big, Hairy, Audacious Goals. Coined by Jim Collins, BHAGs are big ideas, visions for the future. Here is an example:

Gigi Mander, originally from the Philippines, dreams of buying hundreds of acres of farmland for peasant families in Asia or Africa. She would install irrigation systems, provide seed and modern farming equipment, and help them market their crops. This is not just a dream, however. She has a business plan for her BHAG and is actively seeking investors.

Imagination, creativity, planning, persistence, audacity, and courage: These are all needed to put a BHAG into practice.

Do you have a BHAG? How would you make it real?

Source: Adapted from Buchanan, L. (2012a). The world needs big ideas. INC Magazine, 34(9), 57–58.

Emotional Intelligence

The relationship aspects of leadership are also the focus of the work on emotional intelligence (Goleman et al., 2002). From the perspective of emotional intelligence, what distinguishes ordinary leaders from leadership "stars" is that the "stars" consciously address the effect of people's feelings on the team's emotional reality. Inexperienced nurse managers may be less likely to use emotional intelligence than experienced ones (Prufeta, 2017).

How is this done? First, emotionally intelligent leaders recognize and understand their own emotions. When a crisis occurs, emotionally intelligent leaders are able to manage their emotions, channel them, stay calm and clearheaded, and suspend judgment until all the facts are in (Baggett & Baggett, 2005).

Second, emotionally intelligent leaders welcome constructive criticism, ask for help when needed, can juggle multiple demands without losing focus, and can turn problems into opportunities.

Third, emotionally intelligent leaders listen attentively to others, recognize unspoken concerns, acknowledge others' perspectives, and bring people together in an atmosphere of respect, cooperation, collegiality, and helpfulness so they can direct their energies toward achieving the team's goals. "The enthusiastic, caring, and supportive leader generates those same feelings throughout the team," wrote Porter-O'Grady of emotionally intelligent leaders (2003, p. 109).

Moral Leadership

Moral leadership involves deciding that one ought to remain honest, fair, and socially responsible (Bjarnason & LaSala, 2011) under any circumstances. Caring about one's patients and the people who work for you as people as well as employees (Spears & Lawrence, 2004) is part of moral leadership. This can be a great challenge in times of limited financial resources.

Molly Benedict was a team leader on the acute geriatric unit (AGU) when a question of moral leadership arose. Faced with large budget cuts in the middle of the year and feeling a little desperate to figure out how to run the AGU with fewer staff, her nurse manager suggested that reducing the time that UAPs spent ambulating patients would enable UAPs to care for 15 patients, up from the current 10 per UAP. "George," responded Molly, "you know that inactivity has many harmful effects, from emboli to disorientation, especially in our very elderly population. Let's try to figure out how to encourage more self-care and even family involvement in care so the UAPs can still have time to walk patients and prevent their becoming nonambulatory."

Molly based her action on important values, particularly those of providing the highest-quality care possible. Stewart, Holmes, and Usher (2012) urge that caring not be sacrificed at the altar of efficiency (p. 227). This example illustrates how great a challenge that can be for today's nurse leaders. The American Nurses Association (ANA) Code of Ethics (2015) provides the moral compass for nursing practice and leadership (ANA, 2015; Bjarnason & LaSala, 2011). The Code itself does not tell leaders how to behave but provides guidelines for their behavior (Schick-Makaroff & Storch, 2019).

Box 4-2 summarizes a contemporary list of 13 distinctive leadership styles, most of which match up to the eight theories just discussed.

Caring Leadership

Caring leadership in nursing comes from two primary sources: servant leadership and emotional intelligence in the management literature, and caring as a foundational value in nursing (Greenleaf, 2008;

box 4-2

Distinctive Styles of Leadership

1. Adaptive: flexible, willing to change and devise new approaches
2. Emotionally intelligent: aware of their own and others' feelings
3. Charismatic: magnetic personalities who attract people to follow them
4. Authentic: demonstrates integrity, character, and honesty in relating to others
5. Level 5: ferociously pursues goals but gives credit to others and takes responsibility for their mistakes
6. Mindful: thoughtful, analytic, and open to new ideas
7. Narcissistic: doesn't listen to others and doesn't tolerate disagreement but may have a compelling vision
8. No excuse: mentally tough, emphasizes accountability and decisiveness
9. Resonant: motivates others through their energy and enthusiasm
10. Servant: "empathic, aware and healing" (p. 76); leads to serve others
11. Storyteller: uses stories to convey messages in a memorable, motivating fashion
12. Strength-based: focuses and capitalizes on their own and others' talents
13. Tribal: builds a common culture with strong sharing of values and beliefs

Source: Adapted from Buchanan, L. (2012b, June). 13 ways of looking at a leader. INC Magazine, 34(5), 74–76.

McMurry, 2012; Rhodes et al., 2011; Spears, 2010). Although it is uniquely suited to nursing leadership, it is hard to imagine any situation in which an uncaring leader would be preferred over a caring leader.

Servant leaders choose to serve first and lead second, making sure that people's needs within the work setting are met (Greenleaf, 2008). Emotionally intelligent leaders are especially aware of not only their own feelings but others' feelings as well (see Box 4-1). Combining these leadership theories and the philosophy of caring in nursing, you can see that caring leadership is fundamentally people-oriented. The following are behaviors of caring leaders:

- They *respect* their coworkers as individuals.
- They *listen* to other people's opinions and preferences, giving them full consideration.
- They *maintain awareness* of their own and others' feelings.
- They *empathize* with others, understanding their needs and concerns.
- They *develop* their own and their team's capacities.
- They *are competent*, both in leadership and in clinical practice.

As you can see, caring leadership cuts across the leadership theories discussed so far and encompasses some of their best features. An authoritarian leader, for example, can be as caring as a democratic leader (Dorn, 2011). Caring leadership is attractive to many nurses because it applies many of the principles of working with patients and working with nursing staff to the interdisciplinary team.

Still, much of even the caring leadership approach has been derived from theories developed within other disciplines. Many insights from other disciplines are relevant to nursing leadership, which is not surprising given that, across disciplines, we are all studying the behavior of people at work. However, nursing is also concerned with providing care to humans. Leclerc, Kennedy, and Campis (2020) suggest that we need to combine the metrics of traditional, business-oriented leadership (e.g., the number of adverse events that have occurred or the results of patient satisfaction surveys) with the human side of person-centered care to create a human-centered (sic) leadership theory. To further this work, they conducted focus groups with nurse leaders at every level of health-care organizations and looked for attributes from leaders in participants' responses. They found the participants described nursing leaders as . . .

Awakeners: acting as coaches, motivators, and mentors sharing their vision

Connectors: creating a culture of trust, regard, and community

Upholders: embracing humility, fairness, self-awareness, and self-care (Leclerc et al., 2020)

The similarities to caring leadership are strong.

Qualities of an Effective Leader

If leadership is seen as the ability to influence, what qualities must the leader possess in order to be able to do that? Integrity, courage, positive attitude, initiative, energy, optimism, perseverance, generosity, balance, ability to handle stress, and self-awareness are some of the qualities of effective leaders in nursing (Fig. 4.1):

- **Integrity** Integrity is expected of health-care professionals. Patients, colleagues, and employers all expect nurses to be honest, law-abiding, and trustworthy. Adherence to both a code of personal ethics and a code of professional ethics

Qualities

Integrity	Perseverance
Courage	Balance
Initiative	Ability to handle stress
Energy	
Optimism	Self-awareness

Behaviors

Think critically	Set goals, share vision
Solve problems	
Communicate skillfully	Develop self and others

Figure 4.1 Keys to effective leadership.

(ANA Code of Ethics for Nurses: https://www.nursingworld.org/practice-policy/nursing-excellence/ethics/code-of-ethics-for-nurses/, 2015) is expected of every nurse. Would-be leaders who do not exhibit these characteristics cannot expect them of their followers. This is an essential component of moral leadership.

Although an increase in research on nursing leadership has been noted, we continue to use a variety of leadership theories borrowed from other disciplines with none emerging as the best prediction of effective leadership in nursing. The trend appears to be an emphasis on the relationship aspects of nursing (Cummings & Cummings, 2020).

■ **Courage** Sometimes, being a leader means taking some risks. In the story of Billie Thomas, for example, Billie needed some courage to speak to her nurse manager about a deficiency she had observed.

■ **Positive attitude** A positive attitude goes a long way in making a good leader. In fact, many outstanding leaders cite negative attitude as the single most important reason for not hiring someone (Maxwell, 1993, p. 98). Sometimes a leader's attitude is noticed by followers more quickly than are the leader's actions.

■ **Initiative** Good ideas are not enough. To be a leader, you must act on those good ideas. No one will make you do this; this requires initiative on your part.

table 4-3

Winner or Whiner—Which Are You?

A Winner Says:	A Whiner Says:
"We have a real challenge here."	"This is a terrible problem."
"I'll give it my best."	"Can't someone else do it?"
"That's great!"	"That's nice, I guess."
"We can do it!"	"That's not going to work."
"Yes!"	"Maybe. . . ."

Source: Adapted from Holman, L. (1995). Eleven lessons in self-leadership: Insights for personal and professional success. A Lesson in Leadership Book.

■ **Energy** Leadership requires energy. Both leadership and followership are hard but satisfying endeavors that require effort. It is also important that the energy be used constructively.

■ **Optimism** When the work is difficult and one crisis seems to follow another in rapid succession, it is easy to become discouraged. It is important not to let discouragement keep you and your coworkers from seeking ways to resolve the problems. In fact, the ability to see a problem as an opportunity is part of the optimism that makes a person an effective leader. Similar to energy, optimism is "catching." Holman (1995) called this being a *winner* instead of a *whiner* (Table 4-3).

■ **Perseverance** Effective leaders do not give up easily. Instead, they persist, continuing their efforts when others are tempted to stop trying. This persistence often pays off.

■ **Generosity** Freely sharing your time, interest, and assistance with your colleagues is a trait of a generous leader. Sharing credit for successes and support when needed are other ways to be a generous leader (Buchanan, 2013; Disch, 2013).

■ **Balance** In the effort to become the best nurses they can be, some nurses may forget that other aspects of life are equally important. As important as patients and colleagues are, family and friends are important, too. Although school and work are meaningful activities, cultural, social, recreational, and spiritual activities also have meaning. You need to find a balance between work and play.

■ **Ability to handle stress** There is some stress in almost every job. Coping with stress in as positive and healthy a manner as possible helps to conserve energy and can be a model for others. Maintaining balance and handling stress are reviewed in Chapter 13.

■ **Self-awareness** How sharp is your emotional intelligence? People who do not understand themselves are limited in their ability to understand people with whom they are working. They are far more likely to fool themselves than are self-aware people. For example, it is much easier to be fair with a coworker you like than with one you do not like. Recognizing that you like some people more than others is the first step in avoiding unfair treatment based on personal likes and dislikes.

Behaviors of an Effective Leader

From the previous list of leader qualities, it is evident that leadership requires action. The effective leader chooses these actions carefully. Important leadership behaviors include setting priorities, thinking critically, solving problems, respecting people, communicating skillfully, communicating a vision for the future, and developing oneself and others.

■ **Setting priorities** Whether planning care for a group of patients or creating a strategic plan for an organization, priorities continually shift and demand your attention. As a leader, it is important to continually evaluate what you personally need to do, delegate tasks that someone else can do, and estimate how long your top priorities will take you to complete.

■ **Thinking critically** Critical thinking is the careful, deliberate use of reasoned analysis to reach a decision about what to believe or what to do (Feldman, 2002). The essence of critical thinking is a willingness to ask questions and to be open to new ideas or new ways to do things. To avoid falling prey to assumptions and biases of your own or others, ask yourself frequently, "Do I have the information I need? Is it accurate? Am I prejudging the situation?" (Jackson et al., 2004).

■ **Solving problems** Patient problems, paperwork problems, staff problems—these and others occur frequently and need to be solved. The effective leader helps people identify the problems and work through the problem-solving process to find a reasonable solution.

■ **Respecting and valuing the individual** Although people have much in common, each individual has different wants and needs and has had different life experiences. For example, some people really value the psychological reward of helping others; others are more concerned about earning a decent salary. There is nothing wrong with either of these points of view; they are simply different. The effective leader recognizes these differences in people and helps them find the rewards in their work that mean the most to them.

■ **Skillful communication** This includes listening to others, encouraging exchange of information, and providing feedback:

1. *Listening to others* Listening is separate from talking with other people. The only way to find out people's individual wants and needs is to watch what they do and to listen to what they say. It is amazing how often leaders fail simply because they did not listen to what other people were trying to tell them.

2. *Encouraging exchange of information* Many misunderstandings and mistakes occur because people fail to share enough information with each other. The leader's role is to make sure that the channels of communication remain open and that people use them.

3. *Providing feedback* Everyone needs some information about the effectiveness of their performance. Frequent feedback, both positive and negative, is needed so people can continually improve their performance. Some nurse leaders find it difficult to give negative feedback because they fear that they will upset the other person. However, how else can the person know where improvement is needed? Negative feedback can be given in a manner that is neither hurtful nor resented by the individual receiving it. In fact, it is often appreciated. Other nurse leaders, however, fail to give positive feedback, assuming that coworkers will know when they are doing a good job. This is also a mistake because everyone appreciates positive feedback. In fact, for some people, it is the most important reward they get from their jobs.

■ **Communicating a vision for the future** The effective leader has a vision for the future. Blanchard and Miller (2014) call it "one of the privileges and most serious demands of leaders" (p. 35). Communicating this vision to the group and involving everyone in working toward that vision generate the inspiration that keeps people going when things become difficult. Even better, involving people in creating the vision is not only more satisfying for employees but also has the potential to produce the most creative and innovative outcomes (Kerfott, 2000). It is this vision that helps make work meaningful.

■ **Developing oneself and others** Learning does not end upon leaving school. In fact, experienced nurses say that school is just the beginning, that school only prepares you to continue learning throughout your career. As new ways to care for patients are developed, it is your responsibility as a professional to critically analyze them and decide whether they would be better for your patients than current ones. Effective leaders not only continue to learn but also encourage others to do the same. Sometimes, leaders function as teachers. At other times, their role is primarily to encourage others to seek more knowledge.

Becoming a Leader

It is not too soon to begin becoming a leader. Two different approaches to becoming a leader are often suggested (see Table 4-4). The first is learning leadership by doing it: jump right in and take advantage of any leadership opportunities that arise. Ibarra (2015) says that interacting with others as a leader is how you learn to lead. In fact, you become a leader by acting as if you are one (see Table 4-4). The alternative approach is to begin by reflecting on who you are and what you can contribute as a leader. Kethledge and Erwin (2017) suggest that you consciously make time to think and reflect on your leadership. Find a quiet time to do this: Take your lunch outside, go for a run before work, meditate, or just find a quiet place to be alone for a few minutes, thinking about what you are doing. Leaders, they note, can get so caught up in the many activities of a day that they don't have time to think and reflect, to take a broader

table 4-4

On Becoming a Leader: Two Perspectives

Use Outsight	Use Insight
Act, then think about what you did	Think, then act
Learn leadership by doing it	Plan for alone time to think, reflect
Interacting with others shapes your leadership	Solitude is an opportunity to work out solutions to leadership challenges

Source: Ibarra, H. (2015). Act like a leader, think like a leader. Harvard Business Review Press.

view of your situation and to develop the compelling vision that is such a valuable part of what a leader contributes to the group or team. Although seeming to be opposite ideas, these may both be helpful suggestions. Take advantage of opportunities to be a leader, but also find time to stop and think about what is happening around you and how you can make a contribution through your leadership. Owen (2015) notes that learning solely from experience is too random: You could have some very valuable experiences or you could have some very difficult experiences that might discourage you from continuing your efforts. Instead, combine the learning you obtain from books and courses with real-life experience to become a good leader.

Anderson, Manno, O'Connor, and Gallagher (2010) invited five nurse managers from Penn Presbyterian Medical Center who had received top ratings in leadership from their staff to participate in a focus group on successful leadership. They reported that visibility, communication, and the values of respect and empathy were the key elements of successful leadership. The authors quoted participants to illustrate each of these elements (p. 186):

> Visibility: "I try to come in on the off shifts even for an hour or two just to have them see you."
>
> Communication: "Candid feedback"; "A lot of rounding." (Note: This could also be visibility.)
>
> Respect and empathy: "Do I expect you to take seven patients? No, because I wouldn't be able to do it" (punctuation adjusted).

These three key elements draw on components from several leadership qualities and behaviors: skillful communication, respecting and valuing the individual, and energy. Visibility is not as prominent in many of the leadership theories but deserves a place in the description of what effective leaders do.

Followership

Followership and leadership are complementary roles. They are also reciprocal: Without followers, one cannot be a leader. One also cannot be a follower without having a leader either (Lyons, 2002).

Some people associate the term *follower* with a negative image of being very weak, passive, and having less initiative or creativity. Nothing could be further from the reality of a good follower who is essential to accomplishing the work of the group, team, or health-care organization. In fact, Riggio (2020) suggests leaders should value the critical role that followers play in co-constructing good leadership (p. 19).

It is as important to be an effective follower as it is to be an effective leader. In fact, most of us are followers most of the time: members of a team, attendees at a meeting, staff of a nursing care unit, and so forth.

Followership Defined

Followers are those who accept the influence of the leader of a group (Bastardoz & Van Vugt, 2019). They do this in recognition of the need for people to cooperate and coordinate their actions with other members of the group or team in order to get something done. Followership is an important role that everyone in an organization assumes to a greater or lesser degree. Do not underestimate the value of being a good follower. To the contrary, the most valuable follower is a skilled, self-directed professional, one who participates actively in determining the group's direction, invests personal time and energy in the work of the group, thinks critically, and advocates for new ideas (Grossman & Valiga, 2000; Public Broadcasting Service, 2021).

Imagine working on a patient care unit where all staff members, from the unit secretary to the assistant nurse manager, willingly take on extra tasks without being asked (Spreitzer & Quinn, 2001), come back early from coffee breaks if they are needed, complete their patient records on time, support ways to improve patient care, and are proud of the high-quality care they provide. Wouldn't it be wonderful to be a part of that team?

Becoming a Better Follower

There are several things you can do to become a better follower:

- If you discover a problem, inform your team leader or manager right away.
- Even better, include a suggestion for solving the problem in your report.
- Freely invest your interest and energy in your work.
- Be supportive of new ideas and new directions suggested by others.
- When you disagree, explain why.

- Listen carefully and reflect on what your leader or manager says.
- Continue to learn as much as you can about your specialty area.
- Share what you learn.

Being an effective follower not only will make you a more valuable employee but will also increase the meaning and satisfaction that you get from your work.

Bad followers are those who do not do their fair share of the work of the group. They may cut corners, skip over necessary tasks, and undermine the leaders. These and similar behaviors make the group less efficient or effective (Bastardoz & Van Vugt, 2019). In the future, we may teach effective followership as well as effective leadership to all health-care professionals (Riggio, 2020).

Managing Up

Most team leaders and nurse managers respond positively to having staff who are good followers. Occasionally, you will encounter a poor leader or manager who can confuse, frustrate, and even distress you. Here are a few suggestions for handling this:

- Avoid adopting the ineffective behaviors of this individual.
- Continue to do your best work and to contribute leadership to the group.
- If the situation worsens, enlist the support of others on your team to seek a remedy; do not try to do this alone as a new graduate.
- If the situation becomes intolerable, consider the option of transferring to another unit or seeking another position (Deutschman, 2005; Korn, 2004).

There is still more a good follower can do. This is called *managing up*. Managing up is defined as "the process of consciously working with your boss to obtain the best possible results for you, your boss, and your organization" (Zuber & James, quoted by Turk, 2007, p. 21). This is not a scheme to manipulate your manager or to get more rewards than you have earned. Instead, it is a guide for better understanding your manager, what your manager expects of you, and what your manager's own needs might be.

Every manager has areas of strength and weakness. A good follower recognizes these and helps the manager capitalize on areas of strength and compensate for areas of weakness. For example, if your nurse manager is slow in completing quality improvement reports, you can offer to help get them done. However, if your nurse manager seems to be especially skilled in defusing conflicts between attending physicians and nursing staff, you can observe how they handle these situations and ask them how they do it. Remember that your manager is human, a person with as many needs, concerns, distractions, and ambitions as anyone else. This will help you keep your expectations of your manager realistic and reduce the distance between you and your manager.

There are several other ways in which to manage up. U.S. Army General and former Secretary of State Colin Powell said, "You can't make good decisions unless you have good information" (Powell, 2012, p. 42). Keep your manager informed. No one enjoys being surprised, least of all a manager who finds that you have known about a problem (a nursing assistant who is spending too much time in the staff lounge, for example) and not brought it to her attention until it became critical. When you do bring a problem to your manager's attention, try to have a solution to offer. This is not always possible, but when it is, it will be very much appreciated.

Finally, show your appreciation whenever possible (Bing, 2010). Show respect for your manager's authority and appreciation for what your manager does for the staff of your unit. Let others know of your appreciation, particularly those to whom your manager must answer.

Conclusion

To be an effective nurse, you need to be an effective leader. Your patients, peers, and employer are depending on you to lead. Successful leaders never stop learning and growing. John Maxwell (1998), an expert on leadership, wrote, "Who we are is who we attract" (p. xi). To attract leaders, people need to start leading and never stop learning to lead.

The key elements of leadership and followership have been discussed in this chapter. Many of the leadership and followership qualities and behaviors mentioned here are discussed in more detail in later chapters.

Study Questions

1. Why is it important for nurses to be good leaders? What qualities have you observed from nurses that exemplify effective leadership in action? How do you think these behaviors might have improved the outcomes of their patients?

2. Why are effective followers as important as effective leaders?

3. Review the various leadership theories discussed in the chapter. Which ones especially apply to leading in today's health-care environment? Support your answer with specific examples.

4. Select an individual whose leadership skills you particularly admire. What are some qualities and behaviors that this individual displays? How do these relate to the leadership theories discussed in this chapter? In what ways could you emulate this person?

5. As a new graduate, what leadership and followership skills will you work on developing during the first 3 months of your first nursing position? Why?

Case Study to Promote Clinical Judgment

Two new associate-degree graduate nurses were hired for the pediatric unit. Both worked three 12-hour shifts a week, Jan on the day-to-evening shift and Ronnie at night. Whenever their shifts overlapped, they would compare notes on their experience. Jan felt she was learning rapidly, gaining clinical skills, and beginning to feel at ease with her colleagues.

Ronnie, however, still felt unsure of herself and often isolated. "There have been times," she told Jan, "that I am the only registered nurse on the unit all night. The aides and licensed practical nurses (LPNs) are really experienced, but that's not enough. I wish I could work with an experienced nurse as you are doing."

"Ronnie, you are not even finished with your 3-month orientation program," said Jan. "You should never be left alone with all these sick children. Neither of us is ready for that kind of responsibility. And how will you get the experience you need with no experienced nurses to help you? You must speak to our nurse manager about this."

"I know I should, but she's so hard to reach. I've called several times, and she's never available. She leaves all the shift assignments to her assistant. I'm not sure she even reviews the schedule before it's posted."

"You will have to try harder to reach her. Maybe you could stay past the end of your shift one morning and meet with her," suggested Jan. "If something happens when you are the only nurse on the unit, you will be held responsible."

1. In your own words, summarize the problem that Jan and Ronnie are discussing. To what extent is this problem because of a failure to lead? Who has failed to act?

2. What style of leadership was displayed by Jan, Ronnie, and the nurse manager? How effective was their leadership? Did Jan's leadership differ from that of Ronnie and the nurse manager? In what way?

3. In what ways has Ronnie been an effective follower? In what ways has Ronnie not been so effective as a follower?

4. If an emergency occurred and was not handled well while Ronnie was the only nurse on the unit, who would be responsible? Explain why this person or persons would be responsible.

5. If you found yourself in Ronnie's situation, what steps would you take to resolve the problem? Show how the leader characteristics and behaviors found in this chapter support your solution to the problem.

NCLEX®-Style Review Questions

1. An important competency that nurse leaders need to develop in order to lead effectively is the
   1. Ability to be firm and inflexible
   2. Ability to be close-minded and to ignore negative feedback
   3. Ability to communicate effectively with others
   4. Ability to follow orders without questioning them

2. A unit team leader who fails to provide direction to the nursing care team is a(n)
   1. Democratic leader
   2. Laissez-faire leader
   3. Autocratic leader
   4. Situational leader

3. A democratic nurse leader consistently works to
   1. Move the group toward the leader's goals
   2. Make little or no attempt to move the group
   3. Share leadership with the group
   4. Dampen creativity

4. The situational leadership model focuses on
   1. Both followers and the task
   2. The task
   3. The follower
   4. The behavior of others

5. An emotionally intelligent nurse leader
   1. Seeks the emotional support of others
   2. Cannot juggle multiple demands
   3. Works alone without help
   4. Welcomes constructive criticism

6. Transformational nursing leaders have the ability to
   1. Increase the negativity of the team
   2. Work best alone
   3. Define the group's mission and communicate that mission to others
   4. Pay close attention to the weaknesses and shortcomings of others

7. An effective leader will have: **Select all that apply**.
   1. Courage and integrity
   2. A critical mind-set
   3. The ability to set priorities
   4. The ability to provide feedback

8. Effective nurse leaders: **Select all that apply**.
   1. Are also good followers
   2. Effectively work together with shared goals
   3. Never act on their ideas
   4. Have master's degrees

9. Effective followers are those who are
   1. Passive employees
   2. Skilled and self-directed employees
   3. Less valuable employees
   4. Employees who are never supportive of new ideas

10. Autocratic leaders
    1. Postpone decision making as long as possible.
    2. Share leadership with members of the team.
    3. Give orders and make decisions without consulting the team.
    4. Encourage creativity when problem-solving.

The Nurse as Manager of Care

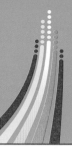

table 5-1

Differences Between Leadership and Management

Leadership	Management
Based on influence and shared meaning	Based on authority
An informal role	A formally designated role
An achieved position	As assigned position
Part of every nurse's responsibility	Usually responsible for budgets and appraising, hiring, and firing people
Requires initiative and independent thinking	Improved by the use of effective leadership skills

Every nurse needs to be a good leader and a good follower. In Chapter 4, we defined *leadership* and *followership* and showed that even as a new nurse, you can be an effective leader. Not everyone needs to be a manager, however, and new graduates are rarely ready to take on management responsibilities. Once you have had time to develop your clinical and leadership skills, then you can begin to think about taking on management responsibilities (Table 5-1).

Management

Are You Ready to Be a Manager?

For most new nurses, the answer to whether they are ready to be a manager is *no*. New graduates who have demonstrated rapid acquisition of clinical skills are sometimes asked to accept a management position. However, if you are approached about this, you should not accept managerial responsibility yet because your managerial skills are still underdeveloped. Equally important, you need to direct your energies to building your own skills, including your leadership skills, before you begin supervising other people and helping them develop their skills.

What Is Management?

The essence of management is getting work done through others. The classic definition of management was Henri Fayol's 1916 list of managerial tasks: planning, organizing, commanding, coordinating, and controlling the work of a group of employees (Wren, 1972). But Mintzberg (1989) argued that managers really do whatever is needed to make sure that employees do their work and do it well. Lombardi (2001) added that two-thirds of a manager's time is spent on people problems. The

rest is taken up by budget work, going to meetings, preparing reports, and other administrative tasks.

Management Theories

There are two major but opposing schools of thought in management: scientific management and the human relations–based approach. As its name implies, the human relations approach emphasizes the interpersonal aspects of managing people, whereas scientific management emphasizes the task aspects.

Scientific Management

Almost 100 years ago, Frederick Taylor argued that most jobs could be done more efficiently if they were analyzed thoroughly (Lee, 1980; Locke, 1982). Given a well-designed task and enough incentive to get the work done, workers will be more productive. For example, Taylor promoted the concept of paying people by the piece instead of by the hour. In health care, the equivalent of what Taylor recommended would be paying by the number of patients bathed or visited at home rather than by the number of hours worked. This creates an incentive to get the most work done in the least amount of time. Taylorism stresses that there is a best way to do a job, which is usually the fastest way to do the job as well (Dantley, 2005).

Work is analyzed to improve efficiency. In health care, for example, there has been much discussion about the time and effort it takes to bring a disabled patient to physical therapy versus sending the therapist to the patient's home or inpatient unit. Reducing staff or increasing the productivity of existing employees to save money are also based on this kind of thinking.

Nurse managers who use the principles of scientific management will pay particular attention to the types of assessments and treatments done on the unit, the equipment needed to do them efficiently, and the strategies that would facilitate more efficient accomplishment of these tasks. Typically, these nurse managers keep careful records of the amount of work accomplished and reward those who accomplish the most.

Human Relations–Based Management

McGregor's theories X and Y provide a good contrast between scientific management and human relations-based management. Similar to Taylorism, Theory X reflects a common attitude among managers that most people do not want to work very

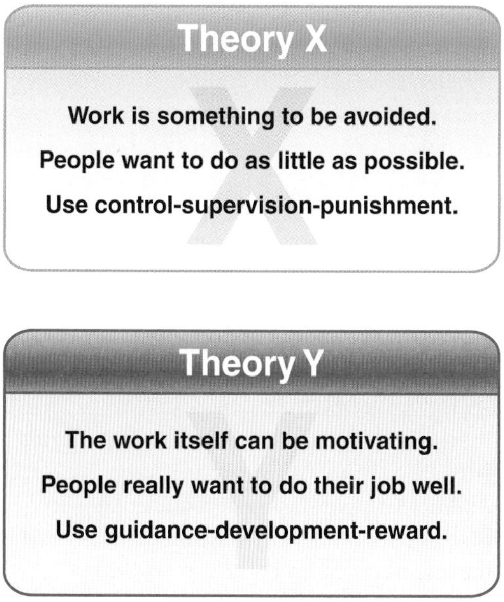

Theory X

Work is something to be avoided.

People want to do as little as possible.

Use control-supervision-punishment.

Theory Y

The work itself can be motivating.

People really want to do their job well.

Use guidance-development-reward.

Figure 5.1 Theory X versus Theory Y.

hard and that the manager's job is to make sure that they do (McGregor, 1960). To accomplish this, according to Theory X, a manager needs to employ strict rules, constant supervision, and the threat of punishment (reprimands, withheld raises, and threats of job loss) to create industrious, conscientious workers.

Theory Y, which McGregor preferred, is the opposite viewpoint. Theory Y managers believe that the work itself can be motivating and that people will work hard if their managers provide a supportive environment. A Theory Y manager emphasizes guidance rather than control, development rather than close supervision, and reward rather than punishment (Fig. 5.1). A Theory Y nurse manager is concerned with keeping employee morale as high as possible, assuming that satisfied, motivated employees will do the best work. Employees' attitudes, opinions, hopes, and fears are important to this type of nurse manager. Considerable effort is expended to work out conflicts and promote mutual understanding to provide an environment in which people can do their best work.

Servant Leadership

The emphasis on people and interpersonal relationships is taken one step further by Greenleaf (2004), who wrote an essay in 1970 that began the servant leadership movement. Similar to transformational

and caring leadership, servant leadership has a special appeal to nurses and other health-care professionals. Despite its name, servant leadership applies more to people in supervisory or administrative positions than to people in staff positions.

The servant leader-style manager believes that people have value as people, not just as workers (Spears & Lawrence, 2004). The manager is committed to improving the way each employee is treated at work. The attitude is "employee first," not "manager first." So managers see themselves as being there for the employee. Here is an example:

Hope Marshall is a relatively new staff nurse at Jefferson County Hospital. When she was invited to be the staff nurse representative on the search committee for a new chief nursing officer, she was very excited about being on a committee with so many managerial and administrative people. As the interviews of candidates began, she focused on what they had to say. All the candidates had impressive résumés and spoke confidently about their accomplishments. Hope was impressed but did not yet prefer one more than the other. Then the final candidate spoke to the committee. "My primary job," he said, "is to make it possible for each nurse to do the very best job he or she can do. I am here to make their work easier, to remove barriers, and to provide them with whatever they need to provide the best patient care possible." Hope had never heard the term *servant leadership*, but she knew immediately that this candidate, who articulated the essence of servant leadership, was the one she would support for this important position.

Qualities of an Effective Manager

Two-thirds of people who leave their jobs say the main reason was an ineffective or incompetent manager (Hunter, 2004). A survey of 3,266 newly licensed nurses found that lack of support from their manager was the nurses' primary reason for leaving their position, followed by a stressful work environment. Following are some of the indicators of their stressful work environment:

- 25% reported at least one needlestick in their first year.
- 39% reported at least one strain or sprain.

■ 62% reported experiencing verbal abuse.

■ 25% reported a shortage of supplies needed to do their work.

These results underscore the importance of having effective nurse managers who can create an environment in which new nurses thrive (Kovner et al., 2007).

Nurse managers hold pivotal positions in hospitals, nursing homes, and other health-care facilities. They report to the administration of these facilities, coordinate with a myriad of departments (the laboratory, dietary, pharmacy, and so forth) and care providers (physicians, nurse practitioners, therapists, and so forth), and supervise a staff that provides care around the clock. They also have a particularly important relationship with their staff. Owen (2015) calls it a "psychological contract" (p. 78) that staff members will do what the manager asks of them, and the manager in turn will be fair and reasonable in regard to assignments, promotions, and evaluations. You can see why managers' effectiveness has considerable influence on the quality of the care provided under their direction (Trossman, 2011).

Consider for a moment the knowledge and skills needed by a nurse manager:

■ Leadership, especially relationship building, teamwork, and mentoring skills

■ Professionalism, including advocacy for nursing staff and support of nursing roles and ethical practice

■ Advanced clinical expertise, including quality improvement and evidence-based practice

■ Human resource management expertise, including staff development and performance appraisals

■ Financial management

■ Coordination of patient care, including scheduling, workflow, work assignments, monitoring the quality of care provided, and documentation of that care (Fennimore & Wolf, 2011; Jones, 2010)

The effective nurse manager possesses a combination of qualities: leadership, clinical expertise, and business sense. None of these alone is enough; it is the combination that prepares an individual for the complex task of managing a unit or team of health-care providers. Consider each of these briefly:

■ **Leadership** All the people skills of the leader are essential to the effective manager.

■ **Clinical expertise** Without possessing clinical expertise oneself, it is very difficult to help others develop their skills and evaluate how well they have done. It is probably not necessary (or even possible) to know everything all other professionals on the team know, but it is important to be able to assess the effectiveness of their work in terms of patient outcomes.

■ **Business sense** Nurse managers also need to be concerned with the "bottom line," with the cost of providing the care that is given, especially in comparison with the benefit received from that care and the funding available to pay for it, whether from private insurance, Medicare, Medicaid, or out of the patient's own pocket. This is a complex task that requires knowledge of budgeting, staffing, and measurement of patient outcomes.

There is some controversy regarding the amount of clinical expertise versus business sense that is needed to be an effective nurse manager. Some argue that a person can be a "generic" manager, that the job of managing people is the same no matter what tasks the individual performs. Others argue that managers must understand the tasks themselves better than anyone else in the work group. Our position is that both clinical skill and business acumen are needed, along with excellent leadership skills.

Behaviors of an Effective Manager

Mintzberg (1989) divided a manager's activities into three categories: interpersonal, decisional, and informational. We use these categories and have added some activities suggested by other authors (Dunham-Taylor, 1995; Montebello, 1994) and from our own observations of nurse managers (Fig. 5.2).

Interpersonal Activities

The interpersonal category is one in which leaders and managers have overlapping concerns. However, the manager has some additional responsibilities that are seldom given to leaders. These include the following:

■ **Networking** As we mentioned earlier, nurse managers are in pivotal positions, especially in inpatient settings where they have contact with virtually every service of the institution as well

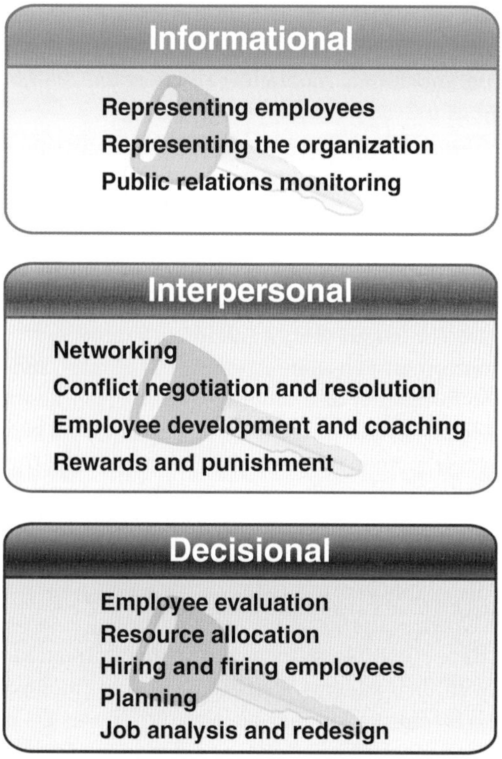

Figure 5.2 Keys to effective management.

as with most people above and below them in the organizational hierarchy. This provides them with many opportunities to influence the status and treatment of staff nurses and the quality of the care provided to their patients. It is important that they "maintain the line of sight," or connection, between what they do as managers, patient care, and the mission of the organization (Mackoff & Triolo, 2008, p. 123). In other words, they need to keep in mind how their interactions with both their staff members and with administration affect the care provided to the patients for whom they are responsible.

- **Conflict negotiation and resolution** Managers often find themselves resolving conflicts among employees, patients, and administration. Ineffective managers often ignore people's emotional side or mismanage feelings in the workplace (Welch & Welch, 2008).

- **Employee development** Managers are responsible for providing for the continuing learning and upgrading of the skills of their employees.

- **Coaching** It is often said that employees are the organization's most valuable asset (Shirey, 2007). Coaching is one way in which nurse managers can share their experience and expertise with the rest of the staff. The goal is to nurture the growth and development of the employee (the "coachee") to do a better job through learning (McCauley & Van Velson, 2004; Shirey, 2007).

Some managers use a directive approach: "This is how it's done. Watch me," or "Let me show you how to do this." Others prefer a problem-solving approach: "How do you think we can improve our outcomes?" or "Let's try to figure out what's wrong here" (Hart & Waisman, 2005).

You can probably see the parallel with democratic and autocratic leadership styles described in Chapter 4. The decision whether to be directive (e.g., in an emergency) or to engage in mutual problem-solving (e.g., when developing a long-term plan to improve patient safety) will depend on the situation.

- **Rewards and punishments** Managers are in a position to provide specific rewards (e.g., salary increases, time off) and general rewards (e.g., praise, recognition) as well as punishments (withhold pay raises, deny promotions).

Decisional Activities

Nurse managers are responsible for making many decisions:

- **Employee evaluation** Managers are responsible for conducting formal performance appraisals of their staff members. Traditionally, formal reviews have been conducted once a year, but people need to know much sooner than that if they are doing well or need to improve. Effective managers are similar to coaches who regularly give their staff feedback (Suddath, 2013).

- **Resource allocation** In decentralized organizations, nurse managers are often given an annual budget for their units and must allocate these resources wisely. This can be difficult when resources are very limited, but it does provide nurse managers with the authority to deploy their resources as needed (Longmore, 2017).

- **Hiring and firing employees** Nurse managers either make the hiring and firing decisions or participate in employment and termination decisions for their units.

■ **Planning for the future** Not only is the day-to-day operation of most units complex and time-consuming, but nurse managers must also look ahead to prepare themselves and their units for future changes in budgets, organizational priorities, and patient populations. They also need to look beyond the four walls of their own organization to become aware of what is happening to their competition and to the health-care system (Kelly & Nadler, 2007).

■ **Job analysis and redesign** In a time of extreme cost sensitivity, nurse managers are often required to analyze and redesign the work of their units to make them as efficient as possible.

Informational Activities

Nurse managers often find themselves in positions within the organizational hierarchy in which they acquire much information that is not available to their staff. They also have much information about their staff that is not readily available to the administration, placing them in a strategic position within the information web of any organization. The effective manager uses this knowledge for the benefit of both the staff and the organization. The following are some examples:

■ **Spokesperson** Nurse managers often speak for the administration when relaying information to their staff members. Likewise, they often speak for staff members when relaying information to administration. You could think of them as central information clearinghouses,

acting as gatherers and disseminators of information to people above and below them in the organizational hierarchy (Shirey et al., 2008, p. 126).

■ **Monitoring** Nurse managers are also expert "sensors," picking up early signs (information) of problems before they grow too big (Shirey et al., 2008). They are expected to monitor the many and various activities of their units or departments, including the number of patients seen, average length of stay, and important patient outcomes such as infection rates, fall rates, and so forth. They also monitor the staff (e.g., absentee rates, tardiness, unproductive time), the budget (e.g., money spent, money left in comparison with money needed to operate the unit), and the costs of procedures and services provided, especially those that are variable such as overtime or disposable versus nondisposable medical supplies (Dowless, 2007).

■ **Reporting** Nurse managers share information with their patients, staff members, and employers. This information may be related to the results of their monitoring efforts, new developments in health care, policy changes, and so forth.

Review Table 5-2 to compare what you have just read about effective nurse managers with descriptions of some of the most common ineffective ("bad management") approaches to being a manager.

The resource allocation, monitoring, and reporting functions became especially important during the COVID-19 pandemic. This health

table 5-2	
Bad Management Styles	
These are the types of managers you do not want to be and for whom you do not want to work.	
Know-it-all	Self-appointed experts on everything, these managers do not listen to anyone else.
Emotionally remote	Isolated from the staff and the work going on, these managers do not know what is going on in the workplace and cannot inspire others.
Purely mean	Mean, nasty, and dictatorial, these managers look for problems and reasons to criticize. They diminish people instead of developing them.
Overly nice	Desperate to please everyone, these managers agree to every idea and request, causing confusion and spending too much money on useless projects.
Afraid to decide	Indecisive managers may announce goals for their unit but fail to be clear about their expectations, assign responsibility, or set deadlines for accomplishment. In the name of fairness, these managers may not distinguish between competent and incompetent or hardworking and unproductive employees, thus creating an unfair reward system.

Source: Based on Schaffer, R. H. (2010, September). Mistakes leaders keep making. Harvard Business Review, 88(9), 87–91; Welch, J., & Welch, S. (2007, July 23). Bosses who get it all wrong. Bloomberg Businessweek, 88(4043); Wiseman, L., & McKeown, A. (2010, May). Bringing out the best in your people. Harvard Business Review, Reprint R1005K, 88(5), 117.

emergency highlighted how important it was to keep staff well supplied with personal protective equipment (PPE) and their units equipped with sufficient respirators and other critical equipment to monitor the effectiveness of the infection control procedures that were put into place and to keep information flowing within the units, throughout the facility, and with the community and public health system.

It is also important for managers to be aware of the mental health consequences of the pressures on staff, which may include depression, anxiety, hyperarousal, burnout, and an inability to function at work. Bringing in extra staff if possible and providing stress management and other support strategies may help staff through such a crisis (Tokac & Razon, 2021; Halcomb et al., 2021).

Becoming a Manager

Not every nurse wants to be a manager; some prefer to follow the path to becoming highly expert clinicians instead. But if you are ready to become a nurse manager and accept a management position, you will find yourself a novice again, this time a novice nurse manager facing a whole new set of challenges. At first you may try to be "all things to all people" with unrealistic expectations of what you can do and become overwhelmed by the number of demands placed on you as a nurse manager. Cox (2017) suggests that new managers learn how to set boundaries, build a new set of constructive relationships with colleagues and mentors (previous friendships may change when your change in status occurs), and undertake extensive personal development to become a good manager. Cox also advises that you give yourself at least a year to become comfortable with your new position and to remember this workplace "serenity prayer": "Grant me the serenity to prioritize the things I can't delegate, the courage to say no when I need to, and the wisdom to know when to go home!" (p. 56).

As you gain experience, you will become a skilled manager, able to optimize the function of your unit and eventually to become a mentor to new nurse managers (Clark-Burg & Alliex, 2017).

Conclusion

Nurse managers have complex, responsible positions in health-care organizations. Ineffective managers may do harm to their employees, their patients, and the organization, whereas effective managers can help their staff members grow and develop as health-care professionals providing the highest-quality care to their patients.

If you have wondered why there are so many conflicting and overlapping theories of leadership and management, it is because management theory is still at an immature (not fully developed) stage as well as being prone to fads (Micklethwait, 2011). Even so, there is still much that is useful in the theories and much to be learned from them.

Study Questions

1. Why should new graduates decline nursing management positions? At what point do you think a nurse is ready to assume managerial responsibilities?

2. Which theory, scientific management or human relations, do you believe is most useful to nurse managers? Explain your choice.

3. Compare servant leadership with scientific management. Which approach do you prefer? Why?

4. Describe your ideal nurse manager in terms of the person for whom you would most enjoy working. Then describe the worst nurse manager you can imagine, and explain why this person would be very difficult to work with.

5. List 10 behaviors of nurse managers and then rank them from least to most important. What rationale(s) did you use in ranking them?

Case Study to Promote Clinical Judgment

Case I

Joe Garcia has been an operating room nurse for 5 years. He is often on call on Saturdays and Sundays, but he enjoys his work and knows that he is good at it.

Joe was called to come in on a busy Saturday afternoon just as his 5-year-old daughter's birthday party was about to begin. "Can you find someone else just this once?" he asked the nurse manager who called him. "I should have let you know in advance that we have an important family event today, but I just forgot. If you can't find someone else, call me back, and I'll come right in." Joe's manager was furious. She said, "I don't have time to make a dozen calls. If you knew that you wouldn't want to come in today, you should not have accepted on-call duty. We pay you to be on call, and I expect you to be here in 30 minutes, not 1 minute later, or there will be consequences."

Joe decided that he no longer wanted to work in that institution. With his 5 years of operating room experience, he quickly found another position in an organization that was more supportive of its staff.

1. What style of leadership and school of management seemed to be preferred by Joe Garcia's manager?

2. What style of leadership and school of management were preferred by Joe?

3. Which of the listed qualities of leaders and managers did the nurse manager display? Which behaviors? Which ones did the nurse manager not display?

4. If you were Joe, what would you have done? If you were the nurse manager, what would you have done? Why?

5. Who do you think was right, Joe or the nurse manager? Why?

Case II

Sung Lee completed her 2-year associate degree in nursing right after high school. Upon graduation, she was offered a staff position at the Harbordale nursing home and rehabilitation center where she had volunteered during high school. Most of her classmates accepted positions in local hospitals, but Sung Lee felt comfortable at Harbordale and had loved her volunteer work there. She thought it would be an advantage to already know many of the staff at Harbordale.

The director of nursing thought it would be best to place Sung Lee on a short-term unit. Most of the patients in the unit were recently discharged from the hospital and still recovering from an acute event such as stroke, injury, or extensive surgery. Sung Lee found her assignment challenging but satisfying. She admired her nurse manager, an experienced clinical nurse leader who became her mentor.

Six months later, the director of nursing called Sung Lee into her office. "Sung Lee," she said, "we are very pleased with your work. You have been a quick learner and very caring nurse. Your colleagues, patients, and physicians all speak well of you."

"Thank you," replied Sung Lee. "I know there's still a lot for me to learn, but I really love my work here."

"You may not be aware of this," continued the director of nursing, "but your nurse manager will be retiring next month. Our policy at Harbordale is to promote from within whenever possible, and I'd like to offer you her position. It's a little soon after graduation, but I'm sure you can handle it."

Sung Lee gasped. "I'm honored that you would consider me for this position. May I have a few days to think it over?"

1. Why did the director of nursing at Harbordale offer the nurse manager position to Sung Lee? If you had been in the director's position, would you have selected Sung Lee for the nurse manager position? Why or why not?

2. If Sung Lee does accept the nurse manager position, how do you think her first month would be? Write a scenario that describes her first month as a nurse manager.

3. If Sung Lee declines this offer, how do you think the director of nursing will respond?

4. Write a list of typical nurse manager roles and responsibilities. For each one, indicate how prepared you are right now to assume each role or responsibility and what you would need to prepare yourself to assume this responsibility.

NCLEX®-Style Review Questions

1. What is the difference between management and leadership?
   1. Management focuses on budget.
   2. Management is an assigned position.
   3. Leadership is not concerned with getting work done.
   4. Leadership is more focused on people.

2. Theory Y emphasizes
   1. Guidance, development, and reward
   2. Leadership, not management
   3. Supervision, monitoring, and reprimands
   4. Evaluation, budgeting, and time studies

3. Servant leadership focuses on
   1. Helping patients care for themselves
   2. Removing incompetent managers
   3. Creating a supportive work environment
   4. Resolving conflicts quickly

4. Effective nurse managers have: **Select all that apply**.
   1. Leadership capabilities
   2. Clinical expertise
   3. Business sense
   4. Budgeting savvy

5. Informational aspects of a nurse manager's job include
   1. Evaluation
   2. Resource allocation
   3. Being a coach
   4. Being a spokesperson

6. When should a new graduate consider taking on management responsibilities?
   1. As soon as they are offered
   2. After developing clinical expertise
   3. After 15 years on the job
   4. Before developing leadership expertise

7. George S. has just become a nurse manager in a long-term care facility. He knows he has a lot to learn—what should he tell his staff?
   1. Nothing; he should pretend he has experience
   2. That he is still learning, too, and values their input
   3. That the staff needs to manage themselves
   4. How little he knows about management

8. Mara Z. wants to become a nurse manager. She has been offered an opportunity to take a nursing management course. Which topic is *most* important for her to learn?
   1. Managing people
   2. Managing the unit's budget
   3. Planning for the future
   4. Redesigning the unit's workflow

9. Scientific management focuses on
   1. Interpersonal relations
   2. Servant leadership
   3. Staff development
   4. Efficiency

10. Which of the following is a major reason why newly licensed nurses resign?
    1. Poor pay scales
    2. Needlestick injuries
    3. Unsupportive management
    4. Lack of advancement opportunities

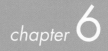
Delegation and Prioritization of Client Care Staffing

OBJECTIVES

After reading this chapter, the student should be able to:

- Define the term *delegation.*
- Define the term *prioritization.*
- Differentiate between delegation and prioritization.
- Define the term *nursing assistive personnel.*
- Discuss the legal implications of making assignments to other health-care personnel.
- Discuss barriers to successful delegation.
- Make appropriate assignments to team members.
- Apply priority-setting guidelines to patient care.

OUTLINE

Elliot, a new graduate, recently completed his orientation. He works from 7 p.m. to 7 a.m. on a busy, monitored neuroscience unit. The client census is 48, making this a full unit. Although there is an associate nurse manager for the shift, Elliot acts as the charge nurse. His responsibilities include receiving and confirming orders; contacting health-care providers with any information or requests; accessing laboratory reports from the computer, reviewing them, and giving them to the appropriate staff members; checking any new medication orders and confirming accuracy on the medication record in the electronic health record (EHR); relieving the monitor technician for dinner and breaks; and assigning staff to dinner and breaks. When Elliot arrives to work, he discovers that one registered nurse (RN) called in sick. His staff tonight consists of two RNs and three nursing assistive personnel (NAP). To complicate matters, the institution just rolled out a new computerized acuity-based staffing model last week, and he needs to enter the complexity level of care for each client. He panics and wants to refuse to take report. After a discussion with the charge nurse from the previous shift, he realizes that refusing to take report is not an option. He sits down to evaluate the acuity of the clients and the capabilities of his staff.

Introduction to Delegation

Delegation is not a new concept. In her book, *Notes on Nursing,* Florence Nightingale (1859) clearly stated: "Don't imagine that if you, who are in charge, don't look to all these things yourself, those under you will be more careful than you are. . . ." She continued by directing, "But then again to look to all these things yourself does not mean to do them yourself. If you do it, it is by so much the better certainly than if it were not done at all. But can you not insure that it is done when not done by yourself? Can you insure that it is not undone when your back is turned? This is what being in charge means. And a very important meaning it is, too. The former only implies that just what you can do with your own hands is done. The latter that what ought to be done is always done. Head in charge must see to house hygiene, not do it herself" (p. 17).

Today, nurses find that more nursing care is needed than there are nurses available to deliver the care. Changes in demographics, improved life expectancy, and newer, more complex therapies continue to generate an increased demand for nursing care. According to a recent McKinsey report (Berlin et al., 2022), the demands on nurses caused by worldwide health issues continue to impact the shortage as many nurses chose to either leave the profession or move out of direct patient care positions to other nursing roles. New directives in health-care law compound this need, requiring nurses to learn how to collaborate and work effectively with other members of the health-care delivery team, particularly NAP. The responsibility to provide safe, effective quality care generates challenges and concerns when RNs delegate duties to NAP. These challenges and concerns are magnified in today's health-care environment of decreasing resources; patients who have complex, chronic conditions; health-care settings with high patient acuity rates; and the use of state-of-the-art technology. RNs need to understand the responsibility, authority, and accountability related to delegation. Decisions must be established on the basic principle of public protection (Mueller & Vogelsmeier, 2013; Puskar et al., 2017; Ver Woert & Hansten, 2020).

Definition of Delegation

In 2005, the American Nurses Association (ANA) and the National Council of State Boards of Nursing (NCSBN) approved papers regarding delegation in nursing practice (NCSBN, 2006). Previously, the ANA (1996) defined *delegation* as the reassigning of responsibility for the performance of a job from one person to another. In 2015, the NCSBN assembled two panels of professionals that represented education, research, and practice. The purpose of the panels was to discuss the delegation research and central issues and evaluate findings from delegation research funded through NCSBN's Center for Regulatory Excellence Grant Program. The goal was to create a set of national guidelines to facilitate and standardize the nursing delegation process. These National Guidelines for Nursing Delegation build on previous work by the NCSBN and the ANA and provide explanations on the responsibilities associated with delegation (NCSBN, 2016).

The NCSBN describes delegation as the transferring of authority. Both the ANA and NCSBN organizations agree that this means the RN has the ability to request another person to perform a task that this individual may not usually be permitted to do. However, RNs maintain accountability for supervising those to whom tasks are delegated (ANA, 2005, 2012a; Mueller & Vogelsmeier, 2013). Nightingale referred to this delegation responsibility when she implied that the "head in charge" does not necessarily carry out the task but still sees that it is completed.

Assignments and Delegation

Making or giving an assignment is not the same as delegation. In an assignment, power is not transferred (the directive to do something that is not necessarily described as part of the job does not occur). Both the NCSBN and the ANA define an *assignment* as the allocation of duties that each staff member is responsible for during a specific work period (NCSBN, 2006; 2016). Assignments relate to situations where an RN directs another individual to do something that the person is already authorized to do. For example, the RN assigns the NAP the responsibility of taking vital signs on three patients. The NAP is already authorized to take vital signs (Siegel et al., 2016). According to the Joint NCSBN and ANA statement (2016), "Delegation is allowing a delegatee to perform a specific nursing activity, skill, or procedure that is beyond the delegatee's traditional role and not routinely performed. This applies to licensed nurses as well as UAP" (p. 6). Therefore, if the RN directed the NAP to check the amount of drainage on a fresh postoperative abdominal dressing, this would be considered delegation because the RN retains responsibility for this action. Matching the skill set of the appropriately educated health-care personnel with the needs of the client and family defines the difference between delegation and assignment (Marquis & Huston, 2021; Weydt, 2010).

The individual state nurse practice acts define the legal boundaries for professional nursing practice (www.ncsbn.org). Individual nursing organizations also set standards of practice for their specialties that fall within the guidelines of the nurse practice acts. Nurses need to understand the guidelines and provisions of their state's nurse practice acts regarding the delegation of patient care (Cipriano, 2010; NCSBN, 2016). However, according to the ANA, specific overlying principles remain firm regarding delegation. These include the following:

■ The nursing profession delineates the scope of nursing practice.
■ The nursing profession identifies and supervises the necessary education, training, and use of ancillary roles concerned with the delivery of direct client care.
■ The RN assumes responsibility and accountability for the provision of nursing care and expertise.
■ The RN directs care and determines the appropriate utilization of any ancillary personnel involved in providing direct client care.
■ The RN accepts assistance from ancillary nursing personnel in delivering nursing care for the client (ANA, 2005, p. 6; ANA, 2012a, p. 7).

Nurse-related principles are also designated by the ANA. These are important when considering what tasks may be delegated and to whom. These principles are:

■ The RN has the duty to be accountable for personal actions related to the nursing process.
■ The RN considers the knowledge and skills of any ancillary personnel to whom aspects of care are delegated.
■ The decision to delegate or assign is based on the RN's judgment regarding the following: the condition of the patient, the competence of the members of the nursing team, and the amount of supervision that will be required of the RN if a task is delegated.
■ The RN uses critical thinking and professional judgment when following the five rights of delegation delineated by the NCSBN (Box 6-1).
■ The RN recognizes that a relational aspect exists between delegation and communication. Communication needs to be culturally appropriate, and the individual receiving the communication should be treated with respect.
■ Chief nursing officers (CNOs) are responsible for creating systems to assess, monitor, verify, and communicate continuous competence requirements in areas related to delegation.
■ RNs monitor organizational policies, procedures, and job descriptions to ensure they are in compliance with the nurse practice act, consulting with the state board of nursing as needed (ANA, 2005, p. 6).

The Five Rights of Delegation

1. Right task
2. Right circumstances
3. Right person
4. Right direction or communication
5. Right supervision or evaluation

Delegation may be direct or indirect. *Direct delegation* is usually "verbal direction by the RN delegator regarding an activity or task in a specific nursing care situation" (ANA, 1996, p. 15). In this case, the RN decides which staff member is capable of performing the specific task or activity. *Indirect delegation* is "an approved listing of activities or tasks that have been established in policies and procedures of the health care institution or facility" (ANA, 1996, p. 15).

Permitted tasks vary from institution to institution and setting to setting. For example, a certified nursing assistant (CNA) performs specific activities designated by the job description approved by the particular health-care institution. CNAs usually take an approved training course and pass an examination indicating they are qualified to perform these skills (NCSBN, 2016). CNAs take direction from both licensed practical/licensed vocational nurses (LPN/LVN) and RNs. Unlicensed assistive personnel (UAPs) or nursing assistive personnel (NAP) may be trained by the institution or take a vocational course to perform specific tasks. These individuals work in a variety of settings. Although the institution delineates tasks and activities, the RN still decides to assign other personnel in specific situations. Take the following example:

> Ms. Ross was admitted to the neurological unit from the neuroscience intensive care unit. She suffered a right hemisphere intracerebral bleed 2 weeks ago and has a left hemiplegia. She has difficulty with swallowing and receives tube feedings through a percutaneous endoscopic transgastric jejunostomy (PEGJ) tube; however, she has been advanced to a pureed diet. She needs assistance with personal care, toileting, and feeding. A physical therapist comes twice a day to get her up for gait training; otherwise, the primary health-care provider wants Ms. Ross in a chair as much as possible.

Assessing this situation, the RN might consider assigning a licensed practical nurse (LPN) to this client. The swallowing problems place the client at risk for aspiration, which means that feeding may present a problem. Based on education and skill level, the LPN is capable of managing the PEGJ tube feeding. However, it may be questionable as to whether the LPN can begin oral feedings. In this case, interprofessional care assistance from speech therapy and evaluation before assigning the LPN is in order (Moss et al., 2016). While assisting with bathing, the LPN can perform range-of-motion exercises to all the client's extremities and assess her skin for breakdown. The LPN also knows the appropriate way to assist the client in transferring from the bed to the chair (LaCharity et al., 2022; Zimmerman & Schultz, 2013).

Supervision

The term *supervisor* implies that an individual holds authority over others (National Labor Relations Act [NLRA], 1935). Although nurses supervise others on a daily basis, they do not necessarily hold "authority" over those they supervise. Therefore, it is important to differentiate between supervision and delegation (Matthews, 2010). According to the NCSBN (2006), "supervision is the provision of guidance and direction, oversight, evaluation and follow-up by the licensed nurse for the accomplishment of a nursing task delegated to nursing assistive personnel" (ANA, 2012, p. 6). Supervision is more direct and requires directly overseeing the work or performance of others. Supervision includes checking with individuals throughout the day to see what activities they completed and what they may still need to finish. When one RN works with another, then supervision is not needed. This is a collaborative relationship and includes consulting and giving advice when needed.

The following gives an example of supervision:

> An NAP has been assigned to take all the vital signs on the unit and give the morning baths to eight patients. Three hours into the morning, the NAP is far behind in the assignment. At this point, it is important that the RN discover the reason the NAP has not been able to complete the assignment. Perhaps one of the clients required more care than expected, or the NAP needed to complete an errand off the unit. Reevaluation of the assignment may be necessary.

Individuals who supervise others also delegate tasks and activities. For example, CNOs often delegate tasks to associate directors. These tasks may include record reviews, unit reports, or client acuities. Certain administrative tasks, such as staff scheduling, may be delegated to another staff member, such as an associate manager. However, the delegator remains accountable for ensuring the activities are completed.

Supervision sometimes entails more direct evaluation of performance, such as performance evaluations and discussions regarding individual interactions with clients and other staff members.

Regardless of where nurses work, they cannot assume that only those in the higher levels of the organization delegate work to other people. New graduates will be responsible at times for delegating some of their work to other nurses, to technical personnel, or to other members of the interprofessional team. Decisions associated with this responsibility often cause some difficulty for new nurses. Knowing each person's capabilities and job description can help you decide which personnel can assist with a task. In all situations, it is important to remember that the patient's safety comes first (Ver Woert & Hansten, 2020).

The Nursing Process and Delegation

Before deciding who should care for a particular client, the nurse needs to assess each client's care requirements, set client-specific goals, and match the skills of the person assigned with the tasks that need to be accomplished *(assessment)*. Thinking this through before delegating helps prevent problems later *(plan)*. Next, the nurse assigns the tasks to the appropriate person *(implementation)*. The nurse must then oversee the care and determine whether client care needs have been met *(evaluation)* (Zimmerman & Schultz, 2013). It is also important for the nurse to allow time for feedback during the day. This enables all personnel to see what has been accomplished and what still needs to be done.

Often, nurses must first coordinate care for groups of clients before delegating tasks to other personnel. Nurses also need to consider their own responsibilities, which may include communicating clearly, assisting other staff members with setting priorities, clarifying instructions, and reassessing the situation.

The Need for Delegation

The 1990s brought rapid change to the health-care environment. These changes, including shorter hospital stays, increased patient acuity, and the intensification of the nursing shortage, have continued well into the 21st century, requiring institutions to hire other personnel to assist nurses with client care (Charett et al., 2020; Marquis & Huston, 2021; McHugh et al., 2013).

Based on the studies by McHugh et al. (2013) and the Institute of Medicine (IOM, 2001, 2010), based on their knowledge, skill set, and level of education, RNs need to provide all care needs to ensure safety and quality in this complex and demanding health-care environment. Although a lofty idea, this system of health-care delivery would be economically prohibitive. For this reason, health-care institutions often use NAP to perform certain patient care tasks.

As the nursing shortage becomes more critical, there is a greater need for institutions to recruit the services of NAPs (ANA, 2002; Bakr, 2021). A survey conducted by the American Hospital Association (AHA) revealed that 97% of hospitals currently employ some type of NAP (Spetz et al., 2008). Because a high percentage of institutions employ these personnel, many nurses believe they know how to work with and safely delegate tasks to them. However, this is not the case. Therefore, many nursing organizations, such as the American Association of Critical Care Nurses (AACN, 2010), the Society of Gastroenterology Nurses (SGNA, 2009), the Association of Rehabilitation Nurses (ARN, 1995, 2017), and the Association for Women's Health, Obstetrics and Neonatal Nurses (AWHONN, 2010), have developed definitions for NAP and criteria regarding their responsibilities. The ANA defines NAP as follows:

Unlicensed assistive personnel/Nursing assistive personnel are individuals who are trained to function in an assistive role to the registered nurse in the provision of patient/client care activities as delegated by and under the supervision of the registered professional nurse. Although some of these people may be certified (e.g., certified nursing assistant [CNA]), it is important to remember that certification differs from licensure. When a task is delegated to an unlicensed person, the professional nurse remains personally responsible for the outcomes of these activities (ANA, 2005).

As work on the unlicensed assistive personnel/nursing assistive personnel (UAP/NAP) issue is ongoing, the ANA updated its position statements in 2012 to define direct and indirect patient care activities that may be performed by UAP/NAP. Included in these updates are specific definitions regarding UAP/NAP and technicians and acceptable tasks (www.nursingworld.org). The ANA continuously updates information based on the changing health-care environment.

Use of the RN to provide all the care a client needs may not be the most efficient or cost-effective use of professional time. More hospitals are moving away from hiring LPNs and utilizing all RN staffing with UAP/NAP. In these facilities, the nursing focus is directed at diagnosing client care needs and carrying out complex interventions.

The ANA cautions against delegating nursing activities that include the foundation of the nursing process and that require specialized knowledge, judgment, or skill (ANA, 1996, 2002, 2005, 2012b). Non-nursing functions, such as performing clerical or receptionist duties, taking trips or doing errands off the unit, cleaning floors, making beds, collecting trays, and ordering supplies, should not be carried out by the highest-paid and most educated member of the team. These tasks are easily delegated to other personnel.

Safe Delegation

In 1990, the NCSBN adopted a definition of *delegation,* stating that delegation is "transferring to a competent individual the authority to perform a selected nursing task in a selected situation" (p. 1). In its publication *Issues* (1995), the NCSBN again presented this definition. Likewise, the ANA Code of Ethics for Nurses (1985) stated, "The nurse exercises informed judgment and uses individual competence and qualifications as criteria in seeking consultation, accepting responsibilities, and delegating nursing activities to others" (p. 1). In 2005, the ANA defined *delegation* as "the transfer of responsibility for the performance of an activity from one individual to another while retaining accountability for the outcome" (p. 4). To delegate tasks safely, nurses must delegate appropriately and supervise adequately (Agency for Healthcare Research and Quality [AHRQ], 2015; Barrow & Sharma, 2021).

In 1997, the NCSBN developed a Delegation Decision-Making Grid (NCSBN, 1997), a tool

---

box 6-2

Seven Components of the Delegation Decision-Making Grid

1. Level of client acuity
2. Level of unlicensed assistive personnel capability
3. Level of licensed nurse capability
4. Possibility for injury
5. Number of times the skill has been performed by the unlicensed assistive personnel
6. Level of decision making needed for the activity
7. Client's ability for self-care

Source: Adapted from the National Council of State Boards of Nursing. (1997). Delegation Decision-Making Grid. National State Boards of Nursing, Inc., 1997 (ncsbn.org).

---

to help nurses delegate appropriately. It provides a scoring instrument for seven categories that the nurse should consider when making delegation decisions. The categories for the grid are listed in Box 6-2.

Scoring the components helps the nurse evaluate the situations, the client needs, and the health-care personnel available to meet the needs. A low score on the grid indicates that the activity may be safely delegated to personnel other than the RN, and a high score indicates that delegation may not be advisable. Figure 6.1 shows the Delegation Decision-Making Grid. The grid is also available on the NCSBN Web site at www.ncsbn.com.

Nurses who delegate tasks to UAP/NAP should evaluate the activities being considered for delegation (Barrow & Sharma, 2021; Hawthorne-Spears & Whitlock, 2016; Keeney et al., 2005; McMullen et al., 2015). The AACN (1990, 2010) recommended considering five factors, which are listed in Box 6-3, in making a decision to delegate.

It is the responsibility of the RN to be well acquainted with the state's nurse practice act and regulations issued by the state board of nursing regarding UAP/NAP (ANA, 2005, 2012b; Hawthorne-Spears& Whitlock 2016; McMullen et al., 2015). State laws and regulations supersede any publications or opinions set forth by professional organizations. As stated earlier, the NCSBN (2016) provides criteria to assist nurses with delegation.

LPNs are trained to perform specific tasks, such as basic medication administration, dressing changes, and personal hygiene tasks. In some states, the LPN, with additional training, may start and monitor intravenous (IV) infusions and administer certain medications.

Elements for Review		Client A	Client B	Client C	Client D
Activity/Task	Describe activity/task:				
Level of Client Stability	Score the client's level of stability: 0. Client condition is chronic/stable/predictable. 1. Client condition has minimal potential for change. 2. Client condition has moderate potential for change. 3. Client condition is unstable/acute/strong potential for change.				
Level of NAP Competence	Score the NAP competence in completing delegated nursing care activities in the defined client population: 0. NAP–expert in activities to be delegated, in defined population 1. NAP–experienced in activities to be delegated, in defined population 2. NAP–experienced in activities, but not in defined population 3. NAP–novice in performing activities and in defined population				
Level of Licensed Nurse Competence	Score the licensed nurse's competence in relation to both knowledge of providing nursing care to a defined population and competence in implementation of the delegation process: 0. Expert in the knowledge of nursing needs/activities of defined client population and expert in the delegation process 1. Either expert in knowledge of needs/activities of defined client population and competent in delegation or experienced in the needs/activities of defined client population and expert in the delegation process 2. Experienced in the knowledge of needs/activities of defined client population and competent in the delegation process 3. Either experienced in the knowledge of needs/activities of defined client population or competent in the delegation process 4. Novice in knowledge of defined population and novice in delegation				
Potential for Harm	Score the potential level of risk the nursing care activity has for the client (risk is probability of suffering harm): 0. None 1. Low 2. Medium 3. High				
Frequency	Score based on how often the NAP has performed the specific nursing care activity: 0. Performed at least daily 1. Performed at least weekly 2. Performed at least monthly 3. Performed less than monthly 4. Never performed				
Level of Decision Making	Score the decision making needed, related to the specific nursing care activity, client (both cognitive and physical status), and client situation: 0. Does not require decision making 1. Minimal level of decision making 2. Moderate level of decision making 3. High level of decision making				
Ability for Self-Care	Score the client's level of assistance needed for self-care activities: 0. No assistance 1. Limited assistance 2. Extensive assistance 3. Total care or constant attendance				
	Total Score				

Figure 6.1 Delegation Decision-Making Grid.

The Factors for Determining if Client Care Should Be Delegated

1. What is the complexity of the client's care needs?
2. How stable is the client's condition?
3. How complex is the client assessment and evaluation of care outcomes?
4. Do infection control procedures exceed those of universal precautions?
5. Will the care provider need special individualized safety precautions?
6. Is special technology involved in the care, and which personnel have the necessary skills to use the technology?

Criteria for Delegation

The purpose of delegation is not to assign tasks to others that you do not want to do yourself. When you delegate to others effectively, the result is you have more time to perform the tasks that only a professional nurse is permitted to do.

In delegating, the nurse must consider both the *ability* of the person to whom the task is delegated and the *fairness* of the task to the individual and the team (Weiss & Tappen, 2015; Weiss et al., 2019). In other words, both the *task aspects* of delegation (Is this a complex task? Is it a professional responsibility? Can this person do it safely?) and the *interpersonal aspects* (Does the person have time to do this? Is the work evenly distributed?) must be considered.

The ANA (2005) has specified tasks that RNs may not delegate because they are specific to the discipline of professional nursing. These activities include initial nursing and follow-up assessments if nursing judgment is indicated (NCSBN, 2016; Zimmerman & Schultz, 2013):

■ Decisions and judgments about client outcomes
■ Determination and approval of a client plan of care
■ Interventions that require professional nursing knowledge, decisions, or skills
■ Decisions and judgments necessary for the evaluation of client care

Task-Related Concerns

The primary task-related concern in delegating work is whether the person assigned to do the task has the ability to complete it. Team priorities and efficiency are also important considerations.

Abilities

To make appropriate assignments, the nurse needs to know the knowledge and skill level, legal definitions, role expectations, and job description for each member of the team. It is equally important to be aware of the different skill levels of caregivers within each discipline because ability differs with each level of education. Additionally, individuals within each level of skill possess their own strengths and weaknesses. Prior assessment of the strengths of each member of the team will assist in providing safe and efficient care to clients. Figure 6.2 outlines the skills of various health-care personnel.

People should not be assigned a task that they do not have the skills or knowledge to perform, regardless of their professional level. Individuals are often reluctant to admit they lack the ability to do something. Instead of seeking help or saying they are not comfortable with a task, they may avoid doing it, delay starting it, do only part of it, or even bluff their way through it, which is a risky choice in health care.

Regardless of the length of time individuals have been in a position, employees need orientation when assigned a new task. Those who seek assistance and advice are showing concern for the team and the welfare of their clients. Requests for assistance or additional explanations should not be ignored, and the person should be praised, not criticized, for seeking guidance (Weiss & Tappen, 2015).

Priorities

The work of a busy unit rarely ends up going as expected. Dealing with sick people, as well as their families, physicians, and other team members, all at the same time, is a difficult task. Setting priorities for the day should be based on client needs, team needs, and organizational and community demands. The values of each may be very different, or even opposed. These differences should be discussed with team members so that decisions can be made based on team priorities.

One way to determine patient priorities is to base decisions on Maslow's hierarchy of needs. Maslow's hierarchy is frequently used in nursing to provide a framework for prioritizing care to meet client needs. The basic physiological needs come first because they are necessary for survival. For example, oxygen and medication administration, IV fluids, and enteral feedings are included in this group.

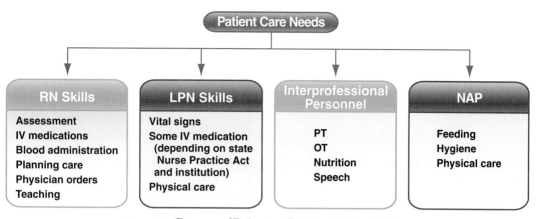

Figure 6.2 Diagram of Delegation Decision-Making Grid.

Identifying priorities and deciding the needs to be met first help in organizing care and in deciding which other team members can meet client needs. For example, nursing assistants can meet many hygiene needs, allowing licensed personnel to administer medications and enteral feedings in a timely manner.

Efficiency

In an efficient work environment, all members of the team know their jobs and responsibilities and work together, similar to gears in a well-built clock. They mesh together and keep perfect time.

The current health-care delivery environment demands efficient, cost-effective care. Delegating appropriately can increase efficiency and save money. Likewise, incorrect delegation can decrease efficiency and cost money. When delegating tasks to individuals who cannot perform the job, the RN must often go back to perform the task.

Although institutions often need to "float" staff to other units, maintaining continuity, if at all possible, is important. Keeping the same staff members on the unit all the time, for example, allows them to develop familiarity with the physical setting and routines of the unit as well as the types of clients the unit services. Time is lost when staff members are reassigned frequently to different units. Although physical layouts may be the same, client needs, unit routines, use of space, and availability of supplies are often different. Time spent to orient reassigned staff members takes time away from delivery of client care. However, when staff members are reassigned, it is important for them to indicate their skill level and comfort in the new setting, as lack of understanding and skill sets impacts patient

safety (AHRQ, 2015). It is just as important for the staff members who are familiar with the setting to identify the strengths of the reassigned person and build on them.

Appropriateness

Appropriateness is another task-related concern. Nothing can be more counterproductive than, for example, floating a coronary care nurse to labor and delivery. More time will be spent teaching the necessary skills than providing safe and effective mother–baby care. Assigning an educated, licensed staff member to perform non-nursing functions to protect safety is also a poor use of personnel.

Relationship-Oriented Concerns

Relationship-oriented concerns include fairness, learning opportunities, health concerns, compatibility, and staff preferences.

Fairness

Fairness requires the workload to be distributed evenly in terms of both the physical requirements and the emotional investment in providing health care. The nurse who is caring for a dying client may have less physical work to do than another team member, but in terms of emotional care to the client and family, that particular nurse may be doing double the work of another staff member.

Fairness also means considering equally all requests for special consideration. The quickest way to alienate members of a team is to be unfair. It is important to discuss with team members any decisions that have been made that may appear unfair to any one of them. Allow the team members to participate in making decisions regarding assignments. Their participation will decrease resentment and increase cooperation. In some health-care institutions, team members make such decisions as a group.

Learning Opportunities

When delegating, the RN needs to consider including assignments that stimulate motivation, learning, and assisting team members to learn new tasks and take on new challenges. A good leader considers helping their team reach their potential. Providing learning opportunities promotes personal development with each team member.

Health Concerns

Some aspects of caregiving jobs are more stressful than others. Rotating team members through the more difficult jobs may decrease stress and allow empathy to increase among the members. Promoting self-care also helps decrease stress and burnout within team members. Special health needs, such as family emergencies or special physical problems of team members, also need to be addressed. If some team members have difficulty accepting the needs of others, the situation should be discussed with the team, bearing in mind the employee's right to privacy when discussing sensitive issues.

Compatibility

No matter how hard nurses may strive to get their team to work together, the individual members may not connect and engage well with each other. Some people work together better than others. Helping people develop better working relationships is part of team building (*TeamSTEPPS*, 2013). Creating opportunities for people to share and learn from each other increases the overall effectiveness of the team.

As the leader, you may be forced to intervene in team member disputes. Many individuals find it difficult to work with others they do not like personally. It sometimes becomes necessary to explain that liking another person is a plus but not a necessity in the work setting and that personal problems have no place in the work environment. For example:

Indigo had been a labor and delivery room supervisor in a large metropolitan hospital for 5 years before she moved to another city. Because a position similar to the one she left was not available, she became a staff nurse at a small local hospital that recently opened its new birthing center. The center included a midwifery birth option. Although Indigo was accustomed to collaborating with midwives, the other nurses on the unit were unfamiliar with this care model. The first day on the job went well, and the other staff members seemed cordial. As the weeks went by, however, Indigo began to have problems getting other staff to help her. No one would offer to relieve her for meals or a break. She noticed that certain groups of staff members always went to lunch together but that she was never invited to join them. She attempted to speak to some of the more approachable coworkers, but she did not get much information. Disturbed by the situation, Indigo went to the nurse manager. The nurse manager listened quietly while Indigo related her experiences. She then asked Indigo to think about the last staff meeting. Indigo realized that she had alienated the staff during the meeting because she had said repeatedly that in "her hospital" things were done in a particular way and voiced criticism of the nurses' behaviors with the midwives. Indigo also realized that instead of asking for help, she was in the habit of demanding it and the nurses resented her "expert" advice on midwifery care. Indigo and the nurse manager discussed the difficulties of her changing positions, moving to a new place, and trying to develop both professional and social ties. Together, they came up with several solutions to Indigo's problem including using Indigo as a resource for the staff on the midwifery care model.

Cultural Considerations

The United States, along with many Western countries, has become more culturally diverse over the last century. Many individuals view this as a challenge as the culturally diverse workforce transforms the workplace. Nurses find themselves within an environment where they confront individuals who are in their most vulnerable positions. They also work in environments with other nurses, professionals, and support staff from cultures that differ from their own culture of origin. For this reason, nurses need to develop a sense of cultural awareness that leads to a better understanding and respect of differences (Greene-Moton & Minkler, 2020).

Staff Preferences

The nursing care environment today differs considerably from the past. Just as patients come from diverse backgrounds, so do members of the nursing profession and support staff (McDaniel, 2021). Considering the preferences of individual team members is important but should not supersede other criteria for delegating responsibly. Allowing team members to always select what they want to do may cause the less assertive members' needs to be unmet. However, if a team member expresses deep moral or ethical concerns regarding the ability to care for a specific patient, this needs to be taken under consideration.

It is important to explain the rationale for decisions made regarding delegation so that all team members may understand the needs of the unit or organization. Box 6-4 outlines basic rights for professional health-care team members. Although written originally for women, the concepts are applicable to all professional health-care providers.

Barriers to Delegation

Many nurses, particularly new ones, have difficulty delegating. The reasons for this include experience issues, licensure issues, legal issues, and quality-of-care issues.

Experience Issues

Many nurses working today graduated during the 1980s, when primary care was the major delivery system. These nurses lacked the education and skill needed for delegation. Nurses educated in the 1970s and before worked in settings with LPNs and nursing assistants, where they routinely delegated tasks. However, client acuity was lower and the care less complex. More expert nurses have considerable delegation experience and can be a resource for younger nurses. New nurses should not be afraid to ask for assistance and guidance in this area.

The added responsibility of delegation creates some discomfort for nurses (Kendall, 2018). Many believe they are unprepared to assume this responsibility, especially in deciding the competency of another person. To decrease this discomfort, nurses need to participate in establishing guidelines for NAP within their institution. The ANA Position Statements on NAP/UAP address this. Table 6-1 lists the direct and indirect client care activities that may be performed by NAP.

Licensure Issues

Although the current health-care environment requires nurses to delegate, many nurses voice concerns about the personal risk regarding their licensure if they delegate inappropriately. The courts have usually ruled that nurses are not liable for the negligence of other individuals, provided that the nurse delegated appropriately. Delegation is within the scope of nursing practice. The art and skill of delegation are acquired with practice.

Legal Issues

State nurse practice acts establish the legal boundaries for nursing practice. Professional nursing organizations define practice standards, and the

---

box 6-4

Basic Entitlements of Nurses in the Workplace

Professionals in the workplace are entitled to:
- Respect from other members of the interprofessional health-care team
- A work assignment that matches skills and education and does not exceed that of other members with the same education and skills set
- Wages commensurate with the job
- Autonomy in setting work priorities
- Ability to speak out for self and others
- A healthy work environment
- Accountability for one's own behaviors
- Act in the best interest of the client
- Be human

Source: Adapted from ANA Resolutions: Workplace Abuse. (2006). American Nurses Association (ANA). Updated in 2015.

---

table 6-1

Direct and Indirect Client Care Activities

Direct Client Care Activities	Indirect Client Care Activities
Assisting with feeding and drinking	Providing a clean environment
Assisting with ambulation	Providing a safe environment
Assisting with grooming	Providing companion care
Assisting with toileting	Providing transportation for noncritical clients
Assisting with dressing	Assisting with stocking nursing units
Assisting with socializing	Providing messenger and delivery services

Source: Adapted from American Nurses Association. (2002). Position statement on utilization of unlicensed assistive personnel/nursing assistive personnel. Author.

policies of the health-care institution create job descriptions and establish policies that guide appropriate delegation decisions for the organization.

Inherent in today's health-care environment is the safety of the client (AHRQ, 2021; Kalisch, 2011; Wagner, 2018). The quality of client care and the delivery of safe and effective care are central to the concept of delegation. RNs are held accountable when delegating care activities to others (Kendall, 2018). This means that they have an obligation to intervene whenever they deem the care provided is unsafe or unethical. It is also important to realize that a delegated task may not be "subdelegated." In other words, if the RN delegated a task to the LPN, the LPN cannot then delegate the task to the NAP, even if the LPN has decided that it is within the abilities of that particular NAP. There may be legal implications if a client is injured because of inappropriate delegation (AHRQ, 2015, 2021; Miller, 2018). Consider the following case:

> In *Hicks v. New York State Department of Health,* a nurse was found guilty of patient neglect because of her failure to appropriately train and supervise the UAP working under her. In this particular situation, a security guard discovered an elderly nursing home client in a totally dark room, undressed and covered with urine and fecal material. The client was partially in his bed and partially restrained in an overturned wheelchair. The court found the nurse guilty of the following: The nurse failed to assess whether the UAP had delivered proper care to the client, and this subsequently led to the inadequate delivery of care (1991).

Quality-of-Care Issues

Nurses have expressed concern regarding the quality of patient care when tasks and activities are delegated to others. Activities typically delegated include turning, ambulating, personal care, and blood glucose monitoring. When these care activities are missed, either delayed or omitted, the probability of untoward and costly outcomes increases (Kalisch, 2011; Kalisch et al., 2009). Failure to carry out these delegated activities appropriately also affects patient safety (IOM, 2001, 2010). Remember Nightingale's words earlier in the chapter, "Don't imagine that if you, who are in charge, don't look to all these things yourself, those under you will be more careful than you are." She added that you do not need to do everything yourself to see that it is done correctly. When you delegate, you control the delegation. You decide to whom you will delegate the task.

Assigning Work to Others

Assigning work can be difficult for several reasons:

1. Some nurses think they must do everything themselves.
2. Some nurses distrust subordinates to do things correctly.
3. Some nurses think that if they delegate all the technical tasks, they will not reinforce their own learning.
4. Some nurses are more comfortable with the technical aspects of patient care than with the more complex issues of patient teaching and discharge planning.

Families and clients do not always see professional activities. Rather, they see direct patient care (Keeney et al., 2005). Nurses believe that when they do not participate directly in client care, they do not accomplish anything for the client. The professional aspects of nursing, such as planning care, teaching, and discharge planning, help to promote positive outcomes for clients and their families. When working with LPNs, knowing their scope of practice helps in making delegation decisions.

Prioritization

Nurses need to know how to effectively prioritize care for their patients. Prioritizing requires making a decision regarding the importance of choosing a specific action or activity from several options (AHRQ, 2015; LaCharity et al., 2022). Sometimes nurses base these choices on personal values; other times, nurses make decisions based on imperatives (Lake et al., 2009). *Prioritization* is defined as "deciding which needs or problems require immediate action and which ones could be delayed until a later time because they are not urgent" (Silvestri, 2008, p. 68; Silvestri & Silvestri, 2020, p. 63). Although it is important to know what to do first, it is just as imperative to understand the result of delaying an action. If postponing the activity may result in an unfavorable outcome, then this activity assumes a level of priority. Within the clinical setting, this process encompasses the ability to visualize the possible client outcomes and foresee potential problems if one task is performed before another (LaCharity et al., 2022).

Nurses focus care based on the intended outcome of the care or intervention. Alfaro- Lefevre (2011, 2017) provides three levels of priority setting:

■ Use the ABCs plus V and L (airway, breathing, circulation, vital signs, and laboratory values). These are the most critical.
■ Address mental status, pain, untreated medical issues, and abnormal laboratory results.
■ Consider long-term health (chronic) problems, health education, rest, and coping (p. 171).

Nurses need to evaluate and assess the situation or need for completion of each task. Certain skills, such as assessment, planning, and evaluating nursing care, always remain within the purview of the RN. Understanding the process for evaluating and setting patient care priorities is essential when coordinating assignments and delegating care to others.

Coordinating Assignments

One of the most difficult tasks for new nurses to master is coordinating daily activities. Often, you have clients for whom you provide direct care while at the same time you must supervise the work of others, such as non-nurse caregivers (NAPs), LPNs, or licensed vocational nurses (LVNs). Although critical (or clinical) pathways, concept maps, and computer information sheets are available to help identify patient needs, these items do not provide a mechanism for coordinating the delivery of care. Developing a personalized worksheet helps prioritize tasks to perform for each patient. Using the worksheets assists the nurse to identify tasks that require the knowledge and skill of an RN and those that can be carried out by NAP.

On the worksheet, tasks are prioritized on the basis of patient need, not nursing convenience. For example, an order states that a patient receives continuous tube feedings. Although it may be convenient for the nurse to fill the feeding container with enough supplement to last 6 hours, it is not the standard practice and may be unsafe for the patient. Instead, the nurse should plan to check the tube feeding every 2 hours.

As for Elliot at the beginning of the chapter, a worksheet will help him determine how to delegate.

First, he needs to decide which patients require the skill sets of an RN. These include receiving and transcribing orders; contacting physicians with information or requests; accessing laboratory reports from the computer, reviewing them, deciding on an action, and giving them to the appropriate staff members; and checking any new medication orders and placing them in the medication administration records. Another RN may be able to relieve the monitor technician for dinner and breaks, and a second RN may be able to assign staff to dinner and breaks. Next, Elliot needs to look at individual patient requirements on the unit and prioritize them. He is now ready to effectively delegate to his staff.

Some activities must be done at a certain time, and their timing may be out of the nurse's control. Examples include medication administration and patients who need special preparation for a scheduled procedure. The following are some tips for organizing work on personalized worksheets to help establish client priorities (Weiss & Tappen, 2015; Weiss et al., 2019):

■ Plan your time around activities that need to occur at a specific time.
■ Do high-priority activities first.
■ Determine which activities are best done in a cluster.
■ Remember that you are responsible for activities delegated to others.
■ Consider your peak energy time when scheduling optional activities.

This list acts as a guideline for coordinating client care. The nurse needs to use critical thinking skills in the decision-making process. Remember that this is one of the ANA nurse-related principlesof delegation (ANA, 2005). For example, activities that are usually clustered include bathing, changing linen, and parts of the physical assessment. Some patients may not be able to tolerate too much activity at one time. Take special situations into consideration when coordinating patient care and deciding who should carry out some of the activities. Remember, however, that even when you delegate, you remain accountable.

Models of Care Delivery

All health-care institutions focus on the intention of delivering safe and effective care while maintaining costs and improving patient and family satisfaction outcomes (Parreira et al., 2021). In order to achieve these goals, organizations implement care delivery methods to achieve them. However, the chosen model needs to fit the organization's vision and mission while considering the availability of human and material resources.

Care delivery models infer how the work is designed, planned, and distributed to nursing and support staff (Parreira et al., 2021). According to Parreria et al., "These models define the way nurses organize and distribute work with the purpose of providing efficient care in an environment where safety issues are a major concern." (p. 2). Management theories through the last two centuries exerted tremendous influence on how health-care organizations select care model delivery systems to meet identified patient/client needs. Functional nursing, team nursing, total client care, and primary nursing are models of care delivery that developed in an attempt to balance the needs of the client with the availability and skills of nurses (DuBois et al., 2013; Parreria et al., 2021). Regardless of the method of assignment or care delivery system, the majority of nursing care is delivered within a group practice model where coordination and continuity of care depend on sharing common practice values and establishing communication (Anthony & Vidal, 2010; Parreria et al., 2021). Nurses need to develop strong delegation and communication skills to successfully follow through with any given model of care delivery. Colleagues and other team members may not always belong to the nurse's culture or country of origin. In today's multicultural environment, nurses also need to develop a cultural awareness of the ethics and values of members of other cultures and subcultures. Without that sensitivity and awareness, conflicts and miscommunication may impact patient safety and inhibit achieving effective outcomes.

Functional Nursing

Functional nursing or task nursing evolved during the mid-1940s because of the loss of RNs who left home to serve in the armed forces during World War II. Before the war, RNs comprised the majority of hospital staffing. Because of the lack of nurses to provide care at home, hospitals used more LPNs or LVNs and NAPs to care for clients.

When implementing functional nursing, the focus is on the task and not necessarily holistic client care. The needs of the clients are categorized by task, and then the tasks are assigned to the "best person for the job." This method takes into consideration the skill set and licensure scope of practice of each caregiver. For example, the RN would perform and document all assessments and administer all IV medications; the LPN or LVN would administer treatments and perform dressing changes. NAP would be responsible for meeting the hygiene needs of clients, obtaining and recording vital signs, and assisting in feeding clients. This method is efficient and effective; however, when implemented, continuity in client care is lost. Many times, reevaluation of client status and follow-up does not occur, and a breakdown in communication among staff occurs (DuBois et al., 2013; Parreria et al, 2021).

Team Nursing

Team nursing grew out of functional nursing. Nursing units often resort to this model when appropriate staffing is unavailable. A group of nursing personnel or a team provides care for a cluster of clients. The manner in which clients are divided varies and depends on several issues: the layout of the unit, the types of clients on the unit, and the number of clients on the unit. The organization of the team is based on the number of available staff and the skill mix within the group (Fernandez et al., 2012). During the pandemic, with a shortage of staff during the time many nurses contracted COVID-19, acute care units found themselves needing to make changes. The shift from the "natural" delivery system existing within the organization to the team method caused an added stress on many staff, particularly those unfamiliar with the method.

In the team approach, an RN assumes the role of the team leader. The team may consist of another RN, an LPN, and NAPs. As fewer LPNs are used within the acute care settings today, a team may consist of one RN and two NAPs. The team leader directs and supervises the team, which provides client care. The team knows the condition and needs of all the clients on the team.

The team leader acts as a liaison between the clients and the health-care provider or physician. Responsibilities include formulating a client plan of care, communicating orders and treatment changes to team members, and solving problems of clients or team members. The nurse manager confers with the team leaders, supervises the client care teams, and, in some institutions, conducts rounds with the health-care providers.

For this method to be effective, the team leader needs strong delegation and communication skills. Communication among team members and the nurse manager avoids duplication of efforts and decreases competition for control of assignments that may not be equal based on client acuity and the skill sets of team members.

Total Patient Care

During the 1920s, total patient care was the original model of nursing care delivery. Much nursing was in the form of private-duty nursing. In this model, nurses cared for patients in homes and in hospitals (Fernandez et al., 2012). Hospital schools of nursing provided students who staffed the nursing units and delivered care under the watchful eyes of nursing supervisors and directors. In this method, one nurse assumes full responsibility for delivering care to a small group of patients (Parreria et al., 2021). This includes acting as a direct liaison among the patient, family, health-care provider, and other members of the health-care team. Today, this model is seen in high-acuity areas such as critical care units; postanesthesia recovery units; and labor, delivery, and recovery (LDR) units. At times, this model requires RNs to engage in non-nursing tasks that might be assumed by NAP.

Primary Nursing

In the 1960s, nursing care delivery models started to move away from team nursing and placed the RN in the role of giving direct patient care. The central principle of this model distributes nursing decision making to the nurses who care for the client. Central to this model are the tenets of relationship building and rapport (Payne & Steakley, 2015; Parreria et al., 2021). As the primary nurse, the RN devises, implements, and maintains responsibility for the nursing care of the patient during the time the patient remains on the nursing unit. The primary nurse, along with associate nurses, gives direct care to the client.

In its ideal form, primary nursing requires an all-RN staff. Although this model provides continuity of care and nursing accountability, staffing is difficult and expensive, especially in today's health-care environment. Some view it as ineffective as other personnel could carry out many tasks that consume the time of the RN. However, many institutions use a dyad form of primary nursing comprised of an RN and an NAP. This model promotes the application of the nursing process and the ability to make decisions based on meeting patient care needs in a holistic manner (Parreria et al., 2021).

Conclusion

The concept of delegation is not new. In today's health-care environment with the need for cost containment, using full RN staffing is unrealistic. Knowing the principles of delegation remains an essential skill for RNs. Personal organizational skills and the ability to prioritize patient care are prerequisites to delegation. Before nurses can delegate tasks to others, they need to identify individual patient needs. Using worksheets, the ABC plus V and L method, and Maslow's hierarchy helps the nurse understand these individual patient needs, set priorities, and identify which tasks can be delegated to others. Using the Delegation Decision-Making Grid helps the nurse delegate safely and appropriately.

Nurses need to be aware of the capabilities of each staff member, show sensitivity to the cultural backgrounds and needs of the staff member, consider the tasks that may be delegated, and identify the tasks that the RN needs to perform. When delegating, the RN uses critical thinking and professional judgment in making decisions. Professional judgment is directed by state nurse practice acts, evidence-based practice, and approved national nursing standards. Institutions develop their own job descriptions for NAP and other health-care professionals, but institutional policies must remain compliant with state nurse practice acts. Although nurses delegate the task or activity, they remain accountable for the delegated decision.

Understanding the concept of delegation helps the new nurse organize and prioritize client care. Knowing the staff and their capabilities simplifies delegation. Utilizing staff members' capabilities creates a pleasant and productive working environment for everyone involved.

Study Questions

1. What are the responsibilities of the professional nurse when delegating tasks to an LPN, LVN, or NAP?

2. What factors need to be considered when delegating tasks?

3. What is the difference between delegation and assignment?

4. What are the nurse manager's legal responsibilities in supervising NAP?

5. Review the scenario on page 90. If you were the nurse manager, how would you have handled Indigo's situation?

6. Define the terms *cultural humility, cultural awareness,* and *cultural sensitivity.* How do these impact delegation?

7. Bring the patient diagnosis census from your assigned clinical unit to class. Using the Delegation Decision-Making Grid, decide which patients you would assign to the personnel on the unit. Give reasons for your decision.

8. What type of nursing delivery model is implemented on your assigned clinical unit? Give examples of the roles of the personnel engaged in client care to support your answer.

Case Study to Promote Clinical Judgment

Julio works at a large teaching hospital in a major metropolitan area. This institution services the entire geographical region, including indigenous people and migrant communities. In addition, because of its reputation, it administers care to international clients and individuals who reside in other states. Similar to all health-care institutions, this one has been attempting to cut costs by using more NAP. Nurses are often floated to other units. Lately, the number of indigenous and foreign clients on Julio's unit has increased. The acuity of these clients has been quite high, requiring a great deal of time from the nursing staff.

Julio arrived at work at 6:30 a.m., his usual time. He looked at the census board and discovered that the unit was filled, and bed control was calling all night to have clients discharged or transferred to make room for several clients who had been in the emergency department (ED) since the previous evening. He also discovered that the other RN assigned to his team called in sick. His team consists of himself and two NAPs, one of which is shared by two teams. He has eight patients on his team:

▪ Two need to be readied for surgery, including preoperative and postoperative teaching, one of whom is a 35-year-old Islamic woman scheduled for a modified radical mastectomy for the treatment of breast cancer.

▪ Three are second-day postoperative clients, two of whom require extensive dressing changes, are receiving IV antibiotics, and need to be ambulated.

▪ One postoperative client is required to remain on total bedrest, has a nasogastric tube to suction as well as a chest tube, is on total parenteral nutrition and lipids, needs a central venous catheter line dressing change, has an IV, is taking multiple IV medications, and has a Foley catheter.

▪ One client is ready for discharge and needs discharge instruction.

▪ One client needs to be transferred to a subacute unit, and a report must be given to the RN of that unit.

Once the latter client is transferred and the other one is discharged, the ED will be sending two clients to the unit for admission.

1. How should Julio organize his day? Set up an hourly schedule.

2. Make a priority list based on the ABC plus V and L method.

3. What type of client management approach should Julio consider in assigning staff appropriately?

4. If you were Julio, which clients or tasks would you assign to your staff? List all of them, and explain your rationale.

5. Using the Delegation Decision-Making Grid, make staff and client assignments.

NCLEX®-Style Review Questions

1. A nurse is helping an NAP provide a bed bath to a comatose patient who is incontinent. Which of the following actions requires the nurse to intervene?
   1. The nursing assistant answers the phone while wearing gloves.
   2. The nursing assistant log-rolls the client to provide back care.
   3. The nursing assistant places an incontinence diaper under the client.
   4. The nursing assistant positions the client on the left side, head elevated.

2. A nurse is caring for a patient who has a pulmonary embolus. The patient is receiving anticoagulation with IV heparin. What instructions should the nurse give the NAP who will help the patient with activities of daily living? **Select all that apply**.
   1. Use a lift sheet when moving and positioning the patient in bed.
   2. Use an electric razor when shaving the patient each day.
   3. Use a soft-bristled toothbrush or tooth sponge for oral care.
   4. Use a rectal thermometer to obtain a more accurate body temperature.
   5. Be sure the patient's footwear has a non-slip sole when the patient ambulates.

3. A nurse is caring for a patient who has chronic obstructive pulmonary disease (COPD) and is 2 days postoperative after a laparoscopic cholecystectomy. Which intervention for airway management should the nurse delegate to an NAP?
   1. Assisting the patient to sit up on the side of the bed
   2. Instructing the patient to cough effectively
   3. Teaching the patient to use incentive spirometry
   4. Auscultating breath sounds every 4 hours

4. A nurse is caring for a patient who is diagnosed with coronary artery disease and sleep apnea. Which action should the nurse delegate to the NAP?
   1. Discuss weight-loss strategies such as diet and exercise with the patient.
   2. Teach the patient how to set up the CPAP machine before sleeping.
   3. Remind the patient to sleep on his side instead of his back.
   4. Administer modafinil (Provigil) to promote daytime wakefulness.

5. A nurse is assigned to care for the following patients. Which patient should the nurse assess first?
   1. A 60-year-old patient on a ventilator for whom a sterile sputum specimen must be sent to the laboratory
   2. A 55-year-old with COPD and a pulse oximetry reading from the previous shift of 90% saturation
   3. A 70-year-old with pneumonia who needs to be started on IV antibiotics
   4. A 50-year-old with asthma who complains of shortness of breath after using a bronchodilator

6. A respiratory therapist performs suctioning on a patient with a closed head injury who has a tracheostomy. Afterward, the NAP obtains vital signs. The nurse should communicate that the NAP needs to report which vital sign value or values immediately? **Select all that apply**.
   1. Heart rate of 96 beats/min
   2. Respiratory rate of 24 breaths/min
   3. Pulse oximetry of 95%
   4. Tympanic temperature of 101.4°F (38.6°C)

7. An experienced LPN is working under the supervision of the RN. The LPN is providing nursing care for a patient who has a respiratory problem. Which activities should the RN delegate to the experienced LPN? **Select all that apply**.
   1. Auscultate breath sounds.
   2. Administer medications via metered-dose inhaler (MDI).
   3. Complete an in-depth admission assessment.
   4. Initiate the nursing care plan.
   5. Evaluate the patient's technique for using MDIs.

8. An assistant nurse manager is making assignments for the next shift. Which patient should the assistant nurse manager assign to a nurse with 6 months of experience and who has been floated from the surgical unit to the medical unit?
   1. A 58-year-old on airborne precautions for tuberculosis (TB)
   2. A 68-year-old who just returned from bronchoscopy and biopsy
   3. A 69-year-old with COPD who is ventilator dependent
   4. A 72-year-old who needs teaching about the use of incentive spirometry

9. The nursing assistant tells a nurse that a patient who is receiving oxygen at a flow rate of 6 L/min by nasal cannula is complaining of nasal passage discomfort. What intervention should the nurse suggest to improve the patient's comfort for this problem?
   1. Suggest that the patient's oxygen be humidified.
   2. Suggest that a simple face mask be used instead of a nasal cannula.
   3. Suggest that the patient be provided with an extra pillow.
   4. Suggest that the patient sit up in a chair at the bedside.

10. The patient with COPD has a nursing diagnosis of ineffective breathing pattern. Which is an appropriate action to delegate to the experienced LPN under your supervision?
    1. Observe how well the patient performs pursed-lip breathing.
    2. Plan a nursing care regimen that gradually increases activity intolerance.
    3. Assist the patient with basic activities of daily living.
    4. Consult with the physical therapy department about reconditioning exercises.

chapter 7

Communicating With Others and Working With the Interprofessional Team

Claude has been working in a busy oncology center for several years. The center uses an interprofessional team approach to client care. Claude manages a caseload of six to eight clients daily, and he believes that he provides safe, competent care and collaborates with other members of the interprofessional team. While Claude was on his way to deliver chemotherapy to a client, the team nutritionist, Sonja, called to him, "Claude, come with me, please."

Claude responded, "Wait one minute. I need to hang the chemo on Mr. Juniper. I will come right after that. Where will you be?"

Sonja responded, "I need you now. There have been changes in Mrs. Alejandro's home care and medication regimen. I am trying to discuss how she needs to change her diet because of the medication changes. I can't seem to explain this to her. She keeps telling me she needs to eat 'cold foods' because she has a 'hot stomach.' You seem to understand her better than I do." Claude stopped what he was doing and went to speak with Sonja and Mrs. Alejandro. While engaged in this conversation, the oncology nurse practitioner (advanced practice provider [APP]) reevaluated Mr. Juniper's laboratory values and physical condition and discontinued Mr. Juniper's chemotherapy order. The APP wrote the order and went on to evaluate other patients without communicating the change to Claude. After Claude finished with Sonja, he returned to Mr. Juniper and proceeded to administer the chemotherapy. That night Mr. Juniper was admitted to the hospital with uncontrollable bleeding and died.

Health-care professionals need to communicate clearly and effectively with each other. When they fail to do so, patient safety is at risk. In this case, the nurse practitioner failed to communicate a change in the patient's status, which resulted in a situation causing the patient's death.

Today's health-care system requires nurses to interact with more than physicians. Health-care providers include advanced practice nurses and physician assistants who work with physicians. Other disciplines involved in direct patient care include pharmacists, dietitians, social workers, physical and occupational therapists, speech-language pathologists, and ancillary unlicensed personnel. Effective communication among all members of the health-care team is essential in the provision of safe patient care. Based on the changes in health care, the report from the Institute of Medicine (IOM), and the move toward an interprofessional model of care delivery, this chapter focuses on communication skills needed to work with members of the interprofessional team and provide information in a multicultural environment.

Communication

People often assume that communication is simply giving information to another person with one person serving as a sender and another as a receiver (Wood, 2016). In fact, giving information is only a small part of communication. Communication models demonstrate that communication occurs on several levels and includes more than just giving information. Communication involves the spoken word as well as the nonverbal message, the emotional state of people involved, outside distractions, and the cultural background that affects their interpretation of the message. Superficial listening often results in misinterpretation of the message. An individual's attitude and personal experience may also influence what is heard and how the message is interpreted. Active listening is necessary if one is to grasp all the levels of meaning in a conversation.

Assertiveness in Communication

Nurses are integral members of the health-care team and often find themselves acting as "navigators" for patients as they guide them through the system. For this reason, nurses need to develop assertive communication skills. Assertive behaviors allow people to stand up for themselves and their rights without violating the rights of others. Assertiveness is different from aggressiveness. People use aggressive behaviors to force their wishes or ideas on others. Assertive communication, in contrast, requires an individual to firmly state a personal position using "I" statements. When working in an interprofessional environment, assertiveness assumes greater importance as nurses need to act as patient advocates to ensure that patients receive safe, effective, and appropriate care. Using assertive communication helps in expressing your ideas and position; however, it does not necessarily guarantee that you will get what you want.

Interpersonal Communication

Communication is an integral part of our daily lives. Most daily communication qualifies as impersonal, such as interactions with salespeople or service personnel. Interpersonal communication is a process that gives people the opportunity to reflect, construct personal knowledge, and develop a sense of collective knowledge about others. Individuals use this form of communication to establish relationships to promote their personal and professional growth. This type of communication remains key to working effectively with others.

Interpersonal communication differs from general communication in that it includes several criteria. First, it is a selective process in that most general communication occurs on a superficial level. Interpersonal communication, in contrast, occurs on a more intimate level. It is a systemic process as it occurs within various systems and among the members within those systems (Wood, 2016). The work of the system influences how we communicate, where we communicate, and the meaning of the communication.

Interpersonal communication is also unique in that the individuals engaged in the communication are unique. It is more than a linear interaction between someone sending a message and another individual receiving that message. Because each person holds a specific role that influences the form and process of the communication, they, in turn, impact the outcome. Finally, interpersonal communication is a dynamic and ongoing process. The communication changes based on the need and the situation.

Transactional models of communication differ from earlier linear models in that the transactional models label all individuals as communicators and not specifically as "senders" or "receivers." They highlight the dynamic process of interpersonal communication and the many roles individuals assume in these interactions. These models also allow for the fact that communication among and between individuals occurs simultaneously as the participants may be sending, receiving, and interpreting messages at the same time (Wood, 2016).

Transactional models acknowledge that noise, which interrupts communication, occurs in all interactions. Noise may assume many forms, such as background conversations within the workplace or even spam or instant messages in the electronic milieu. Transactional models also include the concept of time, as communication among and between individuals changes through time and acknowledges that communication occurs within systems. These systems influence what people communicate and how they relay and process information.

Barriers to Communication Among Health-Care Providers and Health-Care Recipients

Successful interactions among health-care providers and between those providers and their patients require effective communication. Breakdown in communication is attributed to 50% of preventable medical errors (Konsel, 2016). Challenges that impede this communication include low health literacy, cultural diversity, cultural humility of health-care providers, and a lack of interprofessional communication education of providers (Issacson, 2014; Schwartz et al., 2010). In addition, time constraints, patient symptoms, anxiety and embarrassment, and information overload can challenge both the patient's and provider's ability to comprehend the communication (Ali, 2017). Another hindrance to effective communication is implicit or unconscious bias on the part of a communicator (The Joint Commission [TJC], 2016).

Low Health Literacy

Low health literacy is defined as the degree to which an individual can obtain, process, and understand the basic information and services needed to make appropriate health decisions (Osborne, 2018). The IOM reports that approximately 90 million Americans lack the health literacy needed to meet their health-care needs (IOM, 2012). In the United States, the estimated cost of low health literacy is as high as $238 billion (Center for Health Care Strategies, 2013; National Patient Safety Foundation, 2012). Individuals who lack the skills necessary to acquire and use health-care information are less likely to manage their chronic conditions or medication regimens effectively. For this reason, they utilize health-care facilities more frequently and have higher mortality rates.

Cultural Diversity

Nurses work in environments rich in cultural diversity. This diversity exists among both professionals and patients. Culture affects communication in how the content of a message is conveyed, emphasized, and understood. Diverse cultural beliefs, customs, and practices influence both nurse and patient perception of care, as well as the ability for a patient to understand a personal illness and access the needed care (Department of Health and Human Services [HHS], Office of Minority Health, 2013). Understanding the impact that cultural diversity can have will allow you to communicate in an effective, understandable, and respectful way.

Cultural Competence and Humility

Cultural competence and humility affect the way health-care providers interact with each other and with the populations they service. Cultural competence includes a set of similar behaviors, attitudes, and policies that, when joined together, enable individuals or groups to work effectively in cross-cultural situations (HHS, Office of Minority Health, 2013). To practice with cultural competence, health-care professionals need to recognize and relate to how culture is reflected in each other and in the individuals with whom they interface. Cultural humility takes the concept of cultural competency one step further.

We live in a diverse and ethnically rich world, so how do you prepare yourself to care for patients of varying backgrounds during the course of your daily patient care assignment? How does one remain culturally competent when faced with the melting pot of socioeconomic, cultural, and ethnic beliefs that exist in our communities and at the bedside? Tervalon and Murray-Garcia (1998) suggest that cultural humility rather than cultural competence may be a better way to "skillfully and respectfully negotiate cultural, racial, and ethnic diversity in clinical practice" (p. 117). Competence is defined as being able to accomplish something in an efficient manner, whereas cultural humility is an approach that allows us to let go of our personal point of view so that we may consider another's beliefs without bias or stereotype (Issacson, 2014). This ability to accept and understand others creates space for inclusion. Seeing the similarities in cultures and traditions can break down social or systemic barriers that may have prevented the inclusion of groups. In other words, beginning a conversation with the patient to understand what is culturally important to them can remove barriers to effective communication and clinical care.

A nurse greets a young Black man who presents at a very busy inner city emergency department (ED) triage desk. He appears disheveled and angry as he asks for a particular dose of a specific pain medication. The nurse's initial thought is the man is exhibiting drug-seeking behavior; the nurse surmises that the patient is only here for medication and after quick triage tells him to have a seat in the waiting room. During the man's waiting time, he returns to the triage desk and demands to know when he will be seen by a physician. The nurse further decides that this man may be a threat and calls security to come to the waiting room. When the charge nurse hears the commotion, she speaks to the waiting patient and learns that he is from out of town on business and has a history of sickle cell anemia. He had been trying to manage the oncoming crisis and came to the ED for pain medication to tide him over until he could get home. The patient is quickly taken back to be seen by the ED physician. When following up with the triage nurse, the charge nurse learned that the nurse dismissed this patient as a drug addict because he was a young Black male in his 20s, disheveled, and angry. This assessment was based on the nurse's understanding of the community demographics and past experience rather than assessing the patient, reviewing his chief complaint, and exploring his past medical history.

Considerations when engaging a patient and colleagues in conversations concerning care should include (Tervalon & Murray-Garcia, 1998):

- Practice self-reflection to become more aware of your biases and cultural predisposition to remain open to others' points of view.
- Recognize, acknowledge, and respect others' cultural beliefs and practices.
- Acknowledge that many patients perceive that nurses and physicians have power over them.
- Ensure care and engagement with patients is patient focused to ensure that when we engage with a patient, we are in fact learning about one unique individual and that person's beliefs and practices, not a particular culture or ethnic group.

Interprofessional Communication Education of Health-Care Providers

Challenges exist when communicating with professionals in other disciplines. Some difficulties in interprofessional communication are related to the use of concepts and terminology, or jargon, common to one specific discipline but not well understood by

table 7-1	
Barriers to Effective Communication in Health Care	
Low health literacy	Lack of the skills needed to access and use health information
Cultural diversity	Impedes the ability to access, understand, and utilize services and information
Cultural competency of health-care providers	Lack of the ability of health-care providers to identify and consider cultural practices
Communication skills of health-care providers	Health-care providers lack the training needed for communicating with each other (interprofessional communication)

Source: Adapted from Schwartz, F., Lowe, M., & Sinclair, L. (2010). Communication in health care: Consideration and strategies for successful consumer and team dialogue. Hypothesis, 8(1), 1–8.

members of other professions. This interferes with another professional's understanding of the meaning or value of the situation.

Effective and safe health-care delivery requires nurses to be cognizant of these possible barriers to communication with patients and among members of the health-care team (Schwartz et al., 2010). When nurses and other members of the health-care team lack effective communication skills, patient safety is at risk. These barriers are outlined in Table 7-1.

Implicit Bias

Implicit bias refers to attitudes or stereotypes that affect our understanding, actions, and decisions in an unconscious manner (Staats et al., 2015). This bias is formed during a lifetime and contributes to our social behavior. People will make assumptions based on cultural beliefs and traditions as well as their values (Ali, 2017). Oftentimes, these biases are automatic during our interaction with other people and can influence our clinical decision making and even treatment (TJC, 2016). A person's ability to recognize these biases can improve communication with patients and colleagues alike.

Mr. Jones was waiting for the oncoming nurse, whose name was Remy. When Remy arrived, Mr. Jones was surprised to see that he had a male nurse. The unconscious bias here was that Mr. Jones assumed that his nurse would be a woman because only women are nurses and, in his mind, Remy is a girl's name.

Electronic Forms of Communication

Information Systems and E-Mail

Electronic Health Records and Electronic Medical Records

The use of computer technology and documenting in the electronic medical record (EMR) is the norm in today's nursing practice, hospital care institutions, and throughout health care. The Health Information Technology for Economic and Clinical Health (HITECH) Act mandated the use of the electronic health record (EHR) by the year 2015 (Centers for Medicare and Medicaid Services [CMS], 2013a). This organization developed Medicare and Medicaid incentive payment programs to help physicians and health-care institutions transition from traditional record-keeping to the EHR. According to the HHS, "EHR adoption has tripled since 2010, increasing to 44 percent in 2012 and computerized physician order entry has more than doubled (increased 168 percent) since 2008" (CMS, 2013c). In 2015, 84% of all hospitals had a basic form of EHR (Henry et al., 2016).

The goal of computerized record-keeping is to provide safe, quality care to patients. The use of electronic patient records allows health-care providers to retrieve and distribute patient information precisely and quickly. Decisions regarding patient care can be made more efficiently with less waiting time. Errors are reduced, patient safety is increased, and quality is improved. Two examples of improved safety measures are the use of barcode scanning for medication administration and labeling of laboratory samples. Information systems in many organizations also provide opportunities to access current, high-quality clinical and research data to support evidence-based practice (Gartee & Beal, 2012).

Although the terms *EMR* and *EHR* are used interchangeably, they differ in the types of information they contain. EMRs are the computerized clinical records produced in the health-care institution and health-care provider offices. They are considered legal documents regarding patient care within these settings.

The EHR includes summaries of the EMR. EHR documents are shared among varying institutions or individuals such as insurance companies, the government, and the patients themselves (CMS, 2013b). EHRs focus on the total health of a patient extending beyond the data collected in the health-care provider's office. They provide a more inclusive view of a patient's care and are designed to share information with other health-care providers, such as laboratories and specialists, so they contain information from *all the clinicians involved in the patient's care.*

The EMR contains the medical and treatment history of the patients within that specific health-care provider's practice. Some advantages of the EMR compared with paper charts include the ability of the health-care provider to:

- Track data through time.
- Identify which patients need preventive screenings or checkups.
- Monitor patients' status regarding health maintenance and prevention, such as blood pressure readings or vaccinations.
- Evaluate and improve the overall quality of care within the specific practice.

A disadvantage of the EMR is that it does not easily move *out* of the specific provider practice or health-care institution. Recent changes in technology are making the EMR accessible to affiliated health-care providers so that a hospital physician may be able to view a patient's past medical history and recent outpatient visits or test results. These exchanges offer providers access to important patient information drawn from a variety of places where that patient received care, not just within that person's network. This is extremely helpful when caring for patients with chronic conditions or frequent utilization of EDs for basic care. This electronic access to information, however, is not widespread; oftentimes, the patient record needs to be printed or saved to a disc, then delivered by mail to specialists and other members of the care team.

Because security safeguards and firewalls are in place, EHRs also assist in maintaining patient confidentiality when compared with traditional paper systems. Health-care providers and institutions have strict policies in place to enforce processes that protect patient information, which include the use of passwords to limit accessibility to the computerized record and procedures to ensure compliance with federal and state patient privacy and confidentiality standards. Although any breach in confidentiality is unacceptable, this is especially true when famous people, friends, and family are hospitalized. Attempting to access information about a patient not directly under your care in most instances is considered a breach of patient privacy

---

box 7-1

Potential Benefits of Computer-Based Patient Information Systems

- Increased hours for direct patient care
- Patient data accessible at bedside
- Improved accuracy and legibility of data
- Immediate availability of all data to all members of the team
- Increased safety related to positive patient identification, improved standardization, and improved quality
- Decreased medical errors
- Increased staff satisfaction

Source: Adapted from Arnold, J., & Pearson, G. (Eds.). (1992). Computer applications in nursing education and practice. National League for Nursing.

---

and confidentiality and could result in the loss of your job. It is important to remember to never share your password and always log off when stepping away from the computer. Fortunately, many organizations time out a user's access when a computer has been idle for as little as 5 minutes. This helps to protect you and prevent security breaches.

Additional benefits of computerized systems for health-care applications are listed in Box 7-1.

The Computer on Wheels

The advent of the EMR created an unforeseen challenge for nurses. Reinecke (2015) estimates that nurses spend approximately 35% of their shift documenting. Moving to the EMR meant nurses needed to use computers to do their real-time charting; however, computers were located at the nurses' stations away from patients. This in itself created a potential risk to patient safety. Oftentimes, the number of computers available was limited, sometimes making it difficult for nurses to document in a timely manner. Health care's solution to this was the computer on wheels (COW) or workstation on wheels (WOW). This mobile unit freed the nurse from waiting for a computer in the nurses' station and allowed for real-time documentation with the patient. A challenge with this type of technology at the bedside is that nurses can get overly focused on documenting rather than the patient. Things to consider when using a WOW or COW include:

- Make sure that the WOW or COW is either plugged in or that the battery is fully charged.
- Position the WOW or COW in such a way that it is not between you and the patient to ensure eye contact and the genuine nature of your interaction is conveyed to the patient.

■ Log off when leaving the COW or WOW to ensure the security, privacy, and confidentiality of your documentation, especially if the COW or WOW is parked in the hallway.

E-Mail

E-mail has become a communication standard. Organizations use e-mail to communicate both within (intranet) and outside (Internet) of their systems. The same communication principles that apply to traditional letter writing pertain to e-mail. Using e-mail competently and effectively requires good writing skills. Remember, when communicating by e-mail, you are not only making an impression but also leaving a written record (Shea, 2000).

The rules for using e-mail in the workplace are somewhat different than for using e-mail among friends. Much of the humor and wit found in personal e-mail is not appropriate for the work setting. In addition, emoticons are cute but not necessarily appropriate in the work setting.

Professional e-mail may remain informal. However, the message must be clear, concise, and courteous. Avoid common text abbreviations such as "LOL" or "OMG." Think about what you need to say before you write it. Then write it, read it, and reread it. Once you are satisfied that the message is appropriate, clear, and concise, send it.

Many executives read personal e-mail sent to them, which means that it is often possible to contact them directly. Many systems make it easy to send e-mail to everyone at the health-care institution. For this reason, it is important to keep e-mail professional. Remember the "chain of command": Always go through the proper channels.

The fact that you have the capability to send e-mail instantly to large groups of people does not necessarily make sending it a good idea. Be careful if you have access to an all-company mailing list. It is easy to unintentionally send e-mail throughout the system. Consider the following example:

A respiratory therapist and a department administrator at a large health-care institution were engaged in a relationship. They started sending each other personal notes through the company e-mail system. One day, one of them accidentally sent one of these notes to all the employees at the health-care institution. Both employees were terminated. The moral of this story is simple: Do not send anything by e-mail that you would not want published on the front page of a national newspaper or broadcasted on your favorite radio station.

Although voice tone cannot be "heard" in e-mail, the use of certain words and writing styles indicates emotion. A rude tone in an e-mail message may provoke extreme reactions. Follow the "rules of netiquette" (Shea, 2000) when communicating through e-mail. Some of these rules are listed in Box 7-2.

Text Messaging

Text messaging is slowly replacing the phone conversation. It is a pervasive, real-time way to connect with friends, acquaintances, and even coworkers while on the job. Shorthand abbreviations have replaced longer, more commonly used phrases, and although widely accepted as a preferred way of communicating, messages can be misinterpreted because of the absence of voiced emotion and body language.

Secure text messaging has been adopted by many hospitals and health systems. It is an easy way to communicate between the care team and oftentimes allows for more timely care interventions for patients. It is important to learn your organization's policies on the use of secure text messaging to avoid a possible communication breakdown. For example, many organizations support the use of text messaging between teams but prohibit the use of texts as a doctor's order. This means that you might have a text conversation with a patient's physician, at which time the decision to administer a new medication or order a test is made. The physician should then go to the patient's EMR and place the order in real time.

---

box 7-2

Rules of Netiquette

1. If you were face to face, would you say this?
2. Follow the same rules of behavior online that you follow when dealing with individuals personally.
3. Send information only to those individuals who need it.
4. Avoid flaming; that is, sending remarks intended to cause a negative reaction.
5. Do not write in all capital letters; this suggests anger.
6. Respect other people's privacy.
7. Do not abuse the power of your position.
8. Proofread your e-mail before sending it.

Source: Adapted from Shea, V. (2000). Netiquette. Albion.

Generally speaking, there are no laws about texting; however, many employers have policies and procedures that may limit personal cell phone use during work hours. Text messaging is device neutral, which means that texts can be sent to a personal or work-supplied cell phone. Text messages can stay on devices indefinitely, which may leave a patient's protected health information (PHI) unsecured and accessible to unauthorized users (Storck, 2017).

In an attempt to protect patient privacy and confidentiality, secure text messaging is being used in some health-care settings. This secure Health Insurance Portability and Accountability Act (HIPAA)-compliant electronic communication technology allows nurses and other providers to exchange patient information in a timely manner without risk to patient privacy and confidentiality. Usually this is done using appropriate security and password protection. Texting of confidential or patient information should never be done on a private cell phone.

Social Media

John was an experienced registered nurse (RN) who was assigned to take the next admission on his unit. Imagine John's surprise when he entered a room and found a famous movie star! All John could think about was, "Wow! Wait until my friends see this!" He then posted a picture on his Instagram. The next day, John's supervisor called him into the office and fired him for breaching his patient's confidentiality.

Social media is a mainstay in today's society. People post everything from their last meal, to selfies, to pictures of their experiences. Many of these entries are impromptu and lack a filter. Nurses and other health-care professionals are obligated to protect patient privacy and confidentiality at all times. This applies to social media posts as readily as it does the spoken word.

Knowing your state board requirements and national guidelines about patient privacy and media use will help you protect your patient's privacy and your license. The National Council of State Boards of Nursing (NCSBN, 2018) published guidelines on how to avoid disclosing confidential information (Appendix 3). The American Nurses Association (ANA, 2011) offers six tips to avoid breaches of privacy and confidentiality (Box 7-3).

---

box 7-3

Six Tips for Nurses Using Social Media

1. Remember that standards of professionalism are the same online as in any other circumstances.
2. Do not share or post information or photos gained through the nurse–patient relationship.
3. Maintain professional boundaries in the use of electronic media. Online contact with patients blurs boundaries.
4. Do not make disparaging remarks about patients, employers, or coworkers, even if they are not identified.
5. Do not take photos or videos of patients on personal devices, including cell phones.
6. Promptly report a breach of confidentiality or privacy.

Source: American Nurses Association. (2011). 6 tips for nurses using social media. nursebooks.org.

Reporting Patient Information

In today's health-care system, delivery methods involve multiple encounters and patient hand-offs among numerous health-care practitioners who have various levels of education and occupational training. Patient information needs to be communicated effectively and efficiently to ensure that critical information is relayed to each professional responsible for care delivery (O'Daniel & Rosenstein, 2008). If health-care professionals fail to communicate effectively, patient safety is at risk for several reasons: (a) Critical information may not be given, (b) information may be misinterpreted, (c) verbal or telephone orders may not be clear, and (d) changes in status may be overlooked. Medical errors easily occur given any one of these situations.

Hand-Off Communications

The transmission of crucial information and the accountability for care of the patient from one health-care provider to another is a fundamental component of communication in health care. Meant to be a step taken to assure continuity of care, the complexity of the patient's condition or the frequency of transfers involves multiple providers communicating with other professionals in addition to nurses; this situation creates gaps in communication and increases patient safety risk. It is estimated that 80% of serious medical errors are attributed to ineffective or incomplete hand-off communication between members of the health-care team (TJC, 2013). Consider the implications for a teaching hospital where there are more than 4,000 hand-offs every day (TJC, 2017).

Nurses traditionally give one another a "report" whenever they transition a patient to another caregiver or department. Hand-off reports include nurse-to-nurse report given at the change of shift, sometimes called bedside shift report, or during the transfer of a patient from one patient care area to another (e.g., the ED to a medical–surgical unit or to a postacute facility such as a skilled nursing home or acute rehabilitation hospital). One prominent health-care system views the hand-off report as a "handover conducted at the bedside to transfer the patient's trust to the oncoming RN" (UCLA Health, 2012).

In the report, pertinent information related to events that occurred is given to the individuals responsible for providing continuity of care (Box 7-4). Although historically the report has been given face to face, there are newer ways to share information. Many health-care institutions use audiotape, computer printouts, or care summary tabs in the EMR as mechanisms for sharing information. These mechanisms allow the nurses and other providers from the previous shift to complete their tasks and those assuming care to make inquiries for clarification as necessary.

TJC defines the hand-off as not only a transfer of care but an acceptance by the nurse or provider of responsibility for a patient's care. This real-time process is done by effectively communicating specific patient information from one nurse to another to ensure the continuity and safety of patient care (TJC, 2014). In 2009, TJC incorporated "managing hand-off communications" in its national patient safety goals (TJC, 2013). TJC maintains that the report should be organized, concise, and complete, with relevant details so that both the sender and receiver of the report know what is needed for safe patient care. Not every unit or department uses the same process for giving a hand-off report, so organizing your facts or questions assures that the right details are shared between caregivers. The hand-off report process is easily modified according to the pattern of nursing care delivery and the types of patients serviced. Some examples include the intensive care units and EDs where walking rounds are used as a means for giving the report. Another approach is the bedside shift report where the nurse caring for the patient and the oncoming nurse conduct their hand-off report at the bedside with the patient and family. In both examples, nurses gather objective data as one nurse ends a shift and another begins; this allows nurses to discuss and clarify current patient status and set goals for care for the next several hours. However, larger patient care units may find the "walking report" time-consuming and an inefficient use of resources.

It is helpful to take notes or create a worksheet while listening to the report. Many institutions now provide a computerized action plan to assist with gathering accurate and concise information during the hand-off report. This worksheet helps organize the work for the day (Fig. 7.1). As specific tasks are mentioned, the nurse assuming responsibility makes a note of the activity in the appropriate time slot. Patient status, resuscitation status, medications, diagnostic tests, and treatments should be documented. Changes from the prior day or shift should be noted, and any priority interventions and new orders should also be reviewed at this time. During the day, the worksheet acts as a reminder of the tasks that have been completed and of those that still need to be done. Many institutions are

---

box 7-4

Information for Change-of-Shift Report (Hand-Off)

- Identify the patient, including the room and bed numbers.
- Include the patient diagnosis.
- Account for the presence of the patient on the unit. If the patient has left the unit for a diagnostic test, surgery, or just to wander, it is important for the oncoming staff members to know the patient is off the unit.
- Provide the treatment plan that specifies the goals of treatment. Note the goals and the critical pathway steps either achieved or in progress. Personalized approaches can be developed during this time and patient readiness for those approaches evaluated. It is helpful to mention the patient's primary care physician. Include new orders and medications and treatments currently prescribed.

- Document patient responses to current treatments. Is the treatment plan working? Present evidence for or against this. Include pertinent laboratory values as well as any negative reactions to medications or treatments. Note any comments the patient has made regarding the hospitalization or treatment plan that the oncoming staff members need to address.
- Omit personal opinions and value judgments about patients as well as personal or confidential information not pertinent to providing patient care. If you are using computerized information systems, make sure you know how to present the material accurately and concisely.

Name _____ Room # _____ Allergies _____

0700	0800	0900	1000	1100	1200	1300	1400	1500	1600	1700	1800

Name _____ Room # _____ Allergies _____

0700	0800	0900	1000	1100	1200	1300	1400	1500	1600	1700	1800

Name _____ Room # _____ Allergies _____

0700	0800	0900	1000	1100	1200	1300	1400	1500	1600	1700	1800

Figure 7.1 Organization and time management schedule for patient care.

now using electronic tablets or WOWs to allow nurses and other health-care providers to collect, organize, record, and track activities.

Reporting skills improve with practice. When presenting information in a hand-off report, begin by identifying the patient, room number, age, gender, and health-care provider. Also include the admitting as well as current diagnoses. Address the expected treatment plan and the patient's response to any treatments or medications, especially those that may have occurred on your shift or the shift prior. For example, if the patient has had multiple antibiotics and a reaction occurred, or a recent change in pain medication which has affected their sensorium, this information is important and must be relayed to the next nurse. Avoid making value judgments and offering personal opinions about the patient.

Communicating With the Health-Care Provider

The function of professional nurses in relation to their patients' health-care providers is to communicate changes in the patient's condition, share other pertinent information, discuss modifications of the treatment plan, clarify orders, and generally speak out to advocate for their needs. This can be stressful for a new graduate who still has some role insecurity. Having the right information in front of you and using good communication skills are helpful when discussing patient needs, especially in critical situations.

Before calling a health-care provider, make sure that all the information needed is available. The provider may want more clarification about the situation. For example, if calling to report a drop in a patient's blood pressure, be sure to have the list of the patient's medications, the last time the patient received the medications, laboratory results, vital signs, and blood pressure trends. Also be prepared to provide a general assessment of the patient's present status.

Of note, there are times when a nurse calls or pages a physician or health-care provider and the health-care provider does not return the call. This call should be documented in the patient's record. If the provider does not return the call in a reasonable amount of time, or patient safety is in jeopardy, the nurse should follow the chain of command to make sure patient safety is maintained. Involving your immediate supervisor in these situations can allay any concerns you have about escalating communication for your patient's health needs.

ISBARR

Miscommunication contributes to approximately 80% of preventable adverse events, including death, during hospitalization. It is estimated that a typical teaching hospital has more than 4,000 patient hand-offs or handover reports per day (TJC, 2017). Loosely translated, that is 4,000 opportunities for patient harm because of lapses in communication. Given this statistic, both TJC and the Institute for Health Care Improvement (IHI) have mandated that health-care institutions employ a standardized reporting or hand-off system and promote the use of the SBAR technique (Haig et al., 2006; IHI, 2006; Robert Wood Johnson Foundation [RWJF], 2013; TJC, 2013, 2017).

Although originally established by the U.S. Navy as SBAR (Situation, Background, Assessment, and Recommendation) to accurately communicate critical information, the technique was adapted by Kaiser-Permanente as an "escalation tool" to be implemented when a rapid change in patient status occurs or is imminent. This communication technique has recently been updated to ISBARR or ISBAR. ISBARR is an acronym for *I*ntroduction, *S*ituation, *B*ackground, *A*ssessment, *R*ecommendation, and *R*eadback (Enlow et al., 2010; Haig et al., 2006). Another communication tool used to convey timely, accurate information to oncoming nurses is called I PASS the BATON (World Health Organization [WHO], 2011). This mnemonic, short for *I*ntroduction, *P*atient, *A*ssessment, *S*ituation, *S*afety concerns, *B*ackground, *A*ctions, *T*iming, *O*wnership, and *N*ext (actions), outlines the steps taken to ensure timely concise and accurate communication to the oncoming nurse or provider. Whether using SBAR, ISBARR, or I PASS the BATON, these techniques provide a framework for communicating critical patient information in a systemized and organized fashion. These methods focus on the immediate situation so that decisions regarding patient care may be made quickly and safely. The format helps to standardize a communication system to effectively transmit needed information to provide safe and effective patient care. Table 7-2 and Table 7-3 illustrate the ISBARR and I PASS the BATON communication tools, respectively.

The implementation of ISBARR and I PASS the BATON as communication techniques has demonstrated success in reducing adverse events and improving patient safety. It also allows nurses, health-care providers, and members of the interprofessional team to communicate in a collegial and professional manner.

Health-Care Provider Orders and Order Sets

Professional nurses are responsible for accepting and implementing health-care provider orders. It is

table 7-2

ISBARR (*Introduction, Situation, Background, Assessment, Recommendation, and Readback*)

Elements	Description	Example
Introduction	Identification of yourself, your role, and your location	Hello, my name is [name]. I am the nurse at [location] for your patient [name].
Situation	Brief description of the existing situation	Critical laboratory value that needs to be addressed (critical blood gas value, international normalized ratio [INR], etc.)
Background	Medical, nursing, or family information that is significant to the care or patient condition	Patient admitted with a pulmonary embolus and on heparin therapy, receiving oxygen at 4 L via nasal cannula; what steps have been taken?
Assessment	Recent assessment data that indicate the most current clinical state of the patient	Vital signs, results of laboratory values, lung sounds, mental status, pulse oximetry results, electrocardiogram results
Recommendation	Information for future interventions or activities	Monitor patient Change heparin dose Repeat INR Repeat computed tomography or ventilation–perfusion (VQ) scan
Readback	Repeat or restate any new orders or recommendations for clarity	Repeat the recommendations back to the health-care provider or member of the interprofessional health-care team. Repeat the INR and change the heparin dose to 1,500 units; repeat the VQ scan and call with the results.

table 7-3

I PASS the BATON (*Introduction, Patient, Assessment, Situation, Safety concerns, Background, Actions, Timing, Ownership, and Next*)

I	Introduction	Introduce yourself, your role, and the patient's name	Hello, [patient name], my name is [name], and I am the registered nurse who will be caring for you today.
P	Patient	Name, patient identifiers, age, gender, and location	
A	Assessment	Present chief complaint, vital signs, symptoms, and diagnosis	Patient is having abdominal pain; vital signs are temp 98.6°F, pulse 84, BP 150/80, R 24. Pain is in the RUQ, vomited a small amount of green, bilious fluid x2. Admitted for possible small bowel obstruction
S	Situation	Current status, code status, level of uncertainty or certainty, recent changes and response to treatment	Stable, full code, moderate concern because of new onset of vomiting
S	Safety concerns	Critical laboratory values, socioeconomic factors, allergies, and risk assessment (falls, isolation, and others)	Amylase is elevated, no allergies or risk factors identified, good family support
The			
B	Background	Previous episodes, past medical history, current medications, and family history	No prior symptoms of gallstones, history of pancreatitis, family history of diabetes
A	Actions	What has been done and why?	Repeat amylase and chemistry drawn to check for electrolyte imbalance or possible infection. Anti-nausea medication is administered for comfort.
T	Timing	Level of urgency, explicit timing, and prioritization of actions	Patient is stable. Plan is to increase vital signs to every 4 hours, and reevaluate when laboratory results are posted. MD to be notified when laboratory results are in.
O	Owner	Who on the team is responsible (includes patient and family)	RN will monitor the patient and notify MD with change in condition. Laboratory will notify RN and MD when laboratory results are available.
N	Next	Plan of care, anticipated changes, contingency plans	Monitor patient. Possible change may result in surgery.

Source: Adapted from World Health Organization. (2011). Being an effective team player.
Patient safety curriculum guide. Retrieved from http://www.who.int/patientsafety/education
/curriculum/who_mc_topic-4.pdf

important to remember that nurses may only receive orders from physicians, dentists, podiatrists, and APPs such as nurse practitioners who are licensed and credentialed in the state in which they are working. Orders written by medical students need to be countersigned by a physician before implementation.

The four main types of orders are written, telephone, faxed, and electronic. Some health-care institutions are looking into the possibility of receiving health-care provider orders through e-mail and secure texting. These orders include the provider's name, date, and time and provide an electronic record of the order.

Written orders are dated and placed on the appropriate institutional form. The health-care provider gives *telephone orders* directly to the nurse by telephone. Faxed orders come directly from the health-care provider office and need to be initialed by the provider. Telephone orders, e-mail orders, and faxed orders need to be signed when the health-care provider comes to the nursing unit. The *electronic orders* give providers the ability to access the patient record from remote locations, which is slowly eliminating the need for telephone and faxed orders in many institutions. For this reason, health-care institutions may no longer accept telephone, e-mail, or fax orders as the health-care providers because they have direct access to the EMR from remote locations. It is important to verify the institution's policy on telephone, e-mail, and fax orders.

The telephone order needs to be written on the appropriate institutional form, with the time and date noted and the form signed by the nurse. When receiving a telephone order, repeat it back to the provider for confirmation. If the health-care provider is speaking too rapidly, ask the individual to speak more slowly, then repeat the information for confirmation. If a faxed document is unclear, call the health-care provider for clarification. Most institutions require the health-care provider to cosign the order within 24 hours.

Teams

Teams and *teamwork* are everyday terms in today's organizations. Teams bring together the variety of skills, perspectives, and talents that create an effective work environment. Nursing is a "team sport." In other words, nurses bring a specific set of skills and talents and need to work together with other professionals to achieve a common goal. The goal in this case is safe, high-quality patient-centered care. Health-care providers understand that safe, quality patient care thrives in an environment that promotes interprofessional teamwork and collaboration. Not all teams are interprofessional teams, however, and it is important to understand that a team does not necessarily infer collaboration.

In 2004, the IOM revealed that issues surrounding nursing competency contributed in part to ensuring patient safety. TJC (2017) estimates that 68.3% of adverse medical events resulting in patient harm are caused by teamwork failures and, in fact, may have been preventable. The Organization for Associate Degree Nursing (OADN) addressed these concerns and looked at collaboration and teamwork as a way to decrease medical errors and promote safe, high-quality care.

OADN (2021) defined *teamwork* as the ability to perform "effectively within nursing and interprofessional teams, fostering open communication, mutual respect, and shared decision-making to achieve quality patient care." Kalisch and Lee (2011) conducted a study that looked at staffing, teamwork, and collaboration. The study supported the fact that teamwork contributes to safe quality care; however, health-care institutions need to provide adequate staffing to ensure collaboration and teamwork. Health-care institutions that choose to apply for American Nurses Credentialing Center (ANCC) Magnet™ designation must demonstrate how their staffing model promotes teamwork and interprofessional collaboration.

Learning to Be a Team Player

When asking for assistance, nothing is more frustrating to hear than, "Oh, he's not my patient" or "I have my own mess to deal with; I can't help you." A team player states, "I have not seen that patient yet today, but let me help get that information for you," or "How can I be of assistance?"

Every team member brings value to the team through personal strengths and specific skill sets. To develop a strong team, members must treat each other with dignity and respect. They also must understand the role and scope of practice of each discipline. It is important for each member to identify their personal strengths, limitations, and competencies in order to function as a contributing member of the team. Being a team member does not automatically make you a team player.

Team players consistently treat other members with respect, courtesy, and consideration. They demonstrate commitment, understand the team's goals, and support other team members appropriately. They care about the work and purpose of the team and they contribute to its success. Team players with commitment look beyond their own workload and provide support and assistance when and where needed (Nelson & Economy, 2010). The goal in the health-care setting is safe, high-quality patient care.

Building a Working Team

Building a strong team takes time and talent. Assuming that all the team members possess the skill sets that are needed, how do you create an effective, efficient team? Brounstein (2002) identified 10 qualities of an effective team player (Box 7-5). These qualities provide the foundation for a strong professional team.

To build an effective team, first identify the team players and focus on the strengths and weaknesses of each. Teams are usually composed of key stakeholders who have a keen interest in the challenge or opportunity at hand. While building on the strengths, devise a plan to assist team members in addressing their weaknesses. Second, make sure that all members understand the team goal, know their role on the team, and are committed to achieving the desired outcome. In health care, the primary goal is safe, high-quality patient care. Third, act as a role model and exhibit the expected behaviors. Fourth, reward the team for accomplishments and achievements, discuss setbacks, and together create an improvement plan.

---

box 7-5

Ten Qualities of an Effective Team Player

1. Demonstrates dependability
2. Communicates constructively
3. Engages in active listening
4. Actively participates
5. Shares information openly and willingly
6. Supports and offers assistance
7. Displays flexibility
8. Exhibits loyalty to the team
9. Acts as a problem-solver
10. Treats others in a courteous and considerate manner

Source: Adapted from Brounstein, M. (2002). Managing teams for dummies. John Wiley & Sons.

Interprofessional Collaboration and the Interprofessional Team

Although building an interprofessional team seems practical, it requires a commitment and collaboration among members of all the disciplines (O'Daniel & Rosenstein, 2008). The IOM (2010), the National League for Nursing (NLN, 2015), the American Association of Colleges of Nursing (AACN, 2011), and the American Organization of Nurse Executives (AONE, 2012) issued statements supporting collaboration among all members of the health-care team with the purpose of providing safe, effective care and achieving positive patient outcomes. Research demonstrates that the quality of patient care is improved when team members collaborate (Keller et al., 2013). Integrated teams composed of health-care professionals who understand each other's unique roles and functions result in better clinical outcomes and greater patient satisfaction (WHO, 2011). As simple as this concept seems, it takes an integrated and dedicated approach to form a collaborative interprofessional team.

Interprofessional Collaboration

The WHO (2010) defines *interprofessional collaboration* as occurring when "multiple health workers from different professional backgrounds work together with patients, families, caregivers, and communities to deliver the highest quality care (WHO, 2010, p. 7)." Collaboration differs from cooperation. Cooperation means working with someone in the sense of enabling: making them more able to do something (typically by providing information or resources they wouldn't otherwise have). Collaborating (from Latin *laborare*, "to work") requires working alongside someone to achieve something (Martin et al., 2010).

The fundamental difference between collaboration and cooperation is the level of formality in the relationships between agencies and stakeholders. For many years, members of other health-care disciplines cooperated with each other. For example, nurses and physicians cooperated with each other in patient care delivery. However, inequalities existed between the disciplines regarding shared expertise and power (RWJF, 2013).

Collaboration can and should happen every time people come together to solve a problem or establish goals. As a nurse, you will experience collaboration multiple times every work day. Knowing and recognizing the characteristics of collaboration will ready you as a professional nurse. A true collaborative effort comprises the following key components: sharing, partnership, interdependency, and power (O'Brien, 2013). Collaboration assumes that members share responsibility, values, and resources. To engage in partnership, members need to be honest and open with each other, demonstrate mutual trust and respect, and value each other's contributions and perspectives. Members of an interprofessional team are dependent on each other and work with each other to achieve a common goal. Finally, power is shared among the members. The health professionals recognize their own individual scope of practice and skill set while demonstrating an appreciation for the other members' expertise, capabilities, and contributions. They also share in the accountability for the delivery of patient care. This shared effort among health-care professionals helps to coordinate care and promote patient safety and quality of care.

Interprofessional Communication

Breakdowns in verbal and written communication among health-care providers present a major concern in the health-care delivery system. TJC (www.tjc.org) attributes a high percentage of sentinel events to poor communication among health-care providers (2013, 2017). Communication is considered to be a core competency to promote interprofessional collaborative practice. Using a common language among the professions assists in understanding and overcoming barriers to interprofessional communication.

The ISBARR and I PASS the BATON methods were discussed earlier in the chapter. A team-related method of communication, Team STEPPS, developed by the Department of Defense (DoD) and the Agency for Healthcare Research and Quality (AHRQ), is another method. The purpose of this teamwork system is to improve collaboration and communication related to patient safety (AHRQ, 2013). This method includes four skills: leadership,

situation monitoring, mutual support, and communication. The program goals focus on (a) creating highly effective medical teams that optimize the use of information, people, and resources to achieve the best clinical outcomes for patients; (b) increasing team awareness and clarifying team roles and responsibilities; (c) resolving conflicts and improving information sharing; and (d) eliminating barriers to quality and safety. The program is composed of training modules available to health-care institutions.

With the goal of collaboration among health-care professionals to promote continuity of care and facilitate communication, many health-care institutions have created a position known as the "nurse navigator." The function of the navigator is to coordinate patient care by guiding patients through the diagnostic process, educating and supporting patients and families, integrating care with other members of the interprofessional team, and assisting them in making informed decisions (Brown et al., 2012).

Nurses are an integral part of the interprofessional health-care team. Nurses usually have the most contact with the patients and their families. They often find themselves in an advantageous position to observe patient response to treatments and report these back to the interprofessional team. For example:

Mr. Richards, a 68-year-old man, was in a motor vehicle accident and sustained a traumatic brain injury. He had right-sided weakness and dysphagia. The health-care provider requested evaluations and treatment plans from speech pathology, physical therapy, and social services. The speech pathologist conducted a swallow study and determined that Mr. Richards should receive pureed foods for the next 2 days. The RN assigned a licensed practical nurse (LPN) to feed Mr. Richards a pureed lunch. The LPN reported that although Mr. Richards had done well the previous day, he had difficulty swallowing even pureed foods today. The RN immediately notified the speech pathologist, and a new treatment plan was developed.

Building an Interprofessional Team

Effective interprofessional teams include several characteristics and focus on the needs of the patient, not the individual contributions of the team members. Each member understands the characteristics of collaboration and demonstrates a willingness to share, recognize the others' expertise, and participate in open communication. Members of a team are expected to share information through verbal and written communication regularly to ensure safe, timely care for patients. This may be done in different settings, such as daily bedside rounds or more formal team conferences for long-term care planning. The characteristics of an effective interprofessional health-care team are listed in Box 7-6.

Interprofessional teams communicate by engaging in conferences and multidisciplinary patient rounds. These groups begin with the presenter, usually the primary nurse, stating the patient's name, age, and primary diagnosis. Each team member then explains the goal of their discipline, the interventions, and the intended outcomes. The effectiveness of treatment, development of new interventions, and setting of new goals are discussed. All members contribute and participate, demonstrating mutual respect and valuing the expertise of the others including nursing assistive personnel (NAP) as appropriate. A method to oversee the implementation of the plan is devised in order to assess outcomes and make adjustments as needed. The nurse (or nurse navigator) is often the individual who assumes the responsibility for this oversight. The key to a successful interprofessional conference is presenting information in a clear, concise manner and ensuring input from all disciplines and levels of care providers.

Conclusion

The responsibility for delivering and coordinating patient care is an important part of the role of the professional nurse. To accomplish this, nurses need good communication skills. Being assertive without being aggressive and interacting with others in a professional manner enhance the relationships that nurses develop with colleagues, health-care providers, and other members of the interprofessional team.

A major focus of the national safety goals is improved communication among health-care professionals and the development of interprofessional health-care teams. In an effort to improve patient safety, health-care institutions have implemented communication protocols referred to as the SBAR method or Team STEPPS. SBAR sets a specific procedure that reminds nurses how to relay information quickly and effectively to the patient's health-care provider, which ultimately leads to improved patient outcomes. Team STEPPS, developed by the DoD, assists health-care institutions in promoting patient safety through communication and coordination of patient care.

Collaboration and teamwork encourage interprofessional collegial relationships that promote safe quality patient care. Key nursing organizations, the IOM, QSEN, and ANCC Magnet™ criteria address the need for collaboration and teamwork. Nurses act as key players in ensuring interprofessional communication and collaboration in patient care delivery.

Finally, health-care institutions need to be committed to creating an environment that promotes communication and team collaboration. This needs to come from the top down and the bottom up to create an organizational culture that promotes patient safety. Nurses are in a unique position to act as change agents within their organizations by practicing safe, effective patient care; promoting collegial communications; and committing themselves to ensuring effective interprofessional collaboration.

---

box 7-6

Characteristics of Effective Interprofessional Health-Care Teams

1. Members provide care to a common group of patients.
2. Members develop common goals for patient outcomes and work together to achieve the goals.
3. Members have roles and functions and understand their roles and the roles of others.
4. The team develops a mechanism for sharing information.
5. The team creates a system to supervise the implementation of plans, evaluate outcomes, and make adjustments based on the results.

Study Questions

1. This is your first position as an RN, and you are working with an LPN who has been on the unit for 20 years. On your first day, she says to you, "The only difference between you and me is the size of the paycheck." Demonstrate how you would respond to this statement, using assertive communication techniques.

2. A health-care provider orders "Potassium chloride 20 milliequivalents IV over 20 minutes." You realize that this is a dangerous order. How would you approach the health-care provider?

3. A patient is admitted to the same-day surgical center for a breast biopsy. Her significant other, who has just had an altercation with an admissions secretary about their insurance, accompanies her. The patient is met by a nurse navigator who notes that the mammogram and blood work are not in the EMR. The patient's significant other says, "What is wrong with you people? Can't you ever get anything straight? If you can't get the insurance right, and you can't get the diagnostic tests right, how can we expect you to get the surgery right?" How should the nurse navigator assist the patient and her significant other?

4. Your nurse manager asks you to develop an interprofessional team on the unit. This team is to serve as a model for other nursing units. How would you start the process? What qualities would you look for in the team members?

Case Study to Promote Clinical Judgment

Corel Jones is a new nursing assistive personnel (NAP) who has been assigned to your acute rehabilitation unit. Corel is a hard worker; he comes in early and often stays late to finish his work. However, Corel is gruff with the patients, especially with the male patients. If a patient is reluctant to get out of bed, Corel often challenges him, saying, "Hey, let's go. Don't be such a wimp. Move your big butt." Today, you overheard Corel telling a female patient who said she did not feel well, "You're just a phony. You enjoy being waited on, but that's not why you're here." The woman started to cry.

1. You are the newest staff nurse on this unit. How would you handle this situation? What would happen if you ignored it?

2. If you decided to pursue the issue, with whom should you speak? What would you say?

3. What do you think is the reason Corel speaks to patients this way?

NCLEX®-Style Review Questions

1. Jane is a new nurse manager who will be holding her first staff meeting tomorrow. She has learned that the staff members have not been following important patient care policies. What is the most important communication skill that she should use at the meeting?
   1. Talking to the staff
   2. Laughing with them
   3. Listening
   4. Crying

2. As Jane speaks with the team, she learns why the staff members have had difficulty following policies. Which of these would be considered barriers to effective communication?
   1. The charge nurse is unavailable to help the nurses when they have questions about policies.
   2. Some staff are afraid to ask particular charge nurses for help for fear of retribution.
   3. The use of acronyms is confusing to staff members who are new to the unit.
   4. All of the above

3. Bedside shift report is one of the things that Jane reviews at the staff meeting. She stresses the way she would prefer the report to start. Which of these would be the least important to share with the oncoming nurse?
   1. Telling the oncoming nurse what happened on the unit during the shift
   2. Introducing the client and the client's diagnosis to the oncoming nurse
   3. Sharing the nurse's personal opinion of the client
   4. Reviewing new medication orders and the medication administration record (MAR)

4. TJC attributes 80% of all medical errors to
   1. Poor hygiene and hand washing
   2. Poor hand-off communication
   3. Poor work environment
   4. Lack of care

5. Implicit bias affects our understanding in an unconscious manner. A person's ability to recognize these biases can improve communication with patients and colleagues alike. Which of the following statements is true about implicit bias?
   1. Implicit bias forms during a lifetime.
   2. Implicit bias can influence clinical decision making and treatment.
   3. Implicit bias contributes to an individual's social behavior.
   4. All of the above

6. The EMR has many advantages compared with paper charting. It helps track data through time and can help monitor things such as preventative care in primary care practices. Jane is the office nurse in a local practice. She is meeting a new patient for the very first time who informs her that he was recently hospitalized. Jane pulls up the patient's EMR and sees no information regarding his recent hospital stay. How could this have happened?
   1. The patient's discharge was so recent that it is not available yet.
   2. EMRs are usually practice or hospital specific, so the patient's information would not be accessible to Jane.
   3. The patient was hospitalized out of state.
   4. The patient has not signed the necessary consents to give Jane access.

7. Social media is commonly used to update friends and groups on things we have going on in our lives. Health-care organizations routinely use social media to promote medical facts, services, and recognitions. What is important for nurses to remember when deciding to post something work related on a social media site?
   1. Nurses should never post PHI on a social media site.
   2. Stories with good outcomes can be posted to your media page.
   3. Stories and photos can always be shared if the patient's name or face is not visible.
   4. Posting stories on personal time is OK because the nurse is not working.

8. You are working on the trauma unit today, and your new patient with a femur fracture complains of leg pain and seems a little diaphoretic and short of breath. You assess the patient and prepare to contact the surgeon. In preparation for contacting the physician, you
    1. Immediately page the MD; it could be a pulmonary embolism, and time is of the essence. You will give him the particulars when the MD arrives.
    2. Wait for the MD to round on his patient because it should be within the next hour or so.
    3. Medicate the patient for pain and plan to contact the MD when he rounds.
    4. Jot down notes about the situation as it is presented to you, review the patient's history, focus your assessment, and determine what you need for the patient.

9. ISBARR provides a framework for communicating critical client information. ISBARR is an acronym for
    1. Identify, Study, Background, Assess, Recognize, Readback
    2. Issue, Situation, Better, Advise, Refer with Recommendations
    3. Introduce, Situation, Background, Assess, Recommend, Readback
    4. None of the above

10. Who is responsible for accepting, transcribing, and implementing physician orders?
    1. Unit clerk
    2. Medical intern or resident
    3. Professional nurse
    4. Medical assistant

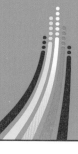

Resolving Problems and Conflicts

Porter O'Grady and Malloch (2016) remind us that "conflict is simply a metaphor for difference" (p. 129). Therefore, it is likely that the pressures and demands of the workplace can often accentuate these differences among people, which can seriously interfere with their ability to work together. Before the COVID-19 pandemic and the murder of George Floyd, various polls and surveys of nurses indicated that the amount of fear, hostility, and unresolved conflict experienced by nurses at work seems to be increasing (Lazoritz & Carlson, 2008; Porter O'Grady & Malloch, 2016; Siu et al., 2008). Since that time, there has been a steady rise in the incidence of hostility experienced by nurses at work, with 59% experiencing verbal abuse from patients and 23% experiencing physical abuse (Robbins & Lesser, 2022). Conflicts with physicians, supervisors, managers, and colleagues can be very stressful and can lead to increased absenteeism, increased turnover, and lower job satisfaction (Moeta & du Rand, 2019; Laschinger et al., 2013; Vivar, 2006). This change in the work environment makes it very important for nurses and nurse leaders to recognize and address conflict in a timely and thoughtful manner. Consider Case 1, which is the first of three that will be used to illustrate how to deal with problems and conflicts.

Conflict

There are no conflict-free work groups (Van de Vliert & Janssen, 2001). Small or large, conflicts are a daily occurrence in the lives of nurses (McElhaney, 1996), and they can interfere with getting work done, as shown in Case 1.

Serious conflicts can be very stressful. Stress symptoms—such as diminished self-confidence, difficulty concentrating, sadness, anxiety, sleep disorders, and withdrawal—and other interpersonal relationship problems can occur. Bitterness, anger, and, in rare occurrences, violence can erupt in the workplace if conflicts are not resolved (see Chapter 13).

Conflict also has a positive side, however. In the process of learning how to manage conflict constructively, people can develop more open, cooperative ways of working together (Tjosvold & Tjosvold, 1995). They can begin to see each other as people with similar needs, concerns, and dreams instead of as competitors or blocks in the way of progress. Being involved in successful conflict resolution can be an empowering experience (Horton-Deutsch & Wellman, 2002).

The goal in dealing with conflict is to create an environment in which conflicts are dealt with in as cooperative and constructive a manner as possible, rather than in a competitive and destructive manner.

Many Sources of Conflict

Why do conflicts occur? The workplace itself can be a generator of conflict. Conflict can be good or bad. Good conflict questions the status quo and can lead to a high level of trust, whereas bad conflict can be perceived as a personal attack and become emotional, which can cloud judgment (Lytle, 2015). Some conflicts are focused on work-related issues such as hospital policies or the coordination of workflow; these are *task-related conflicts* (Kim et al., 2017). Others are primarily interpersonal and stem from communication breakdown related to personal and social issues; these are *relationship-related conflicts* (Kim et al., 2017; Meier et al., 2014).

Power Plays and Competition Between Groups

Differences in status and authority within the health-care team may generate conflicts. For example, physicians often feel that they have authority regarding other members of the team, sometimes causing them to disregard input from other team members (Sun, 2011) or refuse to engage in conflict resolution. The most common problem is disrespect or incivility, but sarcasm, finger-pointing, throwing things, and use of inappropriate language also occur (Lazoritz & Carlson, 2008). In one study of new graduate nurses, 12% reported daily workplace incivility from coworkers, 4.87% reported incivility from supervisors, and 7% reported daily incivility from physicians (Laschinger et al., 2013). The amount of incivility from fellow nurses is especially significant because they are an important source of guidance and support for new graduates.

Incivility, Bullying, Microaggression, and Nurse-to-Nurse Lateral Violence (NNLV)

The American Nurses Association (2015) defines *bullying* as "repeated, unwanted, harmful actions intended to humiliate, offend, and cause distress in the recipient." Bullying involves behavior intended to exert power over another person. It is more than being overly demanding. Workplace bullies often single out one individual as a target, adding a degree of personal malice to their behavior. Their incivility in the form of rude and disrespectful actions may be unintentional or intentional but may still lead to discounting or marginalizing a colleague or patient. An example of incivility could be frequently interrupting a person. Your haste to get your point across could be perceived as rude and could make a colleague feel discounted as a member of the team or even as a person.

Microaggression is defined as a subtle, almost innocuous comment or action that intentionally or unintentionally expresses a prejudiced attitude toward a member of a marginalized group such as a racial minority (Merriam Webster, 2022). The prejudiced attitude may be because of an unconscious bias, leaving perpetrators of the microaggression unaware of their demeaning commentary (Ackerman-Barger et al., 2020).

Regardless of the action taking the form of bullying, incivility, or microaggression, all are forms of workplace violence and the effect on the targeted individual can be devastating. In addition, the cost to the organization is huge. One study estimated the annual cost of nurse workplace violence at approximately $4.3 billion or nearly $250,000 per incident (Embree et al., 2013). Another study reported that nearly 60% of new nurses leave their first job within 6 months because of NNLV (Embree et al., 2013). A Gallup study revealed that one in two adults left their jobs to get away from their manager (Harter & Adkins, 2015). In some settings, nurses feel powerless, trapped by the demands of tasks they must complete, challenged by directives that disregard evidence-supported practice, and frustrated that they cannot provide quality care or correct a situation (Prestia et al., 2017). Conflicts between management and labor unions occur in some workplaces. However, disagreements regarding professional "territory" can occur in any setting. Nurse practitioners and physicians may disagree regarding the scope of nurse practitioner practice, for example. Diversity and disparity issues around racial, social, religious, or gender orientation may create conflicts between caregivers and sometimes with patients and their families (Hall et al., 2015). Examples of disparity experienced in the workplace include things such as sexual harassment and other forms of lateral violence, equal pay for equal work, and inequities in care delivery.

Case 1

Team A and Team B

Team A has stopped talking to Team B. If several members of Team A are out sick, no one on Team B will help Team A with their work. Likewise, Team A members will not take telephone messages for anyone on Team B. Instead, they ask the person to call back later. When members of the two teams pass each other in the hall, they either glare at each other or turn away to avoid eye contact. Arguments erupt when members of the two teams need the same computer terminal or another piece of equipment at the same time.

When a Team A nurse reached for a glucometer at the same moment as a Team B nurse did, the second nurse said, "You've been using that all morning."

"I've got a lot of patients to monitor," was the response.

"Oh, you think you're the only one with work to do?"

"We take good care of our patients."

"Are you saying we don't?"

The nurses fell silent when the nurse manager entered the room.

"Is something the matter?" she asked. Both nurses shook their heads and left quickly.

"I'm not sure what's going on here," the nurse manager thought to herself, "but something's wrong, and I need to find out what it is right away."

We will return to this case later as we discuss workplace problems and conflicts, their sources, and how to resolve them.

Case 1 Team A and Team B.

Increased Workload

Staffing shortages and emphasis on cost reduction have resulted in *work intensification,* a situation in which employees are required to do more in less time (Roch et al., 2014; Willis et al., 2008). The multitasking and prioritization of activities created by unmanageable workloads force nurses to make choices. Common responses are skipping breaks, doing paperwork during lunch, working overtime without pay, and even missed care such as patient teaching or discharge planning (Hessels et al., 2015; Roch et al., 2014). More conflict can arise if nurses believe they are being given inappropriate tasks such as being asked to empty trash or deliver meal trays. This increased workload leaves many nurses conflicted and believing that their employers are taking advantage of them.

Scarcity, Safety, and Security

Limited resources almost inevitably lead to competition to get one's fair share (or more), often resulting in conflict between individuals and between departments (Isosaari, 2011). When cost saving is emphasized and staff members face layoffs, people's economic security is threatened. Inadequate money for pay raises, equipment, supplies, or additional help can increase competition between or among individuals and departments as they scramble to grab their share of what little is available. Even crowded conditions in a busy nurses' station can increase interpersonal tension and lead to battles regarding scarce work space (McElhaney, 1996). Scarcity and resource depletion can threaten the safety and security of the work environment and be a source of considerable stress and tension, which may create underlying conflict (Kim et al., 2017).

Cultural Differences

Language differences and implicit attitudes or bias may make communication challenging (Hall et al., 2015). Cultural differences can stem from individuals or an organization. Some of these cultures emphasize the importance of the individual, whereas others may emphasize the importance of the group (Osterberg & Lorentsson, 2010). Different beliefs about how hard a person should work, what constitutes productivity, and even what it means to arrive at work "on time" can lead to conflicts if they are not reconciled.

Ethical Conflicts

Moral distress occurs when nurses encounter a situation that violates their personal or professional ethics, especially when others ignore it or pretend it is not a concern (Lachman et al., 2012). Examples of such conflicts are feeling pressured to record care that was not given, taking a shortcut by failing to fully explain a procedure before obtaining patient consent, or acquiescing to an order to deliver futile care to the terminally ill or injured. The pandemic has contributed to the moral distress of some nurses because of the futility of patient care. A particular frustration voiced to this author by a critical care nurse during the Delta surge was the profound sadness and frustration that she felt when caring for her unvaccinated COVID-19 patients, knowing that their illness and eventual deaths were preventable.

When Conflict Occurs

Conflict can occur at any level and involve any number of people. On the individual level, conflict can occur between two people on a team, in different departments, or between a staff member and a patient or family member. On the group level, conflict can occur between two teams (as in Case 1), two departments, or two different professional groups (e.g., between nurses and social workers regarding who is responsible for advance care planning). Conflict can also occur between two organizations (e.g., when two home health agencies compete for a contract with a large hospital). The focus in this chapter is primarily on the first two levels: among individuals and groups of people within a health-care organization.

Health-care oriented workplaces have been especially resistant to effective conflict management in the past, but several forces are reducing this resistance. The Institute of Medicine (IOM) report *To Err Is Human* (IOM, 1999) exposed serious threats to patient safety because of preventable errors and made it clear that problems need to be resolved, not buried. The Joint Commission (TJC) added several standards that focus on improved staff communication and problem resolution (TJC, 2018). "Improve staff communication" remains on TJC's 2022 national list of patient safety goals to ensure patient and staff safety (TJC, 2022). Nurses also find themselves in patient care situations where an ethical

box 8-1

Signs That Conflict Resolution Is Needed

- You feel very uncomfortable in a situation.
- Members of your team are having trouble working together.
- Team members stop talking with each other.
- Team members begin "losing their cool," attacking each other verbally.

Source: Adapted from Patterson, K., Grenny, J., McMillan, R., & Switzler, A. (2003, March 18). Crucial conversations: Making a difference between being healed and being seriously hurt. Vital Signs, 13(5), 14–15.

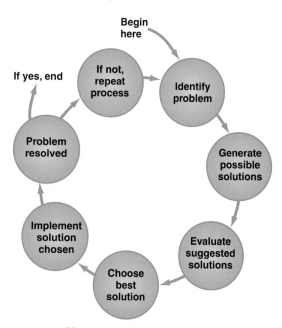

Figure 8.1 The process of resolving a problem.

response might cause some conflict about which they cannot remain silent if this puts a patient at risk. Developing competency in dealing with conflict is an important leadership skill (Kritek, 2011). Box 8-1 lists situations in which conflict resolution is needed.

Resolving Problems and Conflicts

Win, Lose, or Draw?

Some people think about problems and conflicts that occur at work in the same way they think about a basketball game or tennis match: Someone has to win and someone has to lose. However, there are some problems with this sports comparison. First, the aim of conflict resolution is to work together more effectively, not to win. Second, if people really do lose, they are likely to feel bad about it. Therefore, they may spend their time gearing up to win the next round rather than concentrating on their work. A win–win result in which both sides gain some benefit is the best resolution (Haslan, 2001). Sometimes people cannot reach agreement (consensus) but can recognize and accept their differences and get on with their work (McDonald, 2008).

Other Conflict Resolution Myths

Many people think of what can be "won" as a fixed amount: "I get half, and you get half." This is the *fixed pie* myth of conflict resolution (Thompson & Fox, 2001). Another erroneous assumption is called the *devaluation reaction:* "If the other side is getting what they want, then it has to be bad for us" (Thompson & Nadler, 2000). These erroneous beliefs can be serious barriers to the achievement of a mutually beneficial conflict resolution.

When disagreements first arise, *problem-solving* may be sufficient. If the situation has already developed into a full-blown conflict, however, *negotiation,* either informal or formal, of a settlement may be necessary.

Problem Resolution

The use of the problem-solving process in patient care should be familiar. The same approach can be used when issues arise between staff members on your unit. The goal is to find a solution that is acceptable to everyone involved. The process illustrated in Figure 8.1 includes identifying the issue, generating solutions, evaluating the suggested solutions, choosing what appears to be the best solution, implementing that solution, evaluating the extent to which the problem has been resolved, and, finally, concluding either that the problem has been resolved or that it will be necessary to repeat the process to find a better solution.

Identify the Problem or Issue

Early recognition of conflict and intervention are important in the patient care environment. The impact of tension and stress can lead to emotional exhaustion, mistrust, and disruptive behavior that can compromise patient care (Kim et al., 2017). It can also contribute to the ability to deliver optimal care and may even compromise patient safety (Christie & Jones, 2013). Once a conflict is identified, it is important to address the participants in a nonthreatening manner and ask them what they want (Sportsman, 2005). If the issue is not emotionally charged, they may be able to give a direct answer. Other times, however, some discussion and exploration of the issues will be necessary before the real problem emerges. "It would be nice," wrote Browne and Keeley, "if what other people were really saying was always obvious, if all their essential thoughts were clearly labeled for us . . . and if all knowledgeable people agreed about answers to important questions" (Browne & Keeley, 1994, p. 5). Of course, this is not what usually happens.

Getting to the root cause of conflict can be time-consuming because issues may be deep-seated and driven by more than the situation at hand (Girardi, 2015a). People are often vague about what their real concern is; sometimes they are genuinely uncertain about what the real problem is. Strong personal beliefs, physical exhaustion, miscommunication, and ambiguity around scope of practice or a policy are factors affecting conflict, all of which can divert our attention away from patient care priorities (Kim et al., 2017). All this needs to be sorted out so that the problem is clearly identified and a solution can be sought.

Generate Possible Solutions

Here, creativity is especially important. Try to discourage people from using old solutions for new problems. It is natural for people to try a solution that has already worked well; however, previously successful solutions may not work in the future. Creative problem-solving requires that the team understand and define the problem they are solving, generate new ideas about the problem, and, finally, find and act on the best solution (Markham, 2017).

There are a variety of techniques that can help a team find an innovative solution, such as brainwriting, a variation on brainstorming (Markham, 2017). Bring the group together to discuss the problem, give them paper, and then, before discussing solutions, ask each of them to write down as many solutions as they can imagine, then list the ideas. This approach gives everyone a chance to formulate their individual ideas before the discussion begins, which reduces the chances of people subconsciously anchoring themselves to the influence of early ideas (Greenfield, 2014). Then give everyone a chance to consider each suggestion on its own merits.

Review Suggested Solutions and Choose the Best Solution

An open-minded evaluation of each suggestion is needed, but accomplishing this is not always easy. Some groups get "stuck in a rut," unable to "think outside the box." Other times, groups find it difficult to separate the suggestion from its source. On an interdisciplinary team, for example, the status of the person who made the suggestion may influence whether the suggestion is judged to be useful. Yet the best suggestions often come from those closest to the problem (McChrystal, 2012), such as the care assistants who spend the most time with their patients. Whose solution is most likely to be the best one, the physician's or the unlicensed assistant's? A suggestion should be judged on its merits, not its source. Which of the suggested solutions is most likely to work? Usually, it is the combination of suggestions that leads to the best solutions (Greenfield, 2014).

Implement the Solution Chosen

The true test of any suggested solution is how well it actually works. Once a solution has been implemented, it is important to give it time to work. Impatience sometimes leads to premature abandonment of a good solution.

Evaluate: Is the Problem Resolved?

Not every problem is resolved successfully on the first attempt; sometimes it is because the root cause of the conflict was not clearly identified. If the problem has not been resolved, then the process needs to be resumed with even greater attention to what the real problem is and how it can be resolved successfully. Consider the following situation in which problem-solving was helpful (Case 2).

A new nurse manager asked Ms. Deloitte to meet with her to discuss the problem. The following is a summary of their problem-solving:

- **The issue** Ms. Deloitte wanted to take her vacation from the end of December through early January. Making the assumption that she was going to be permitted to go, she had purchased nonrefundable tickets. The policy prohibits vacations during the holiday schedule, which begins on December 20 and ends on January 5 this year. The former nurse manager had not enforced this policy with Ms. Deloitte, but the new nurse manager thought it fair to enforce the policy with everyone, including Ms. Deloitte.

Case 2

The Vacation

Francine Deloitte has been a unit secretary for 10 years. She is prompt, efficient, accurate, courteous, flexible, and productive—everything a nurse manager could ask for in a unit secretary. When nursing staff members are very busy, she distributes afternoon snacks or sits with a family for a few minutes until a nurse is available. There is only one issue on which Ms. Deloitte is insistent and stubborn: taking her 2-week vacation over the Christmas and New Year holidays. This is forbidden by hospital policy, but every nurse manager has allowed her to do this because it is the only special request she ever makes and because it is the only time she visits her family during the year.

A recent reorganization of the administrative structure had eliminated several layers of nursing managers and supervisors. Each remaining nurse manager was given responsibility for two or three units. The new nurse manager for Ms. Deloitte's unit refused to grant her request for vacation time at the end of December. "I can't show favoritism," she explained. "No one else is allowed to take vacation time at the end of December." Assuming that she could have the time off as usual, Francine had already purchased a nonrefundable ticket for her visit home. When her request was denied, she threatened to quit. On hearing this, one of the nurses on Francine's unit confronted the new nurse manager saying, "You can't do this. We are going to lose the best unit secretary we've ever had if you do."

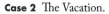

Case 2 The Vacation.

- **Possible solutions**
  1. Ms. Deloitte resigns.
  2. Ms. Deloitte is fired.
  3. Allow Ms. Deloitte to take her vacation as planned.
  4. Allow everyone to take vacations between December 20 and January 5 as requested.
  5. Allow no one to take a vacation between December 20 and January 5.
- **Evaluate suggested solutions** Ms. Deloitte preferred solutions 3 and 4. The new nurse manager preferred 5. Neither wanted 1 or 2. They could agree only that none of the solutions satisfied both of them, so they decided to try again.
- **Second list of possible solutions**
  1. Reimburse Ms. Deloitte for the cost of the tickets.
  2. Allow Ms. Deloitte to take one last vacation between December 20 and January 5.
  3. Allow Ms. Deloitte to take her vacation during Thanksgiving instead.
  4. Allow Ms. Deloitte to begin her vacation on December 26 so that she would work on Christmas Day but not on New Year's Day.
  5. Allow Ms. Deloitte to begin her vacation earlier in December so that she could return in time to work on New Year's Day.
- **Choose the best solution** As they discussed the alternatives, Ms. Deloitte confirmed that she could change the day of her flight without a

penalty. The nurse manager said she could support solution 5 on the second list if Ms. Deloitte understood that she could not take vacation time between December 20 and January 5 in the future. Ms. Deloitte agreed to this.
- **Implement the solution** Ms. Deloitte returned on December 30 and worked both New Year's Eve and New Year's Day.
- **Evaluate the solution** The rest of the staff members had been watching the situation very closely. Most believed that the solution had been fair to them as well as to Ms. Deloitte. Ms. Deloitte thought she had been treated fairly. The nurse manager believed both parties had found a solution that was fair to Ms. Deloitte but still reinforced the manager's determination to enforce the vacation policy.
- **Resolved, or resume problem-solving?** Ms. Deloitte, staff members, and the nurse manager all thought the problem had been solved satisfactorily.

Negotiating an Agreement Informally

When a disagreement has become too big, too complex, or too heated for problem resolution to be successful, a more elaborate process may be required to resolve it. On evaluating Case 1, the nurse manager decided that the tensions between Team A and Team B had become so great that negotiation would be necessary.

The Informal Negotiation Process

- Scope the situation. Ask yourself:
  What am I trying to achieve?
  What is the environment in which I am operating?
  What problems am I likely to encounter?
  What does the other side want?
- Set the stage.
- Conduct the negotiation.
- Set the ground rules.
- Clarify the problem.
- Make your opening move.
- Continue with offers and counteroffers.
- Agree on the resolution of the conflict.

The process of negotiation is a complex one that requires careful thought beforehand and considerable skill in its implementation. Box 8-2 is an outline of the most essential aspects of negotiation. Case 1 is used to illustrate how it can be done.

Scope the Situation

For a strategy to be successful, it is important that the entire situation be understood thoroughly. Walker and Harris (1995) suggested asking three questions:

1. **What am I trying to achieve?** The nurse manager in Case 1 is very concerned about the tensions between Team A and Team B. She wants the members of these two teams to be able to work together in a cooperative manner, which they are not doing at the present time.
2. **What is the environment in which I am operating?** The members of Teams A and B were openly hostile to each other. The overall climate of the organization, however, was benign. The nurse manager knew that teamwork was encouraged and that her actions to resolve the conflict would be supported by the administration.
3. **What problems am I likely to encounter?** The nurse manager knew that she had allowed the problem to go on too long. Even physicians, social workers, and visitors to the unit were getting caught up in the conflict. Team members were actively encouraging other staff to take sides, making it clear that "if you're not with us, you're against us." This made people from other departments very uncomfortable because they had to work with both teams. The nurse manager knew that resolution of the conflict would be a relief to many people.

It is important to ask one additional question in preparation for negotiations.

4. **What does the other side want?** In this situation, the nurse manager was not certain what either team really wanted. However, she realized that she needed this information before she could begin to negotiate. Rather than assume, it would be important that the nurse manager hear what each team wanted in their own words.

Set the Stage

When a conflict such as the one between Teams A and B has gone on for some time, the opposing sides are often unwilling to meet to discuss the problem. A typical response to conflict is avoidance; if allowed to fester, unaddressed conflict can lead to mistrust and a "climate of fear" (Girardi, 2015b, p. 62), staff disengagement, and the formation of alliances to create a sense of safety (Girardi, 2015b). This avoidance prevents an exchange of information between the two groups (Sun, 2011). If this occurs, it may be necessary to confront them with direct statements designed to open communication between the two sides, challenging them to seek resolution of the situation. At the same time, it is important to avoid any suggestion of blame because this provokes defensiveness.

To confront Teams A and B with their behavior toward one another, the nurse manager called them together at the end of the day shift. "I am very concerned about what I have been observing," she told them. "It appears to me that our two teams are working against each other." She continued with some examples of what she had observed, taking care not to mention names or blame anyone for the problem. She was also prepared to take responsibility for having allowed the situation to deteriorate before taking this much-needed action.

Conduct the Negotiation

As indicated earlier, conducting a negotiation requires a great deal of skill.

1. **Manage the emotions** When people are very emotional, they have trouble thinking clearly. Acknowledging these emotions is essential to negotiating effectively (Fiumano, 2005). When faced with a highly charged situation, do not respond with added emotion. Take time out if you need to get your own feelings under

control. Then find out why emotions are high (watch both verbal and nonverbal cues carefully) and refocus the discussion on the issues. Allow disagreements to be expressed. Those who are willing to voice their differences play an important role in helping the group move toward resolution of the problem. The leader's role is to encourage group members to listen to and consider these differences, the first step in moving toward resolution of the conflict (Sarkar, 2009). Without effective leadership to prevent disagreements, emotional outbursts, and personal attacks, a mishandled negotiation can worsen a situation. With effective leadership, the conflict may be resolved (Box 8-3).

2. **Set ground rules** Members of Teams A and B began throwing accusations at each other as soon as the nurse manager made her statement. The nurse manager stopped this quickly and said, "First, we need to set some ground rules for this discussion. Everyone will get a chance to speak but not all at once. Please speak for yourself, not for others. And please do not make personal remarks or criticize your coworkers. We are here to resolve this problem, not to make it worse." She had to remind the group of these ground rules several times during the meeting.

3. **Clarification of the problem** The nurse manager wrote a list of problems raised by team members on a chalkboard. As the list grew longer, she asked the group, "What do you see here? What is the real problem?" The group remained silent. Finally, someone said, "We don't

have enough people, equipment, or supplies to get the work done." The rest of the group nodded in agreement, thereby clarifying the problem to be solved.

4. **Opening move** Once the problem is clarified, it is time to obtain everyone's agreement to seek a way to resolve the conflict. In a more formal negotiation, you may make a statement about what you wish to achieve. This first statement sets the stage for the rest of the negotiation (Suddath, 2012). For example, if you are negotiating a salary increase, you might begin by saying, "I am requesting a 10% increase for the following reasons. . . ." Of course, your employer will probably make a counteroffer, such as, "The best I can do is 3%." These are the opening moves of a negotiation.

5. **Continue the negotiations** The discussion should continue in an open, nonhostile manner. Each side's concerns may be further explained and elaborated. Additional offers and counteroffers are common. As the discussion continues, it is helpful to emphasize areas of agreement as well as disagreement so that both parties are encouraged to continue the negotiations (Tappen, 2001).

Agree on a Resolution of the Conflict

After much testing for agreement, elaborating each side's positions and concerns, and making offers and counteroffers, the people involved should finally reach an agreement.

The nurse manager of Teams A and B led them through a discussion of their concerns related to working with severely limited resources. The teams soon realized that they had a common concern and that they might be able to help each other rather than compete with each other. The nurse manager agreed to become more proactive in seeking resources for the unit. "We can simultaneously seek new resources and develop creative ways to use the resources we already have," she told the teams. Relationships between members of Team A and Team B improved remarkably after this meeting. They learned that they could accomplish more by working together than they had ever achieved separately.

Formal Negotiation: Collective Bargaining

There are many varieties of formal negotiations, from real estate transactions to international peace treaty negotiations. A formal negotiation process

---

box 8-3

Tips for Leading the Discussion

- Create a climate of comfort.
- Let others know the purpose is to resolve a problem or conflict.
- Freely admit your own contribution to the problem.
- Begin with the presentation of facts.
- Recognize your own emotional response to the situation.
- Set ground rules.
- Do not make personal remarks.
- Avoid placing blame.
- Allow each person an opportunity to speak.
- Do speak for yourself but not for others.
- Focus on solutions.
- Keep an open mind.

Source: Adapted from Patterson, K., Grenny, J., McMillan, R., & Surtzler, A. (2003, March 18). Crucial conversations: Making a difference between being healed and being seriously hurt. Vital Signs, 13(5), 14–15.

of special interest to nurses is collective bargaining, which is highly formalized because it is governed by laws and contracts called *collective bargaining agreements.*

Collective bargaining involves a formal procedure governed by labor laws, such as the National Labor Relations Act in the United States. Non-profit health-care organizations were added to the organizations covered by these laws in 1974. Once a union or professional organization has been designated as the official bargaining agent for a group of nurses, a contract defining such important matters as salary increases, benefits, time off, unfair treatment, safety issues, and promotion of professional practice is drawn up. This contract governs employee–management relations within the organization.

A collective bargaining contract is a legal document that governs the relationship between management and staff, who are represented by the union (for nurses, it may be the nurses' association or another health-care workers' union). The contract may cover some or all of the following:

- **Economic issues** Salaries, shift differentials, length of the workday, overtime, holidays, sick leave, breaks, health insurance, pensions, and severance pay.
- **Management issues** Promotions, layoffs, transfers, reprimands, grievance procedures, and hiring and firing procedures.
- **Practice issues** Adequate staffing, standards of care, code of ethics, safe working environment, other quality-of-care issues, and staff development opportunities.

Better patient–nurse staffing ratios, more reasonable workloads, opportunities for professional development, and better relationships with management are among the most important issues for practicing nurses (Budd et al., 2004).

Case 3 is an example of how collective bargaining agreements can influence the outcome of a

---

Case 3

Collective Bargaining

The chief executive officer (CEO) of a large home health agency in a southwestern resort area called a general staff meeting. She reported that the agency had grown rapidly and was now the largest in the area. "Much of our success is due to the professionalism and commitment of our staff members," she said. "With growth comes some problems, however. The most serious problem is the fluctuation in patient census. Our census peaks in the winter months when seasonal residents are here and troughs in the summer. In the past, when we were a small agency, we all took our vacations during the slow season. This made it possible to continue to pay everyone his or her full salary all year. However, given pressures to reduce costs and the large number of staff members we now have, we cannot continue to do this. We are very concerned about maintaining the high quality of patient care currently provided, but we have calculated that we need to reduce staff by 30 percent over the summer in order to survive financially."

The CEO then invited comments from the staff members. The majority of the nurses said they wanted and needed to work full-time all year. Most supported families and had to have a steady income all year. "My rent does not go down in the summer," said one. "Neither does my mortgage payment or the grocery bill," said another. A small number said that they would be happy to work part-time in the summer if they could be guaranteed full-time employment from October through May. "We have friends who would love this work schedule," they added.

"That's not fair," protested the nurses who needed to work full-time all year. "You can't replace us with part-time staff." The discussion grew louder and the participants more agitated. The meeting ended without a solution to the problem. Although the CEO promised to consider all points of view before making a decision, the nurses left the meeting feeling very confused and concerned about the security of their future income. Some grumbled that they probably should begin looking for new positions "before the ax falls."

The next day the CEO received a telephone call from the nurses' union representative. "If what I heard about the meeting yesterday is correct," said the representative, "your plan is in violation of our collective bargaining contract." The CEO reviewed the contract and found that the representative was correct. A new solution to the financial problems caused by the seasonal fluctuations in patient census would have to be found.

Case 3 Collective Bargaining.

conflict between management and staff in a health-care organization.

The Pros and Cons of Collective Bargaining

Some nurses believe it is unprofessional to belong to a union. Others point out that physicians and teachers are union members and that the protections offered by a union outweigh the downside. There is no easy answer to this question.

Probably the greatest advantages of collective bargaining are the protection of the right to fair treatment and the availability of a written grievance procedure that specifies both the employee's and the employer's rights and responsibilities if an issue arises that cannot be settled informally (Forman & Merrick, 2003). Another advantage is salary: Nurses working under a collective bargaining agreement can earn as much as 28% more than those who do not (Pittman, 2007).

The greatest disadvantage of using collective bargaining as a way to deal with conflict is that it clearly separates management from staff, often creating an adversarial relationship. Any nurses who make staffing decisions may be classified as supervisors and, therefore, may be ineligible to join the union, separating them from the rest of their colleagues (Martin, 2001). The result is that management and staff are treated as opposing parties rather than as people who are trying to work together to provide essential services to their patients. The collective bargaining contract also adds another layer of rules and regulations between staff members and their supervisors. Because management of such employee-related rules and regulations can take almost a quarter of a manager's time (Drucker, 2002), this can become a drain on a nurse manager's time and energy.

Conclusion

Conflict is inevitable, especially within any large, diverse group of people in a complex system, such as health care, who are trying to work together. However, conflict does not have to be destructive, nor does it have to be an entirely negative experience. If it is handled skillfully, proactive response to conflict can stimulate people to learn more about each other, strengthen relationships, and encourage a collaborative approach to problem-solving. Resolving a conflict, when done well, can lead to improved working relationships, more creative methods of operation, and higher productivity.

Study Questions

1. Debate the question of whether conflict is constructive or destructive. How can good leadership affect the outcome of a conflict?

2. Give an example of how each of the seven sources of conflict listed in this chapter can lead to a serious problem. Then discuss ways to prevent the occurrence of conflict from each of the seven sources.

3. What is the difference between problem resolution and negotiation? Under what circumstances would you use one or the other?

4. Identify a conflict (actual or potential) in your clinical area and explain how either problem resolution or negotiation could be used to resolve it.

5. In what ways does collective bargaining increase conflict? How does it help resolve conflict?

Case Study to Promote Clinical Judgment

A not-for-profit hospice center in a small community received a generous gift from the grateful family of a patient who had died recently. The family asked only that the money be "put to the best use possible."

Everyone in this small facility had an opinion about the "best" use for the money. The administrator wanted to renovate the old, rundown headquarters. The financial officer wanted to put the money in the bank "for a rainy day." The chaplain wanted to add a small chapel to the building.

The nurses wanted to create a food bank to help the poorest of their clients. The social workers wanted to buy a van to transport clients to health-care provider offices. The staff agreed that all the ideas had merit, and that all the needs identified were important ones. Unfortunately, there was enough money to meet only one of them.

The more the staff members discussed how to use this gift, the more insistent each group became that their idea was best. At their last meeting, it was evident that some were becoming frustrated and that others were becoming angry. It was rumored that a shouting match between the administrator and the financial officer had occurred.

1. In your analysis of this situation, identify the sources of the conflict that are developing in this facility.

2. What kind of leadership actions are needed to prevent the escalation of this conflict?

3. If the conflict does escalate, how could it be resolved?

4. Which idea do you think has the most merit? Why did you select the one you did?

5. Try role-playing a negotiation among the administrator, the financial officer, the chaplain, a representative of the nursing staff, and a representative of the social work staff. Can you suggest a creative solution?

NCLEX®-Style Review Questions

1. The purpose of learning how to negotiate conflict is to
   1. Eliminate conflict entirely
   2. Resolve conflicts more effectively
   3. Win
   4. Reduce stress

2. Differences in status and authority within the health-care team can generate conflict. What is the most common cause of conflict?
   1. Disrespect and incivility
   2. Inappropriate language and sarcasm
   3. Blaming and finger pointing
   4. Physical violence

3. The hospital has recently reorganized; therefore, several departments were closed. The patient census on the unit has increased. The staff have always had a strong team spirit, but the nurse manager knows that workflow changes can cause conflict. What can the nurse manager do to reduce the possibility of conflict among her team?
   1. Monitor the quality of patient care.
   2. Ensure that supplies and equipment are readily available.
   3. Assess the equity of nursing assignments.
   4. All of the above

4. The nursing and respiratory departments both experienced job cuts. The nurse manager notices that members of his staff are having more trouble getting a fast response from a respiratory therapist. What source of conflict is probably operating here?
   1. Union–management conflict
   2. Interpersonal problem
   3. Cultural differences
   4. Work intensification

5. What is the most desirable result of a problem resolution?
   1. Win–lose
   2. Lose–lose
   3. Win–win
   4. None of the above

6. What is brainwriting?
   1. A strategy to encourage the free flow of ideas
   2. A mutually beneficial negotiation result
   3. A winning approach to formal negotiation
   4. A devaluation reaction to negotiation

7. Florence has two team members who continually criticize each other despite being told to stop. Which approach is the most appropriate for this situation?
   1. Refer each of them for employee counseling.
   2. Engage in problem resolution.
   3. Bring in a union representative.
   4. Engage in a formal negotiation process.

8. Which of the following issues may be addressed in a collective bargaining agreement?
   1. Shift differentials
   2. Safe working environment
   3. Grievance procedures
   4. All of the above

9. Nursing management and the nursing union are having differences on several issues. There may be a need for negotiation. Which of the following is a serious disadvantage to using collective bargaining to resolve this conflict?
   1. Protecting the right to fair treatment
   2. Creating an adversarial relationship between staff and management
   3. Lacking professionalism on the part of the collective bargaining unit members
   4. Failing to uphold important standards of care

10. If an informal negotiation session becomes too highly emotional, what should the nurse manager do?
    1. Let the feelings flow.
    2. Cancel the negotiation.
    3. Deal with the feelings first.
    4. Tell them to ignore the feelings and deal with the issues.

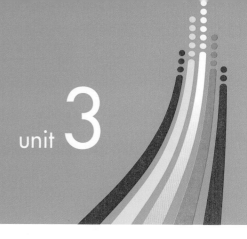

unit 3

Health-Care Organizations

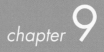

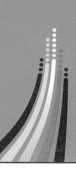

chapter 9

Organizations, Power, and Professional Empowerment

OBJECTIVES

After reading this chapter, the student should be able to:

- Recognize the various ways in which health-care organizations differ.
- Explain the importance of organizational culture.
- Define power and empowerment.
- Identify sources of power in a health-care organization.
- Describe several ways in which nurses can be empowered.

OUTLINE

The topics in this chapter—organizations, power, and empowerment—are not as remote from a nurse's everyday experience as you may first think. Although it is difficult to focus on these "big picture" factors when caught up in the busy day-to-day work of a staff nurse, they have a significant effect on you and your practice, as you will see in this chapter. Consider two scenarios, which are analyzed in the following examples:

Scenario 1

In school, Hazel Rivera had always received high praise for the quality of her nursing care plans. "Thorough, comprehensive, systematic, holistic—beautiful!" was the comment she received on the last one she wrote before graduation.

Now Hazel is a staff nurse on a busy orthopedic unit. Although her time to write comprehensive care plans during the day is limited, Hazel often stays after work to complete them. Her friend Carla refuses to stay late with her. "If I can't complete my work during the shift, then they have given me too much to do," she said.

At the end of their 3-month probationary period, Hazel and Carla received written evaluations of their progress and comments about their value to the organization. To Hazel's surprise, her friend Carla received a higher rating than she did. Why?

Scenario 2

The nursing staff of the critical care department of a large urban hospital formed an evidence-based practice group about a year ago. They had made many changes in their practice based on reviews of the research on several different procedures, and they were quite pleased with the results.

"Let's look at the bigger picture next month," their nurse manager suggested. "We should consider the research on different models of patient care. We might get some good ideas for our unit." The staff nurses agreed. It would be a nice change to look at the way they organized patient care in their department.

The nurse manager found a wealth of information on different models for organizing nursing care. They finally decided that a separate geriatric intensive care unit made sense because

a large proportion of their patient population was in their 70s, 80s, and 90s.

Several nurses volunteered to form an ad hoc committee to design a similar unit for older patients within their critical care department. When the plan was presented, both the nurse manager and the staff thought it was excellent. The nurse manager offered to present the plan to the vice president for nursing, and the staff eagerly awaited the vice president's response.

However, the nurse manager returned with discouraging news. The vice president did not support their concept and said that, although they were free to continue developing the idea, they should not assume that it would ever be implemented. What happened?

Were the disappointments experienced by Hazel Rivera and the critical care department staff predictable? Could they have been avoided? Without a basic understanding of organizations and the part that power plays in health-care institutions, people are doomed to be continually surprised by the response to their well-intentioned efforts. As you read this chapter, you will learn why Hazel Rivera and the staff of the critical care department were disappointed.

This chapter begins by looking at some of the characteristics of the organizations in which nurses work and how these organizations operate. Then it focuses on the subject of power within organizations: What it is, how it is obtained, and how nurses can be empowered.

Understanding Organizations

One of the attractive features of nursing as a career is the wide variety of settings in which nurses can work. From rural migrant health clinics to organ transplant units in an academic medical center, nurses' skills are needed wherever there are concerns about people's health. Relationships with patients may extend for months or years, as they do in school health or in nursing homes, or they may be brief and never repeated, as often happens in doctors' offices, operating rooms, and emergency departments (EDs).

Types of Health-Care Organizations

Although some nurses work as independent practitioners, as consultants, or in the corporate world, most nurses are employed by health-care organizations. These organizations can be classified into three types on the basis of their sponsorship and financing:

1. **Private not-for-profit** Many health-care organizations were founded by civic, charitable, or religious groups. Many of today's hospitals, long-term care facilities, home-care services, and community agencies began this way. Some have been in existence for generations. Although they need sufficient money to pay their staff and expenses, as not-for-profit organizations, they do not have to generate a profit in addition to meeting expenses.
2. **Public** Government-operated health service organizations range from county public health departments to complex medical centers, such as those operated by the Veterans Administration, a federal agency. These organizations provide care to people who might have limited access elsewhere because of things such as health insurance limitations.
3. **Private for-profit** Increasing numbers of health-care organizations are operated for profit, similar to other businesses. These include large hospital and nursing home chains, health maintenance organizations, and many free-standing centers that provide special services, such as surgical and diagnostic centers.

The differences between these categories have become blurred for several reasons:

■ All compete for patients, especially for patients with health-care insurance or the ability to pay their own health-care bills.
■ All experience the effects of cost constraints.
■ All may provide services that are eligible for government reimbursement, particularly Medicaid and Medicare funding, if they meet government standards.

Organizational Characteristics

The size and complexity of many health-care organizations make them difficult to understand. One way to begin is to find a metaphor or image that describes their characteristics. Morgan (1997) suggested using animals or other familiar images to describe an organization. For example, an aggressive organization that crushes its competitors is similar to a bull elephant, whereas a timid organization in danger of being crushed by that bull elephant is similar to a mouse. Using a different kind of image, an organization adrift without a clear idea of its future in a time of crisis could be described as a rudderless boat on a stormy sea, whereas an organization with its sights set clearly on exterminating its competition could be described as a guided missile. Regardless of the image, organizations are dynamic in that they are adaptive, interconnected, and affected by the external environment and internal factors (Institute of Medicine [IOM], 2001).

Organizational Culture

People seek stability, consistency, and meaning in their work. An organizational culture is an enduring set of shared values, beliefs, and assumptions (Cameron & Quinn, 2006). It is taught (often indirectly) to new employees as the "right way" or "our way" to provide care and relate to one another. As with the cultures of societies and communities, it is easy to observe the superficial aspects of an organization's culture, but much of it remains hidden from the casual observer. Perera and Peiro (2012) note that "the real values of an organization are those that actually govern its behavior and decision-making processes, whether they are formally stated or not" (p. 752). Edgar Schein, a well-known scholar of organizational culture, identified three levels of organizational culture:

1. **Artifact level** Visible characteristics such as patient room layout, paint colors, lobby design, logo, directional signs, and so on
2. **Espoused beliefs** Written goals, philosophy of the organization
3. **Underlying assumptions** Unconscious but powerful beliefs and feelings, such as a commitment to cure every patient, no matter the cost (Schein, 2004)

Organizational cultures differ greatly. Some are very traditional, preserving their well-established ways of doing things even when these processes no longer work well. Others, in an attempt to be progressive, chase the newest management fad or buy the latest high-technology equipment. Some are warm, friendly, and open to new people and new ideas. Others are cold, defensive, and indifferent or even hostile to the outside world (Tappen, 2001). These very different organizational cultures have a powerful effect on employees and the people served by the organization. Organizational culture shapes people's behavior, especially their responses to each other, which is a particularly important factor in health care.

Culture of Safety

The way in which a health-care organization's operation affects the safety of both patients and staff has been a subject of much discussion. The shared values, attitudes, and behaviors that are directed to preventing or minimizing patient harm despite complex and hazardous work have been called the culture of safety (Agency for Healthcare Research and Quality [AHRQ], 2016, 2019; Vogus & Sutcliffe, 2007). Key features of an organization's safety culture include:

- Acknowledgement of the organizational risk and a commitment to consistent, safe operations
- Maintenance of a blame-free environment where errors and near misses are reported by staff without fear of reprimand or punishment
- Multidisciplinary and interprofessional collaboration to solve patient and environmental safety issues
- Commitment to providing resources necessary to address safety concerns

Other aspects important to creating a culture of safety include a vigilance in detecting and eliminating error-prone situations and an openness to questioning existing systems and to changing them to prevent errors (AHRQ, 2016; Armstrong & Laschinger, 2006; Vogus & Sutcliffe, 2007).

It is not easy to change an organization's culture. In fact, Hinshaw (2008) points out we are trying to create a culture of safety at a particularly difficult time, given the shortages of nurses and other resources within the health-care system (Connaughton & Hassinger, 2007).

Nursing shortages are credited with medical errors, higher rates of failure to rescue, and mortality rates as well as increased nurse burnout and job dissatisfaction (Haddad et al., 2022). Nurses with an increased workload caused by staffing shortages may not be well prepared or feel valued by their employer or colleagues. They may feel left out of key decisions about organizing patient care, and suffer fatigue and burnout, all of which can lead to medical error. Increased workload and stress have been found to increase adverse events by as much as 28% (Redman, 2008; Weissman et al., 2007). Clearly, organizational factors can contribute either to an increase in errors or to protecting patient safety.

Care Environments

The environment in which care is provided is closely related to patient safety. A care environment that is healthy and supportive of nurse work is essential to ensure the delivery of safe, high-quality patient care. In fact, patients face less risk of failure to rescue or death in better care environments (see Aiken et al., 2008). What constitutes a better, more supportive care environment? Collegial relationships with physicians, skilled nurse managers with high levels of leadership ability, emphasis on staff development, and quality of care are important factors (Press Ganey, 2017). Mackoff and Triolo (2008) offer a list of factors that contribute to the excellence and longevity (low turnover) of nurse managers:

- **Excellence** Always striving to be better, refusing to accept mediocrity
- **Meaningfulness** Being very clear about the purpose of the organization (serving the poor, healing the environment, protecting abused women, for example)
- **Regard** Understanding the work people do and valuing it
- **Learning and growth** Providing mentors, guidance, and opportunities to grow and develop

Identifying an Organization's Culture

The culture of an organization is intangible; you cannot see it or touch it, but you will know if you violate one of its norms. To learn about the culture of an organization when you are applying for a new position or trying to familiarize yourself with your new workplace, visit its Web site and read the mission, vision, and values. First, do the things you learn about the organization align with the things that are important to you and your practice? Can you see them in action when observing staff? An easy way to know is to ask people who are familiar with the organization or work there to describe it in a few words. For example, the vision statement for an academic medical center in California is "to heal humankind, one patient at a time, by improving health, alleviating suffering, and delivering acts of kindness" (UCLA Health, 2009). Entering the lobby of UCLA Health, what would you expect to see that would convey that staff are committed to this vision? Asking staff about workloads, their participation in decision making, and examples of nursing's role in ensuring patient safety and good nursing care are ways that you could learn more about them.

Does it matter in what type of organization you work? The answer, emphatically, is yes. What does the organization value? For example, the extreme value placed on "busyness" in hospitals (i.e., being seen doing something at all times) can lead to manager actions such as floating a staff member to a "busier" unit if that individual is found reading a new research study or looking up information on the Internet (Scott-Findley & Golden-Biddle, 2005). Even more important, a hospital or skilled nursing facility with a positive, supportive work environment is not only a better place for nurses to work but also safer for patients, whereas an organization that ignores threats to patient safety endangers both its staff and those who receive their care.

Once you have grasped the totality of an organization in terms of its overall culture, you are ready to analyze it in a little more detail, particularly its goals, structure, and processes.

Organizational Goals

Try answering the following question:

Question Every health-care organization has just one goal, which is to keep people healthy, restore them to health, or assist them in dying as comfortably as possible, correct?

Answer The statement is only partially correct. Most health-care organizations have a mission statement similar to this but also have several other goals, not all of which are directed to providing excellent patient care.

Does this answer surprise you? What other goals might a health-care organization have? Following are some examples:

■ **Survival** Organizations have to maintain their own existence. Many health-care organizations are cash-strapped, causing them to limit hiring, streamline work, and reduce costs, putting enormous pressure on their staff (Roark, 2005). The survival goal is threatened when reimbursements are reduced, competition increases, the organization fails to meet standards, or patients are unable to pay their bills (Trinh & O'Connor, 2002).

■ **Growth** Chief executive officers (CEOs) typically want their organizations to grow by expanding into new territories, adding new services, and bringing in new patients.

■ **Profit** For-profit organizations are expected to return some profit to their owners. Not-for-profit organizations, however, have to be able to pay their bills to avoid falling into debt while continuing to maintain and purchase high-cost pharmaceuticals, medical equipment, and supplies. This is sometimes difficult to accomplish.

■ **Status** Many CEOs also want their health-care organization to be known as the best in its field, for example, by having the best transplant unit, having the shortest wait time in the ED, having world-renowned physicians, providing "the best nursing care in the community" (Frusti et al., 2003), providing gourmet meals, or having the most attractive birthing rooms in town.

■ **Dominance** Some organizations also want to drive others out of the health-care business or acquire them, surpassing the goal of survival and moving toward dominance of a particular market by driving out the competition.

Problems can arise if the mission statement of a health-care organization is not well aligned (i.e., in agreement) with the day-to-day actions of its leaders. This disconnect can reduce morale, lead to gaps in the quality of care provided, and tarnish its image in the community (Nelson, 2013). The disconnect between these goals may have profound effects on every one of the organization's employees, nurses included. For example, return to the story of Hazel Rivera. Why did she receive a less favorable rating than her friend Carla?

After comparing ratings with those of her friend Carla, Hazel asked for a meeting with her nurse manager to discuss her evaluation. The nurse manager explained the rating: Hazel's care plans were very well done, and the nurse manager genuinely appreciated Hazel's efforts to make them so. The problem was twofold. First, Hazel was unable to complete her work within her shift, which made the manager question Hazel's time management skills. Second, because her care planning extended into the next shift, she had to be paid overtime for this work according to the union contract, which reduced salary dollars that the nurse manager would have available when the patient care load was especially high. "The corporation is very strict about staying within the budget," she said. "In fact, my rating is higher when I don't use up all of my budgeted overtime hours." When Hazel asked what she could do to improve her rating, the nurse manager offered to help her streamline the care plans and manage her time better so that the care plans could be done during her shift.

Staff nurses can contribute to the accomplishment of organizational goals. This begins with recognition that there is a *connection* between the work they do and achievement of the organization's goals. An example would be to reduce unplanned readmissions of recently discharged patients. To contribute to achieving this goal, nurses can include patients and their families in discharge planning and patient education to better prepare patients to care for themselves when they go home. This is a *specific action* to be taken, a change in practice that nurses can integrate into patient care. Monthly *reports* on changes in the rate of unplanned hospital readmissions provide information about the progress made toward achieving the goal. *Recognition* of this progress motivates them to continue these efforts (Berkow et al., 2012).

Structure

The Traditional Approach

Almost all health-care organizations have a hierarchical structure of some kind (Box 9-1). In a traditional hierarchical structure, employees are ranked from the top to the bottom, as if they were on the steps of a ladder (Fig. 9.1). The number of people on the bottom rungs of the ladder is almost always much greater than the number at the top. The president or CEO is usually at the top of this ladder, whereas the housekeeping and maintenance crews are usually at the bottom. Nurses fall somewhere in the middle of most health-care organizations, higher than the cleaning people,

aides, and technicians; parallel with therapists; but lower than physicians and administrators. The organizational structure of a small ambulatory care center in a horizontal form is illustrated in Figure 9.2.

The people at the top of the ladder have authority to issue orders, spend the organization's money, and hire and fire people. Much of this authority is delegated to people below them, but they retain the right to reverse a decision or regain control of these activities whenever they deem necessary.

The people at the bottom have little authority but do have other sources of power. They usually play no part in deciding how money is spent or who will be hired or fired but are responsible for carrying out the directions issued by people above them on the ladder. Their primary source of power is the importance of the work they do: If there was no one at the bottom, most of the work would not get done.

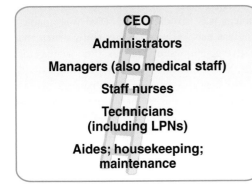

Figure 9.1 The organizational ladder.

CEO

Administrators

Managers (also medical staff)

Staff nurses

Technicians (including LPNs)

Aides; housekeeping; maintenance

---

box 9-1

What Is a Bureaucracy?

Although it seems as if everyone complains about "the bureaucracy," not everyone is clear about what a bureaucracy really is. Max Weber defined a *bureaucratic organization* as having the following characteristics:

- **Division of labor** Specific parts of the job to be done are assigned to different individuals or groups. For example, nurses, physicians, therapists, dietitians, and social workers all provide portions of the health care needed by an individual.
- **Hierarchy** All employees are organized and ranked according to their level of authority within the organization. For example, administrators and directors are at the top of most hospital hierarchies, whereas aides and maintenance workers are at the bottom.
- **Rules and regulations** Acceptable and unacceptable behavior and the proper way to carry out various tasks are defined, often in writing. For example, procedure books, policy manuals, bylaws, statements, and memos prescribe many types of behavior, from acceptable isolation techniques to vacation policies.
- **Emphasis on technical competence** People with certain skills and knowledge are hired to carry out specific parts of the total work of the organization. For example, a community mental health center has psychiatrists, social workers, and nurses to provide different kinds of therapies and clerical staff to do the typing and filing.

Some bureaucracy is characteristic of the formal operation of every organization, even the most deliberately informal, because it promotes smooth operations within a large and complex group of people.

Source: Etzioni, A. (1964). Modern organizations. Prentice-Hall, Englewood Cliffs, NJ. Adapted from Chapter 5.

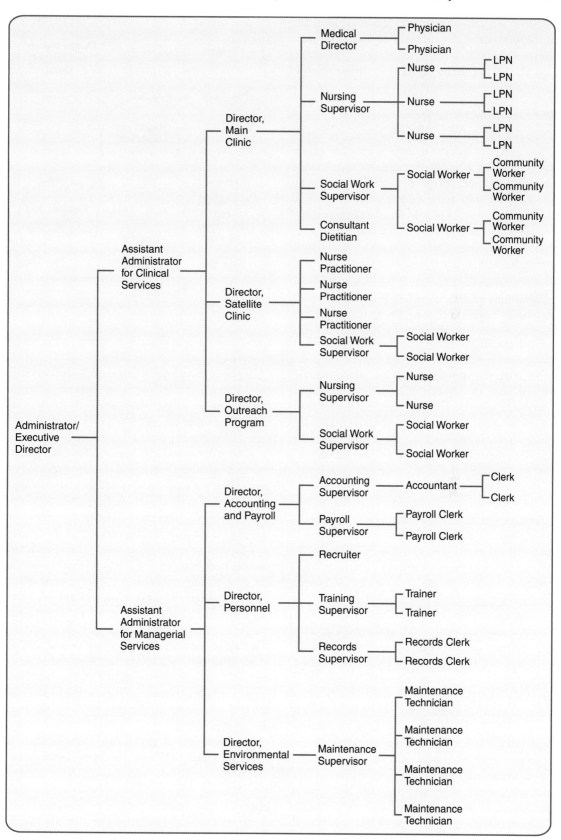

Figure 9.2 Table of organization of an ambulatory care center. *Source: Adapted from DelBueno, D. J. (1987). An organizational checklist. Journal of Nursing Administration, 17(5), 30–33. https://doi.org/10.1097/00005110-198705000-00008*

Some amount of bureaucracy is characteristic of the formal operation of every organization, even the most deliberately informal, because it promotes smooth and consistent operations within a large and complex group of people.

More Innovative Structures

There is much interest in restructuring organizations, not only to save money but also to make the best use of a health-care organization's most valuable resource, its people. This begins with knowing the jobs those people need to do and then hiring the right people. Leaders may involve frontline nurses and staff in the interview process to gain different perspectives on a candidate's strengths and a better understanding of their philosophy on patient care and nursing practice. Organizations must be sure to provide their employees with the resources they need to function, which includes the kind of leadership that can inspire the staff and unleash their creativity (Krout, 2021; Rosen, 1996).

Increasingly, people recognize that organizations need to be both efficient and adaptable. Organizations need to be prepared for uncertainty, for rapid changes in their environment, and for quick, creative responses to these challenges. In addition, they need to provide an internal climate that not only allows but also motivates employees to work to the best of their ability.

Innovative organizations have adapted an increasingly *organic* structure that is more dynamic, more flexible, and less centralized than the static traditional hierarchical structure (Yourstone & Smith, 2002). In these organically structured organizations, many decisions are made by the people who will implement them, not by their bosses.

The organic network emphasizes increased flexibility of the organizational structure (Fig. 9.3), decentralized decision making, and autonomy for working groups and teams. Rigid unit structures are reorganized into autonomous teams that consist of key stakeholders made up of professionals from different departments and disciplines. Each team is given a specific task or function (e.g., an intravenous team, a hospital infection control team, and a child protection team in a community agency). The teams are responsible for their own self-correction and self-control, although they may also have a designated leader. Together, team members make decisions about work assignments and how to deal

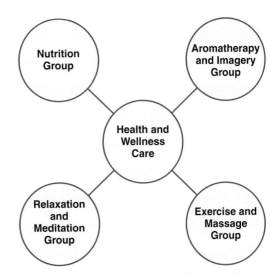

Figure 9.3 An organic organizational structure for a nontraditional wellness center. *Source: Based on Morgan, A.(1993). Imaginization: The art of creative management. Sage.*

with problems that arise. In other words, the teams supervise and manage themselves.

Supervisors, administrators, and support staff have different functions in an organic network. Instead of spending their time directing and controlling other people's work, they become planners and resource people. They are responsible for providing the conditions required for the optimal functioning of the teams, and they are expected to ensure that the support, information, materials, and funds needed to do the job well are available to the teams. They will oftentimes describe themselves as responsible for removing barriers so that teams may stay focused on the work at hand. They also act as coordinators between the teams so that the teams are cooperating rather than blocking each other, working toward the same goals, and not duplicating effort. The story of the critical care department staff is an example of a manager's effort to involve the staff in improving care delivery on the unit. It is important for the manager to help the team ensure that changes recommended at the unit level are aligned with the goals of the organization. How could this manager have better prepared the staff during their work?

The structure of health-care organizations is changing rapidly. For example, many formerly independent organizations are considering joining together into accountable care organizations that provide a continuum of care, from primary care to inpatient care and long-term care, for the people they serve. The goal is to provide the best-quality care by eliminating redundancies and keeping costs under control (Evans, 2013).

Processes

Organizations have formal processes for getting things done and informal ways to get around the formal processes (Perrow, 1969). The *formal* processes are the written policies and procedures present in all health-care organizations. The *informal* processes are not written and often not discussed. They exist in organizations as a kind of "shadow" organization that is harder to see but equally important to recognize and understand (Purser & Cabana, 1999).

The informal route is often much simpler and faster to use than the formal one. Because the informal ways of getting things done are seldom discussed (and certainly not a part of a new employee's orientation), it may take some time for you to figure out what they are and how to use them. Once you know they exist, they may be easier for you to identify. The following is an example:

Jocylene noticed that Harold seemed to get STAT x-rays done on his patients faster than she did. At lunch one day, Jocylene asked Harold why that happened. "That's easy," he said. "The people in x-ray feel unappreciated. I always tell them how helpful they are. Also, if you call and let them know that the patients are coming, they will get to them faster." Harold has just explained an informal process to Jocylene.

Here is another example:

Community Hospital recently installed a new electronic health record (EHR) system. Both the laboratory and the ED already had computerized record systems, but these old systems did not interface with the new hospital-wide system. Eventually, they would transition to the new system as well, but in the meantime, they had to continue sharing information across departments. To do this, they created "workarounds," going back to paper reports that had to be sent to nursing units (Clancey, 2010). Although Community Hospital was officially paperless, the informal system had to develop a workaround during the transition to a hospital-wide EHR.

Sometimes, people are unwilling to discuss the informal processes. However, careful observation of the most experienced "system-wise" individuals in an organization will eventually reveal these processes. This will help you do things as efficiently as they do.

A word of caution, however: Sometimes workarounds are the result of a systems problem that has been overlooked or not escalated to a department or leader who can facilitate a necessary change. Leaving a workaround in place might not be the best thing to do, especially if it could lead to an error. Recognizing them and socializing them with your colleagues and supervisors is important.

Power

There are times when one's attempts to influence others are overwhelmed by other forces or individuals. Where does this power come from? Who has it? Who does not?

In the earlier section on hierarchy, it was noted that although people at the top of the hierarchy have most of the *authority* in the organization, they do not necessarily have all of the *power*. In fact, the people at the bottom of the hierarchy also have some sources of power. This section explains how this can be true. First, power is defined, and then the sources of power available to people on the lower rungs of the ladder are considered.

Definition

Power is the ability or capacity to influence other people despite their resistance. Using power, one person or group can impose its will on another person or group (Haslam, 2001). The use of power can be positive, as when the nurse manager gives a staff member an extra day off in exchange for working an extra weekend, or negative, as when a nurse administrator transfers a "bothersome" staff nurse to another unit after that staff nurse pointed out a physician error (Sepasi et al., 2016).

Sources

Isosaari (2011) calls organizations "systems of power" (p. 385). There are numerous sources of power; many of them are readily available to nurses, but some of them are not. The following is a list derived primarily from the work of French, Raven, and Etzioni (Barraclough & Stewart, 1992; Isosaari, 2011):

- **Authority** The power granted to an individual or a group to control resources and decision making by virtue of position within the organizational hierarchy
- **Reward** The promise of money, goods, services, recognition, or other benefits
- **Control of information** The special knowledge an individual is believed to possess; as Sir Francis Bacon said, "Knowledge is power" (Bacon, 1597, quoted in Fitton, 1997, p. 150)
- **Coercion** The threat of pain or of some type of harm, which may be physical, economic, or psychological

Power at Lower Levels of the Hierarchy

There is power at the bottom of the organizational ladder as well as at the top. Patients also have sources of power (Bradbury-Jones et al., 2007). Various groups of people in a health-care organization have different types of power available to them:

- *Managers* are able to reward people with salary increases, promotions, and recognition. They can also cause economic or psychological pain for the people who work for them, particularly through their authority to evaluate and fire people but also through the way they make assignments, grant days off, and so on.
- Considerable power regarding health-care decisions is associated with health-care professionals: Their guidance is not often questioned by *patients* (Fredericks et al., 2012). The patient-centered care movement is directed to redistributing this power, involving patients and their families in decisions about their health care. For the most part, patients have not exerted the potential power that they possess. If patients refused to use the services of a particular organization, that organization would eventually cease to exist. Although patients can reward health-care workers by praising them to their supervisors, they can also cause problems by complaining about them.
- *Assistants and technicians* may also appear to be relatively powerless because of their low positions in the hierarchy. Imagine, however, how the work of the organization (e.g., hospital, nursing home) would be impeded if all the nursing aides failed to appear one morning.

- *Registered nurses* have expert power and authority regarding licensed practical nurses, aides, and other personnel by virtue of their position in the hierarchy. They are critical to the operation of most health-care organizations and could cause considerable trouble if they refused to work or withhold their expertise, which presents another source of nurse power.

Fralic (2000) offered a good example of the power of information that nurses have always had: Florence Nightingale showed very graphically in the 1800s that far fewer wounded soldiers died when her nurses were present, and many more died when they were not. Think of the power of that information. Immediately, people were saying, "What would you like, Miss Nightingale? Would you like more money? Would you like a school of nursing? What else can we do for you?" She had solid data, she knew how to collect it, and she knew how to interpret and distribute it in terms of things that people valued (p. 340).

Empowering Nurses

This final section looks at several ways in which nurses, either individually or collectively, can maximize their power and increase their feelings of empowerment.

Power is the actual or potential ability to "recognize one's will even against the resistance of others," according to Max Weber (quoted in Mondros & Wilson, 1994, p. 5). *Empowerment* is a psychological state, a feeling of competence, control, and entitlement. Given these definitions, it is possible to be powerful and yet not feel empowered. *Power* refers to ability, whereas *empowerment* refers to feelings. Both are of importance to nursing leaders and managers.

Feeling empowered includes the following:

- **Self-determination** Feeling free to decide how to do your work
- **Meaning** Caring about your work, enjoying it, and taking it seriously
- **Competence** Confidence in your ability to do your work well
- **Impact** Feeling that people listen to your ideas, that you can make a difference (Spreitzer & Quinn, 2001)

The following contribute to nurse empowerment:

- **Decision making** Control of nursing practice within an organization

- **Autonomy** Ability to act on the basis of one's knowledge and experience (Manojlovich, 2007)
- **Manageable workload** Reasonable work assignments
- **Reward and recognition** Appreciation, both tangible (raises, bonuses) and intangible (praise), received for a job well done
- **Fairness** Consistent, equitable treatment of all staff (Spence & Laschinger, 2005)

The opposite of empowerment is *disempowerment*. Inability to control one's own practice leads to frustration and sometimes failure. Work overload and lack of meaning, recognition, or reward produce emotional exhaustion and burnout (Spence & Laschinger, 2005). Nurses, similar to most people, want to have some power and to feel empowered. They want to be heard, to be recognized, to be valued, and to be respected. They do not want to feel unimportant or insignificant to society or to the organization in which they work.

Participation in Decision Making

The amount of power available to or exercised by a given group (e.g., nurses) *within* an organization can vary considerably from one organization to the next. Three sources of power are particularly important in health-care organizations:

- **Resources** The money, materials, and human help needed to accomplish the work
- **Support** Authority to take action without having to obtain permission
- **Information** Patient care expertise and knowledge about the organization's goals and activities of other departments

In addition, nurses also need access to *opportunities*: opportunities to be involved in decision making, to be involved in vital functions of the organization, to grow professionally, and to move up the organizational ladder (Sabiston & Laschinger, 1995). Without these, employees cannot be empowered (Bradford & Cohen, 1998). Nurses who are part-time, temporary, or contract employees are less likely to feel empowered than full-time permanent employees, who generally feel more secure in their positions and connected to the organization (Kuokkanen & Katajisto, 2003). Managers and higher-level administrators can take actions to empower nursing staff by providing these opportunities.

Nursing Professional (Shared) Governance

Nursing practice councils are an effective, although not simple, way to share decision making (Brody et al., 2012). "Professional or shared governance is a nursing practice model designed to ensure staff nurse participation in decision-making related to their professional practice and the delivery of nursing care. This structure includes everything from unit-based practice to health system-wide councils which include Professional Development, Quality, Practice, and Executive or Coordinating Councils." (Porter O-Grady & Malloch, 2016). These councils set standards for patient safety, diversity, staffing, career ladders, evaluations, promotion, and similar items. In many cases, the adoption of a shared governance model requires a change in the organization (Currie & Loftus-Hills, 2002; Moore & Wells, 2010).

Genuine sharing of decision making can be difficult to accomplish in some organizations, partly because managers are reluctant to relinquish control or to trust their staff members to make wise decisions. Yet Hess (2017) reminds us that "nursing shared governance is an organizational innovation invented by nurse managers that gives staff nurses legitimate control over their practice and extends their influence into areas previously controlled by managers" (p. 1). Having some control regarding one's work and the ability to influence decisions are essential to empowerment (Manojlovich & Laschinger, 2002). Thus, genuine empowerment of the nursing staff cannot occur without this sharing. For example, if staff members cannot control the budget for their unit, they cannot implement a decision to replace aides with registered nurses without approval from higher-level management. If they want increased autonomy in decision making about the care of individual patients, they cannot do so if opposition by another group, such as physicians, is given greater credence by the organization's administration.

Return to the example of the staff of the critical care department. Why did the vice president for nursing tell the nurse manager that the plan would not be implemented?

Actually, the vice president for nursing thought the plan had some merit. She believed that the proposal to create a geriatric intensive care unit could save money, provide a higher quality of patient care, and result in increased nursing staff satisfaction. However, the critical care department was the centerpiece of the hospital's agreement with a nearby medical school. In this agreement, the medical school provided the services of highly skilled intensivists in return for the learning opportunities afforded their students. In its present form, the nurses' plan would not allow sufficient autonomy for the medical students, a situation that would not be acceptable to the medical school. The vice president knew that the board of trustees of the hospital believed their affiliation with the medical school brought a great deal of prestige to the organization and that they would not allow anything to interfere with this relationship.

"If shared governance were in place here, I think we could implement this or a similar model of care," she told the nurse manager.

"How would that work?" she asked.

"If we had shared governance, the nursing practice council would review the plan and, if they approved it, forward it to a similar medical practice council. Then committees from both councils would work together to figure out a way for this to benefit everyone. It wouldn't necessarily be easy to do, but it could be done if we had real collegiality and agreement between the professions. I have been working toward this model but haven't convinced the rest of the administration to put it into practice yet. Perhaps we could bring this up at the next nursing executive meeting. I think it is time I shared my ideas on this subject with the rest of the nursing staff."

In this case, the organizational goals and processes existing at the time the nurses developed their proposal did not support their idea. However, the vice president could see a way for it to be accomplished in the future. Implementation of genuine shared governance would make it possible for the critical care nurses to accomplish their goal.

Professional Organizations

Although the purposes of the American Nurses Association (ANA) and other professional organizations are discussed in Chapter 15, these organizations are considered here specifically in terms of how they can empower nurses.

A collective voice, expressed through these organizations, can be stronger and is more likely to be heard than one individual voice. By joining together in professional organizations, nurses make their viewpoint known and their value recognized more widely. The power base of nursing professional organizations is derived from the number of members and their expertise in health matters.

Why there is power in numbers may need some explanation. Large numbers of active, informed members of an organization represent large numbers of potential voters to state and national legislators, most of whom wish to be remembered favorably in forthcoming elections. Large groups of people also have a "louder" voice: They can write more letters, speak to more friends and family members, make more telephone calls, and generally attract more attention than small groups can.

Professional organizations can empower nurses in several ways:

- Collegiality, the opportunity to work with peers on issues of importance to the profession
- Commitment to improving the health and well-being of the people served by the profession
- Representation at the state or province and national level when issues of importance to nursing arise
- Enhancement of nurses' competence through publications and continuing education
- Recognition of achievement through certification programs, awards, and the media

Collective Bargaining

Similar to professional organizations, collective bargaining uses the power of numbers, in this case for the purpose of equalizing the power of employees and employer, to improve working conditions, gain respect, increase job security, and have greater input into collective decisions (empowerment) and pay increases (Tappen, 2001). It can provide nurses with a stronger "voice," providing support and reducing fearfulness in speaking out about concerns (Seago et al., 2011). It also may reduce staff turnover (Porter et al., 2010; Temple et al., 2011).

When people join for a common cause, they can exert more power than when they attempt to bring about change individually. Large numbers of people have the potential to cause more psychological or economic pain to an "opponent" (the employer in the case of collective bargaining) than an individual can. For example, the resignation of one nursing assistant or one nurse may cause a temporary problem, but it is usually resolved rather quickly by hiring another individual. If 50 or 100 aides or nurses call in "sick" or resign, however, the organization can be paralyzed and will have much more difficulty replacing these essential workers. Collective bargaining takes advantage of this power in numbers.

An effective collective bargaining contract can provide considerable protection to employees. However, the downside of collective bargaining (as with most uses of coercive power) is that it may encourage conflict rather than cooperation between employees and managers, an "us" against "them" environment (Haslam, 2001). Many nurses are also concerned about the effect that going out on strike might have on their patients' welfare and on their own economic security. Most administrators and managers prefer to operate within a union-free environment (Hannigan, 1998). Others are able to develop cooperative working relationships with their collective bargaining units, finding ways to work within the restrictions of a union contract and work together toward shared goals. For example, a nursing labor management partnership, part of a hospital-wide labor management partnership, was developed at Mt. Sinai Medical Center in New York (Porter et al., 2010). The mission of this partnership was for nurses and management to work together to achieve "unprecedented excellence" in patient care and create a positive work environment (p. 273). By respecting each other's differences and searching for common ground, nursing management and nursing union leaders worked together on shared goals such as reduction of nosocomial (caused by hospitalization) pressure ulcers by 75% in 2 years.

Another example of collaboration is from Shands Jacksonville Medical Center in Jacksonville, Florida. Nursing management wanted to institute a clinical ladder whereby nurses could achieve higher pay and higher clinical levels by completing certain requirements, such as obtaining a higher degree, conducting a research study, or working on implementing an evidence-based change in practice. Because a traditional clinical ladder would conflict with the union's efforts to achieve pay equity, however, the achievements were instead rewarded with bonuses for staff that did not affect their annual salaries (Lawson et al., 2011). It was a good way to achieve a win–win outcome for all involved.

Enhancing Expertise

Most health-care professionals, including nurses, are empowered to some extent by their professional knowledge and competence. You can take steps to enhance your competence, thereby increasing your sense of empowerment (Fig. 9.4):

■ Participate in interdisciplinary team conferences and patient-centered conferences on your unit.

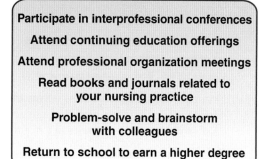

Participate in interprofessional conferences

Attend continuing education offerings

Attend professional organization meetings

Read books and journals related to your nursing practice

Problem-solve and brainstorm with colleagues

Return to school to earn a higher degree

Figure 9.4 How to increase your expert power.

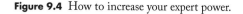

■ Participate in continuing education offerings to enhance your expertise.
■ Attend local, regional, and national conferences sponsored by relevant nursing and specialty organizations.
■ Read journals and books in your specialty area.
■ Participate in nursing research projects related to your clinical specialty area.
■ Discuss with colleagues in nursing and other disciplines how to handle a difficult clinical situation.
■ Observe the practice of experienced nurses.
■ Return to school to earn a bachelor's degree and higher degrees in nursing.

You can probably think of more, but this list at least gives you some ideas. You can also share your knowledge and experience with other people. This means not only using your knowledge to improve your own practice but also communicating what you have learned to your colleagues in nursing and other professions. It also means letting your supervisors know that you have enhanced your professional competence. You can share your knowledge with your patients, empowering them as well. You may even reach the point at which you have learned more about a particular subject than most nurses have and want to write about it for publication or as a poster submission at a local or national nursing symposium.

Conclusion

Although most nurses are employed by health-care organizations, too few have taken the time to analyze the operation of their employing health-care organization and the effect it has on their practice. Understanding organizations and the power relationships within them will increase the effectiveness of your leadership.

Study Questions

1. Describe the organizational characteristics of a facility in which you currently have a clinical assignment. Include the following: the type of organization, its organizational culture, its structure, and its formal and informal goals and processes.

2. Define power, and describe how power affects the relationships between people of different disciplines (e.g., nursing, medicine, physical therapy, housekeeping, administration, finance, social work) by citing examples in a health-care organization.

3. Discuss ways in which nurses can become more empowered. How can you use your leadership skills to do this?

Case Study to Promote Clinical Judgment

Tanya Washington will finish her associate's degree nursing program in 6 weeks. Her preferred clinical area is pediatric oncology, and she hopes to become a pediatric nurse practitioner one day. Tanya has received two job offers, both from urban hospitals with large pediatric units. Because several of her friends are already employed by these facilities, she asked them for their thoughts.

"Central Hospital is a good place to work," said one friend. "It is a dynamic, growing institution, always on the cutting edge of change. Any new idea that seems promising, Central is the first to try it. It's an exciting place to work."

"City Hospital is also a good place to work," said her other friend. "It is a strong, stable institution where traditions are valued. Any new idea must be carefully evaluated before it is adopted. It's been a pleasure to work there."

1. How would the organizational culture of each hospital affect a new graduate?

2. Which organizational culture do you think would be best for a new graduate, Central's or City's?

3. Would your answer differ if Tanya were an experienced nurse?

4. What do you need to know about Tanya before deciding which hospital would be best for her?

5. What else would you want to know about the two hospitals?

NCLEX®-Style Review Questions

1. If you are employed at a hospital owned by a corporation listed on the stock market, in which category does your facility belong?
   1. Publicly (government) supported
   2. Voluntary, not-for-profit
   3. For-profit
   4. All of the above

2. Creating a culture of safety requires organizational commitment to preventing harm. Which of the following is not a key feature of a culture of safety?
   1. Provision of adequate resources to provide care and service
   2. Use of interprofessional collaboration to solve problems and assess risk
   3. Adherence to staffing ratios
   4. Encouragement of the reporting of errors and near misses

3. Organizational culture is best defined as
   1. The stated vision and mission of an organization
   2. Policies and procedures
   3. The type of décor that was chosen for the facility
   4. An enduring set of shared values and beliefs

4. Communities and regulatory agencies continually challenge hospitals, skilled nursing facilities, and home health companies to enhance, improve, or change care delivery and the care environment to ensure safe, high-quality care. Which factors are important in improving a hospital's care environment?
   1. Adequate staffing
   2. Collegial relationships among staff
   3. Emphasis on staff development
   4. All of the above

5. Which of the following is a characteristic of a bureaucratic organization?
   1. Organic structure
   2. Flexible teams
   3. Rigid unit structures
   4. Self-correction and self-control

6. What is the best explanation of authority?
   1. It is position dependent.
   2. It is based upon the ability to lead others.
   3. It is expertise-driven.
   4. It resides primarily in the clients served.

7. There are numerous sources of power in an organization. Several are available to nurses. Which one is not?
   1. Authority
   2. Reward
   3. Control of information
   4. Coercion

8. Nurses who feel empowered can make significant contributions to a health-care organization. Feeling empowered includes feeling as if you make a difference, that colleagues value your opinion, and that your voice is important. What is essential to nurse empowerment?
   1. Belonging to a professional organization
   2. Participating on a unit practice council
   3. Having reasonable work assignments
   4. Taking part in a rewards and recognition program

9. You have been asked to serve on your unit practice council. This is an important role and one that you are excited to perform. What should you know about professional governance so that you are prepared for this work? Professional governance in nursing involves
   1. Working longer hours
   2. Attending a lot of meetings
   3. Having nurses set nursing standards for daily practice
   4. Changing the organization's culture

10. Several of your colleagues are going to join the ANA. You know the annual dues are a little more than you can afford right now, but you want to learn more. Your friends think that joining the ANA will help empower them. How do professional organizations empower nurses?
    1. They represent nurses in the political arena.
    2. They equalize power between employees and staff.
    3. They provide opportunities for promotion.
    4. They provide health insurance.

chapter 10

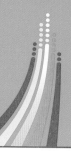

Organizations, People, and Change

When asked the theme of a nursing management conference, a top nursing executive answered, "Change, change, and more change." Whether it is called innovation, turbulence, or change, change is constant in the workplace today. Mismanaging change is common. In fact, as many as three out of four major change efforts fail (Cameron & Quinn, 2006; Hempel, 2005; Shirey, 2012), often because of resistant staff or a resistant organizational culture. This chapter discusses how people respond to change, how you can lead change, and how you can help people cope with change when it becomes difficult.

Change

A Natural Phenomenon

"Being scared by change doesn't help" (Carter, quoted by Safian, 2012, p. 97). Change is a part of everyone's lives. People have new experiences, meet new people, and learn something new. People grow up, leave home, graduate from college, begin a career, and perhaps start a family. Some of these changes are milestones, ones for which people have prepared and have anticipated for some time. Many are exciting, leading to new opportunities and challenges. Some are entirely unexpected, sometimes welcome and sometimes not. When change occurs too rapidly or demands too much, it can make people uncomfortable, or even anxious or stressed.

Macro and Micro Change

The "ever-whirling wheel of change" (Dent, 1995, p. 287) in health care seems to spin faster every year. Medicare and Medicaid cuts, large numbers of people who are uninsured or underinsured, organizational restructuring and downsizing, and staff shortages are major concerns. Increasingly diverse patient populations, rapid advances in technology, and new research findings necessitate frequent changes in nursing practice (Boyer, 2013; Cornell et al., 2010; Rodts, 2011). When first introduced, managed care had a tremendous impact on the provision of health care, and the recent legislative changes affecting the Patient Protection and Affordable Care Act (PPACA) may revolutionize health-care delivery yet again (Leonard, 2012; Webb & Marshall, 2010). Such changes sweep through the health-care system, affecting patients and caregivers alike. They are the *macro-level* (large-scale) changes that affect virtually every health-care facility.

A change may be local (confined to one nursing care unit, for example) or organization-wide. The change may be small, affecting just one specific care practice or one aspect of system operation, or sweeping, revolutionizing the structure and operation of the entire organization. Finally, the change may be implemented gradually or happen swiftly (Chreim & Williams, 2012).

A series of small-scale changes to improve care on a pediatric care unit is described by MacDavitt (2011):

> The team used a two-phase approach, designing the change in Phase I and implementing it in Phase II. One of the changes was the initiation of bedside rounding including family members if they were available. Most of the pediatricians were enthusiastic supporters. However, the pulmonologists were more resistant, agreeing to test it first with only one patient and then increasing the number by one each day. This had to begin all over again the next week when there was a new attending pulmonologist. The team persisted, patiently working through each new rotation of attending pulmonologists. Families were enthusiastic about the bedside rounds and complained if they didn't happen. This was critical to successful implementation of bedside rounds.

Change anywhere in a system creates ripples across the system (Parker & Gadbois, 2000). Every change that occurs at the system (organization or macro) level filters down to the *micro level*, to nursing units, teams, and individuals. Nurses, colleagues in other disciplines, and patients are participants in these changes. The micro level of change is the primary focus of this chapter.

New graduates may find themselves given responsibility for helping to bring about change. The following change-related activities are examples of the kinds of changes in which they might be asked to participate:

■ Introducing a new technical procedure
■ Implementing evidence-based practice guidelines
■ Contributing to discussions on new policies for staff evaluation and promotion
■ Participating in quality improvement and patient safety initiatives
■ Preparing for surveys and safety inspections

Change and the Comfort Zone

Stages of Change

The basic stages of the change process originally described by Kurt Lewin in 1951 are *unfreezing, change*, and *refreezing* (Lewin, 1951; SafeStart 2022; Schein, 2004).

- *Unfreezing* involves actions that create readiness to change.
- *Change* is the implementation phase, the actions needed to put the change into effect.
- *Refreezing* is the restabilizing phase during which the change that was made becomes a regular part of everyday functions.

Similarly, people's emotional response to a proposed change will go through several stages. The first response to a proposed change is often shock or denial, particularly when the change is seen as a disruption of the present routine. As efforts to bring about the change proceed, staff may respond with frustration, anger, and fear at times, especially if they fear losing their jobs. Eventually, they will recognize that the change is occurring or will occur and acceptance usually develops if the fear, anger, and frustration are addressed. The goal is to achieve the commitment of those who are involved in it (SafeStart, 2022).

An ideal response to change, one leaders and managers hope to achieve, is change engagement which is defined by Albrecht and colleagues (2020, p. 4) as an enduring and passionate psychological state characterized by genuine enthusiasm and willingness to support, adopt, and promote the change.

Imagine a work situation that is basically stable. People are generally accustomed to each other, have a routine for doing their work, know what to expect, and know how to deal with whatever problems arise. They are operating within their "comfort zone" (Farrell & Broude, 1987; Lapp, 2002). A change of any magnitude is likely to move people out of this comfort zone into discomfort. This move out of the comfort zone is called *unfreezing* (Fig. 10.1). For example:

Many health-care institutions offer nurses the choice of weekday or weekend work. Given these choices, nurses with school-age children are likely to find their comfort zone on weekday shifts. Imagine the discomfort they would experience if they were transferred to weekends. Such a change would rapidly unfreeze their usual routine and move them into the discomfort zone. They might have to find a new babysitter or begin a search for a new child-care center that is open on weekends. An alternative would be to establish a child-care center where they work. Yet another alternative would be to find a position that offers more suitable working hours.

Whatever alternative they chose, the nurses were being challenged to find a solution that enabled them to move into a new comfort zone. To accomplish this, they would have to find a consistent, dependable source of child care suited to their new schedule and to the needs of their children and then refreeze their situation. If they did not find a satisfactory alternative, they could remain in an unsettled state, in a discomfort zone, caught in a conflict between their personal and professional responsibilities.

As this example illustrates, what seems to be a small change can greatly disturb the people involved in it. The next section considers the many reasons why change can be unsettling and why change provokes resistance.

Resistance to Change

People resist change for a variety of reasons that vary from person to person and situation to situation. You might find that one patient-care technician is delighted with an increase in responsibility, whereas another is upset about it. Some people are eager to make changes; others prefer the status quo (Hansten & Washburn, 1999). Managers may find that one change in routine provokes a

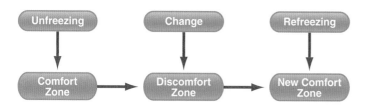

Figure 10.1 The change process. *Source: Based on Farrell, K., & Broude, C. (1987). Winning the change game: How to implement information systems with fewer headaches and bigger paybacks. Breakthrough Enterprises; and Lewin, K. (1951). Field theory in social science: Selected theoretical papers. Harper & Row.*

storm of protest and that another is hardly noticed. Why does this happen? We will first consider why people may be ready for change and why they may resist change.

Preference for Certainty

An interesting research study on nurses' preferred information-processing styles suggests that nurse managers were more receptive to change than their staff members (Kalisch, 2007). Nurse managers were found to be innovative and decisive, whereas staff nurses preferred "proven" approaches and were resistant to change. Nursing assistants, unit secretaries, and licensed practical nurses were also unreceptive to change, adding layers of people who formed a "solid wall of resistance" to change. Kalisch suggests that helping teams recognize their preference for certainty (as opposed to change) will increase their receptivity to necessary changes in the workplace.

Speaking to People's Feelings and Attitudes

Although both thinking and feeling responses to change are important, Kotter (1999) says that the heart of responses to change lies in the emotions surrounding it. He suggests that a *compelling story* will increase receptivity to change more than a carefully crafted analysis of the need for change. It is more likely to create that sense of urgency needed to stimulate change (Braungardt & Fought, 2008; Shirey, 2011). How is this done? The following are some examples of appeals to feelings:

- Instead of presenting statistics about the number of people who are readmitted because of poor discharge preparation, providing a story may be more persuasive. For example, you can tell the staff about a patient who collapsed at home the evening after discharge because he had not been able to control his diabetes post-surgery. Trying to break his fall, he fractured both wrists and needed surgical repair. With broken wrists, he is now unable to return home or take care of himself.
- Even better, videotape an interview with this man, letting him tell his story and describe the repercussions of poor preparation for discharge.
- Drama may also be achieved through visual display. A culture plate of pathogens grown from swabs of ventilator equipment and patient room furniture is more attention-getting than an

infection control report. A display of disposables with price tags attached used for just one patient is more memorable than an accounting sheet listing the costs.

- Few training programs designed to change attitudes and reduce assumptions and biases against others, whether colleagues or patients, have been demonstrated to be effective (Murrar & Brauer, 2019). Rather, using narration, whether a demonstration, recorded story, or spoken narrative, has "unique power" (Murrar & Brauer, 2019) to persuade (i.e., to reduce negative attitudes).

The purpose of these activities is to present a compelling image that will affect people emotionally, increasing their receptivity to change and moving them into a state of readiness to change (Kotter, 1999).

Sources of Resistance

Resistance to change comes from three major sources: technical concerns, relationship to personal needs, and threats to a person's position and power (Araujo Group, n.d.).

Technical Concerns

The change itself may have *design flaws*. Resistance may be based on concerns about whether the proposed change is really a good idea.

> The Professional Practice Committee of a small hospital suggested replacing a commercial mouthwash with a mixture of hydrogen peroxide and water in order to save money. A staff nurse objected to this proposed change, saying that she had read a research study several years ago that found peroxide solutions to be an irritant to the oral mucosa (Tombes & Gallucci, 1993). A later review of the research noted that this depended on the concentration used (Hossainian et al., 2011). Fortunately, the chairperson of the committee recognized that this objection was based on technical concerns and requested a thorough study of the evidence before instituting the change. "It's important to investigate the evidence supporting a proposed change thoroughly before recommending it," she said.

A change may provoke resistance for *practical* reasons. For example, if the barcodes on patients' armbands are difficult to scan, nurses may develop a way to work around this safety feature by taping a duplicate armband to the bed or to a clipboard, defeating the electronically monitored medication system (Englebright & Franklin, 2005).

Personal Needs

Change oftentimes requires individuals to take risks that may or may not be perceived as positive by others in the organization—staff and managers alike (Porter O'Grady & Malloch, 2016). Change can create anxiety, much of it related to what people fear they might lose (Berman-Rubera, 2008; Johnston, 2008). This discomfort can cause some individuals to play it safe rather than threaten their current situation. Human beings have a hierarchy of needs, from the basic physiological needs to the higher-order needs for belonging, self-esteem, and self-actualization (Fig. 10.2). Maslow (1970) observed that the more basic needs (those lower on the hierarchy) must be at least partially met before a person is motivated to seek fulfillment of the higher-order needs.

Change may make it more difficult for people to meet any or all of their needs. It may actually threaten safety and security needs. For example, if a massive downsizing occurs and a person's job is eliminated, needs ranging from having enough money to pay for food and shelter to opportunities to fulfill one's career potential are likely to be threatened.

In other cases, the threat is subtler and may be harder to anticipate. For example, an institution-wide reevaluation of the effectiveness of the advanced practice role would be a great concern to a staff nurse who is working toward accomplishing a lifelong dream of becoming an advanced practice nurse in oncology. Reorganization that reassigns some staff members to different units could challenge the belonging needs of those who leave their peers and must establish relationships on the new unit.

Perceived injustice of the change is also likely to generate resistance. If the change favors one group over another, for example, those not favored may be very resistant and morale is likely to suffer. On the other hand, a fair, just change is likely to gain support. For example, if nursing staff in the OR (operating room) have a 1-hour lunch break, staff in the recovery room having only a half hour lunch break are likely to become resentful, even if the OR nurses rarely take the full hour.

Position and Power

Once gained within an organization, status, power, and influence are hard to relinquish. This applies to people anywhere in the organization, not just those at the top. For example:

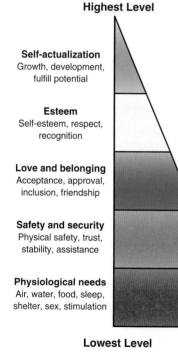

Highest Level

Self-actualization
Growth, development,
fulfill potential

Esteem
Self-esteem, respect,
recognition

Love and belonging
Acceptance, approval,
inclusion, friendship

Safety and security
Physical safety, trust,
stability, assistance

Physiological needs
Air, water, food, sleep,
shelter, sex, stimulation

Lowest Level

Figure 10.2 Maslow's hierarchy of needs. *Source: Based on Maslow, A. H. (1970). Motivation and personality. Harper & Row.*

A clerk in the surgical suite had been preparing the operating room schedule for many years. Although his supervisor was expected to review the schedule before it was posted, she rarely did so because the clerk was skillful in balancing the needs of various parties, including some very demanding surgeons. When the supervisor was transferred to another facility, her replacement decided that she had to review the schedules before they were posted because they were ultimately her responsibility. The clerk became defensive. He tried to avoid the new supervisor and posted the schedules without her approval. This surprised her. She knew the clerk did this well and did not think that her review of them would be threatening.

Why did this happen? The supervisor had not realized the importance of this task to the clerk. The opportunity to tell others when and where they could perform surgery gave the clerk a sense of importance and even a feeling of power. The supervisor's insistence on reviewing his work reduced the importance of his position. What seemed to the new supervisor to be a very small change in routine had provoked surprisingly strong resistance because it threatened the clerk's sense of importance and power.

Recognizing Resistance

Resistance may be *active* or *passive* (Heller, 1998). It is easy to recognize resistance to a change when it is expressed directly. When a person says to you, "That's not a very good idea," "I'll quit if you schedule me for the night shift," or "There's no way I'm going to do that," there is no doubt you are encountering resistance. Active resistance can take the form of outright refusal to comply, writing memos that destroy the idea, quoting existing rules that make the change difficult to implement, or encouraging others to resist.

When resistance is less direct, however, it can be difficult to recognize unless you know what to look for. Passive approaches usually involve avoidance: canceling appointments to discuss implementation of the change, being "too busy" to make the change, refusing to commit to changing, agreeing to it but doing nothing to change, and simply ignoring the entire process as much as possible (Table 10-1). Once resistance has been recognized, action can be taken to lower or even eliminate it.

Lowering Resistance

A great deal can be done to lower people's resistance to change. Strategies fall into four categories: sharing information, disconfirming currently held beliefs, providing psychological safety, and dictating (forcing) change (Tappen, 2001).

table 10-1

Resistance to Change

Active	Passive
Attacking the idea	Avoiding discussion
Refusing to change	Ignoring the change
Arguing against the change	Refusing to commit to the change
Organizing resistance of other people	Agreeing but not acting

Sharing Information

Much resistance is simply the result of misunderstanding a proposed change. Sharing information about the proposed change can be done on a one-to-one basis, in group meetings, or through written materials distributed to everyone involved via print or electronic means.

Disconfirming Currently Held Beliefs

Disconfirming current beliefs is a primary force for change (Schein, 2004). Providing evidence that what people are currently doing is inadequate, incorrect, inefficient, or unsafe can increase people's willingness to change. For example, Lindberg and Clancy (2010) note a widespread belief in the inevitability of health-care–associated infections, that they are unfortunate but unavoidable. To implement a successful campaign to reduce infection rates, this myth would have to be dispelled. The dramatic presentations described in the section on receptivity help to disconfirm current beliefs and practices. The following is a less dramatic example but still persuasive:

Jolene was a little nervous when her turn came to present information to the clinical practice committee on a new enteral feeding procedure. Committee members were very demanding: They wanted clear, evidence-based information presented in a concise manner. Opinions and generalities were not acceptable. Jolene had prepared thoroughly and had practiced her presentation at home until she could speak without referring to her notes. The presentation went well. Committee members commented on how thorough she was and on the quality of the information presented. To her disappointment, however, no action was taken on her proposal.

Returning to her unit, she shared her disappointment with the nurse manager. Together, they used the unfreezing–change–refreezing process as a guide to review the presentation. The nurse manager agreed that Jolene had thoroughly reviewed the information on enteral feeding. The problem, she explained, was that Jolene had not attended to the need to unfreeze the situation. Jolene realized that she had not given the committee a compelling reason for change. Had she put any emphasis on the high risk of contamination and resulting gastrointestinal disturbances of the procedure currently in use, they might have welcomed the need for change. Instead, she had left members of the committee still comfortable with current practice. At the next meeting, Jolene presented additional information on the risks associated with the current enteral feeding procedures. This disconfirming evidence was persuasive. The committee accepted her proposal to adopt the new, lower-risk procedure.

Without the addition of the disconfirming evidence, it is likely that Jolene's proposed change would never have been implemented. The *inertia* (tendency to remain in the same state rather than to move toward change) exhibited by the clinical practice committee is not unusual (Pearcey & Draper, 1996).

Providing Psychological Safety

As indicated earlier, a proposed change can threaten people's basic needs. Resistance can be lowered by reducing that threat, leaving people feeling more comfortable with the change. Each situation poses different kinds of threats and, therefore, requires different actions to reduce the levels of threat; the following is a list of useful strategies to increase psychological safety:

■ Express approval of people's interest in providing the best care possible.
■ Recognize the competence and skill of the people involved.
■ Provide assurance (if possible) that no one will lose their position because of the change.
■ Suggest ways in which the change can provide new opportunities and challenges (new ways to increase self-esteem and self-actualization).
■ Involve as many people as possible in the design or plan to implement change.
■ Provide opportunities for people to express their feelings and ask questions about the proposed change.
■ Allow time for practice and learning of any new procedures before a change is implemented.

Dictating Change

This is an entirely different approach to change. People in authority in an organization can simply require people to make a change in what they are doing or can reassign people to new positions (Porter-O'Grady, 1996). This may not work well if

there are ways for people to resist, however, such as in the following situations:

■ When passive resistance can undermine the change
■ When high motivational levels are necessary to make the change successful
■ When people can refuse to obey the order without negative consequences

The following is an example of an unsuccessful attempt to dictate change:

A new, as yet insecure nurse manager believed that her staff members were taking advantage of her inexperience by taking more than the two 15-minute coffee breaks allowed during an 8-hour shift. She decided that staff members would have to sign in and out for their coffee breaks and their 30-minute meal break. Staff members were outraged by this new policy. Most had been taking fewer than 15 minutes for coffee breaks or 30 minutes for lunch because of the heavy care demands of the unit. They refused to sign the coffee break sheet. When asked why they had not signed it, they replied, "I forgot," "I couldn't find it," or "I was called away before I had a chance." This organized passive resistance was sufficient to overcome the nurse manager's authority. The nurse manager decided that the coffee break sheet had been a mistake, removed it from the bulletin board, and never mentioned it again.

For people in authority, dictating a change often seems to be the easiest way to institute change: Just tell people what to do, and do not listen to any arguments. There is risk in this approach, however. Even when staff members do not resist authority-based change, overuse of dictates can lead to a passive, dependent, unmotivated, and unempowered staff. Providing high-quality patient care requires staff members who are actively engaged, motivated, and highly committed to their work.

Leading Change

Now that you understand how change can affect people and have learned some ways to lower their resistance to change, consider what is involved in taking a leadership role in successful implementation of change.

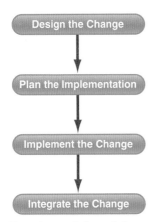

Figure 10.3 Four phases of planned change.

The entire process of bringing about change can be divided into four phases: designing the change, deciding how to implement the change, carrying out the actual implementation, and following through to ensure the change has been integrated into the regular operation of the facility (Fig. 10.3).

Designing the Change

This is the starting point. The first step in bringing about change is to craft the change carefully. Not every change is for the better: Some fail because they are poorly conceived in the first place.

Ask yourself the following questions:

- What are we trying to accomplish?
- Is the change necessary?
- Is the change technically correct?
- Will it work?
- Is this change a better way to do things?

There is rarely a time when chief nursing officers are not concerned about doing everything they can to retain their most skilled, experienced nurses. Part of the customary efforts to retain experienced staff is to conduct an exit interview whenever a skilled nurse resigns. On many occasions, the results of exit interviews are filed away without any further review and analysis, resulting in a great loss of information (Rieley, 2015). Simply learning why nurses in care facilities are leaving can provide insights into the concerns of staff and the types of changes that may provide a higher level of retention.

The lesson here is to encourage people to talk about the changes planned, to express their doubts, and to provide their input (Fullan, 2001). Those who do are usually enthusiastic supporters later in the process and less likely to be among those who resign from their positions.

Planning

All the information presented previously about sources of resistance and ways to overcome that resistance should be taken into consideration when deciding how to implement a change.

For large-scale change, it is often helpful to appoint a champion, even an additional co-champion, to lead the innovation, help staff to prepare for the change, and monitor progress (Staren et al., 2010).

The environment in which the change will take place is another factor to consider when assessing resistance to change. This includes the amount of change occurring at the same time and the past history of change in the organization. Is there goodwill toward change because it has gone well in the past? Or have other changes gone badly? Bad experiences with previous changes can generate ill will and resistance to additional change (Maurer, 2008). There may be external pressure to change because of the competitive nature of the health-care market. In other situations, government regulations may either make it difficult to bring about a desired change or may force a change.

Almost everything you have learned about effective leadership is useful in planning the implementation of change: communicating the vision, motivating people, involving people in decisions that affect them, dealing with conflict, eliciting cooperation, providing coordination, and fostering teamwork. Consider all of these when formulating a plan to implement a change. Remember that people have to move out of their comfort zone to get them ready to change.

Implementing the Change

You are finally ready to embark on a journey of change and innovation that has been carefully planned. Consider the following factors:

- **Magnitude** Is it a major change that affects almost everything people do, or is it a minor one?
- **Complexity** Is this a difficult change to make? Does it require new knowledge and skill? How much time will it take to acquire them?
- **Pace** How urgent is this change? Can it be done gradually, or must it be implemented immediately?

■ **Stress** Is this the only change that is taking place, or is it just one of many? How stressful are these changes? How can you help people keep their stress at tolerable levels?

A simple change, such as introducing a new type of thermometer, may be planned, implemented, and integrated easily into everyone's work routine. A complex change, such as redesigning the care delivery model on a unit, may require testing the new system, evaluating what works and what does not, and adapting the system before it works well in your facility.

For example, a new nurse manager, after observing staff deliver care on the unit, noticed that they were struggling to deliver care in the manner in which they were accustomed. This was because of several resignations. Staff were frustrated, and the manager was desperate to find a solution for the patients and the staff who cared for them. At the next staff meeting, the manager asked the staff to share their challenges and ideas to improve the work environment to improve care. The team identified three big dissatisfiers that were barriers to caring for their patients: (1) transporting patients off the floor for therapy delayed care, especially because some patients were not safe to leave at therapy without an aide; (2) the unit was very big, 40 beds on each of two corridors, which made assignments physically taxing; and (3) there was no continuity of care for patients from shift to shift. Brainstorming to find solutions ensued, and the team decided on three solutions: (1) replace the unit waiting area with a satellite gym so most patients would not have to leave the unit for therapy, (2) break the unit into four discrete teams, and (3) design a self-scheduling model that assigned the same staff to the same team and ensured that one person on each shift had worked the day before so that the patients always saw a familiar face. The success of this initiative was based on involving the key stakeholders, the manager's ability to present a compelling argument for the change, and the team's ownership of the change.

Some discomfort is likely to occur with almost any change, and it is important to keep it within tolerable limits. Involving the staff in the problem-solving and planning can reduce the threat of change and associated stress. You can exert some pressure to make people pay attention to the change process, but not so much pressure that they are overstressed. In other words, you want to raise the heat enough to get them moving but not so much that they boil over (Heifetz & Linsky, 2002).

Integrating the Change

This is the refreezing phase of change. After the change has been made, make sure that everyone has moved into a new comfort zone. Ask yourself:

■ Is the change well integrated into everyday operations and routines?
■ Is it working well?
■ Are people comfortable with it?
■ Is it well accepted? Is there any residual resistance that could still undermine it?

It may take some time before a change is fully integrated into everyday routines. As Kotter noted, change "sticks" when, instead of being the new way to do something, it has become "the way we always do things around here" (1999, p. 18).

Personal Change

The focus of this chapter is on leading others through the process of change. However, if you are leading change, you "have to be willing to change yourself" (Olivier, quoted by Suddath, 2012, p. 85). Choosing to change may be an important part of your development as a leader.

Hart and Waisman (2005) used the story of the caterpillar and the butterfly to illustrate personal change:

> Caterpillars cannot fly. They have to crawl or climb to find their food. Butterflies, on the other hand, can soar above an obstacle. They also have a different perspective on their world because they can fly. It is not easy to change from a caterpillar to a butterfly. Indeed, the transition (metamorphosis) may be quite uncomfortable and involves some risk. Are you ready to become a butterfly?

The process of personal change is similar to the process described throughout this chapter: first, recognize the need for change, then learn how to do things differently, and then become comfortable with the "new you" (Guthrie & King, 2004). A more detailed step-by-step process is given in Table 10-2. You might, for example, decide that you need to

table 10-2

Which Stage of Change Are You In?

While studying how smokers quit the habit, Dr. James Prochaska, a psychologist at the University of Rhode Island, developed a widely influential model of the "stages of change." What stage are you in? See if any of the following statements sound familiar.

Typical Statement	Stage	Risks
"As far as I'm concerned, I don't have any problems that need changing."	1 Precontemplation	You are in denial. You probably feel coerced by other people who are trying to make you change. But they are not going to shame you into it—their meddling will backfire.
"I guess I have faults, but there's nothing that I really need to change."	("Never")	
"I've been thinking that I wanted to change something about myself."	2 Contemplation	Feeling righteous because of your good intentions, you could stay in this stage for years. But you might respond to the emotional persuasion of a compelling leader.
"I wish I had more ideas on how to solve my problems."	("Someday")	
"I have decided to make changes in the next 2 weeks."	3 Preparation	This "rehearsal" can become your reality. Some 85% of people who need to change their behavior for health reasons never reach this stage or progress beyond it.
"I am committed to joining a fitness club by the end of the month."	("Soon")	
"Anyone can talk about changing. I'm actually doing something about it."	4 Action	It is an emotional struggle. It is important to change quickly enough to feel the short-term benefits that give a psychic lift and make it easier to stick with the change.
"I am doing okay, but I wish I was more consistent."	("Now")	
"I may need a boost right now to help me maintain the changes I've already made."	5 Maintenance	Relapse. Even though you have created a new mental pathway, the old pathway is still there in your brain, and when you are under a lot of stress, you might fall back on it.
"This has become part of my day, and I feel it when I don't follow through."	("Forever")	

Source: Adapted from Deutschman, A. (2005b). What state of change are you in? Retrieved from www.fastcompany .com/52596/which-stage-change-are-you

stop interrupting people when they speak with you. Or you might want to change your leadership style from laissez-faire to participative.

Is a small change easier to accomplish than a radical change? Perhaps not. Deutschman (2005a) reports research that suggests radical change might be easier to accomplish because the benefits are evident much more quickly.

An extreme example: On the individual level, many people could avoid a second coronary bypass or angioplasty by changing their lifestyle, yet 90% do not do so. Deutschman compares the typical advice (exercise, stop smoking, eat healthier meals) with Ornish's radical vegetarian diet (only 10% of calories from fat). After 3 years, 77% of the patients who went through this extreme change had continued these lifestyle changes. Why? Ornish suggests several reasons: (a) After several weeks, people felt a change—they could walk or have sex without pain; (b) information alone is not enough—the emotional aspect is dealt with in support groups and through meditation, relaxation, yoga, and aerobic exercise; and (c) the motivation to pursue this change is redefined—instead of focusing on fear of death, which many find too frightening, Ornish focuses on the joy of living, feeling better, and being active without pain.

A large-scale, revolutionary change from fragmented, provider-centered care to fully integrated patient-centered primary care is described by Chreim and Williams (2012). A family practice with eight physicians saw 9,000 patients a year. Some of the care they provided (well baby care, for example) overlapped with (duplicated) the public health nurses' care. To integrate care would require radical changes in the system, including electronic sharing of patient records; paying physicians per patient per year (called capitation) instead of per

table 10-3	
Five Myths About Changing Behavior: An Alternative Perspective	
Myth	**Reality**
1. Crisis is a powerful impetus for change.	Ninety percent of patients who have had coronary bypasses do not sustain changes in their unhealthy lifestyles, which worsens their heart disease and threatens their lives.
2. Change is motivated by fear.	It is too easy for people to deny the bad things that might happen to them. Compelling, positive visions of the future are a stronger inspiration for change.
3. The facts will set us free.	Our thinking is guided by narratives, not facts. When a fact does not fit people's conceptual "frames"—the metaphors used to make sense of the world—people reject the fact. Change is best inspired by emotional appeals rather than factual statements.
4. Small, gradual changes are easier to make and sustain.	Radical changes may be easier because they yield benefits quickly.
5. People cannot change because the brain becomes "hardwired" early in life.	Brains have extraordinary "plasticity," meaning that people can continue learning throughout life—assuming they remain active and engaged.

Source: Adapted from Deutschman's Fact Take: Five Myths About Changing Behavior. Deutschman, A. (2005a/May). Change or die. Fast Company, 94, 52–62.

visit; and moving physicians, nurses, and others to shared locations. After 4 years, patient satisfaction was higher and more patients received preventive services such as Pap smears or blood pressure checks. Collaboration and teamwork among providers increased. Chreim and Williams noted that there had been considerable motivation to change, and the provincial government supported the change. "What is best for the patient" (p. 227) became a shared value and motivation. There were many difficulties to overcome, including frustration with developing and learning how to use the electronic information system, deciding how to share tasks such as diabetes education, and limited physical space to co-locate care providers. Perseverance when encountering barriers and setbacks and the ability to tolerate uncertainty were essential in implementing this large-scale change successfully.

The traditional approach to change is turned on its head: A major change appears easier to accomplish than a minor change, and people are not stressed but feel better making the change. Deutschman's list of five commonly accepted myths about change that have been refuted by new insights from research summarizes this approach (Table 10-3).

It remains to be seen whether these new insights on changing behavior are useful outside of these special situations.

Conclusion

Change is an inevitable part of living and working. How people respond to change, the amount of stress it causes, and the amount of resistance it provokes can be influenced by good leadership. Handled well, most changes can become opportunities for professional growth and development rather than just additional stressors with which nurses and their clients have to cope.

Study Questions

1. Why is change inevitable? What would happen if no change at all occurred in health care?

2. Why do people resist change? Why do nursing staff members seem particularly resistant to change?

3. How can leaders overcome resistance to change?

4. Describe the process of implementing a change from beginning to end. Use an example from your clinical experience to illustrate this process.

Case Study to Promote Clinical Judgment

A large health-care corporation recently purchased a small, 50-bed rural nursing home. A new vice president of nursing was brought in to replace the former one, who had retired after 30 years. The vice president addressed the staff members at the reception held to welcome her. "My philosophy is that you cannot manage anything that you haven't measured. Everyone tells me that you have all been doing an excellent job here. With my measurement approach, we will be able to analyze everything you do and become more efficient than ever." The nursing staff members soon found out what the new vice president meant by her measurement approach. Every bath, medication, dressing change, episode of incontinence care, feeding of a resident, or trip off the unit had to be counted, and the amount of time each activity required had to be recorded. Nurse managers were required to review these data with staff members every week, questioning any time that was not accounted for. Time spent talking with families or consulting with other staff members was considered time wasted unless staff members could justify the "interruption" in their work. No one complained openly about the change, but absenteeism rates increased. Personal day and vacation time requests soared. Staff members nearing retirement crowded the tiny personnel office, overwhelming the sole benefits manager with their requests to "tell me how soon I can retire with full benefits." The vice president of nursing found that shortage of staff was becoming a serious problem and that no new applications were coming in, despite the fact that this rural area offered few good job opportunities.

1. What evidence of resistance to change can you find in this case study?

2. What kind of resistance to change did the staff members exhibit?

3. Why did staff members resist this change?

4. If you were a staff nurse at this facility, how do you think you would have reacted to this change in administration?

5. How do you think the director of nursing handled this change? What could the nurse managers and staff nurses have done to improve the situation?

6. How could the new administrator have made this change more acceptable to the staff?

NCLEX®-Style Review Questions

1. Which of the following is a macro-level change?
   1. Shift in Medicare payment policies
   2. Change in shift differentials
   3. Opening a new unit
   4. Changing visiting hours

2. Which of the following best describes what is most likely to be within a nurse's comfort zone?
   1. A new assignment
   2. Tasks the nurse has done many times
   3. Change to a different shift
   4. Addition of several new tasks

3. How can you increase your staff's receptivity to an important change in procedures?
   1. Assign the new procedure to the newest staff member.
   2. Apologize for making their work more complicated.
   3. Provide them with a booklet on preparing for change.
   4. Give them time to learn the new procedure.

4. A new nurse manager plans to implement a new scheduling process. This was met with resistance from the staff who were very happy with the current scheduling process. How can the nurse manager lower their resistance to this change?
   1. Tell the staff that their concerns about the new schedule are unfounded and plan to post the new schedule.
   2. Share information about the new schedule and discuss its impact on the unit.
   3. Post the schedule and deal with staff on an individual basis.
   4. Ask the staff to come up with an alternative for the nurse manager's consideration.

5. There has been a sudden increase in catheter-associated urinary tract infections that must be addressed on Jane's unit. What is the best way for Jane to persuade the staff to implement a new Foley catheter care protocol?
   1. Tell them the change has been ordered by the administration.
   2. Present statistics proving the need to change.
   3. Tell a compelling story about why change is needed.
   4. Explain the importance of the change in simple terms.

6. What type of resistance to a change is the hardest to overcome?
   1. The resistance that comes from inertia ("We always do it this way.")
   2. Active resistance to changing a preferred procedure
   3. Passive resistance to an unpopular change
   4. Resistance based upon fear of losing one's job

7. When is it most appropriate to dictate (order) change?
   1. When the change is very complicated
   2. In an emergency
   3. When resistance is very high
   4. If the change is unimportant

8. In which of the following situations would a personal change probably be the hardest to make?
   1. When the need is immediate
   2. If the benefits will be realized years from now
   3. When the reward is immediate
   4. If it is change that keeps you in your comfort zone

9. When designing a technical change, which of the following should be considered?
   1. Will it work better than the old way?
   2. Is this change needed?
   3. Is there a simple way to do this?
   4. All of the above

10. Which of the following is the best indication that a change has been integrated?
    1. When no one talks about it anymore
    2. If adoption occurred rapidly
    3. When resistance turns from active to passive
    4. When a full year has passed since the change was introduced

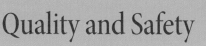

Quality and Safety

Overview

You are entering professional nursing at a time when issues pertaining to the safety and quality of care provided in the U.S. health-care system have come to the forefront of our attention. Considering the potential impact of decisions nurses make every day in managing patient care at the bedside, it may seem natural to assume that these decisions are always based on creating a safe and effective environment for every patient. Patients place their lives in nurses' hands and trust them to be knowledgeable and to use good judgment when making decisions about their care. However, this is not always the case; errors do occur, and there are times when the quality of care provided could be improved. As a registered nurse (RN), you will participate daily in activities necessary to support safety and quality initiatives at the bedside. You will also be asked to contribute to improving safety and quality in your organization and even in the health-care system. To do this, you need to understand that we work within a system, which means that whenever there is a breakdown anywhere in the system, there is risk for error. This chapter discusses health-care safety and quality, presents reasons for errors, and offers ways nurses can help to create a culture of safety to reduce errors and improve the safety and quality of the care provided.

Safety and Quality in Health Care

Safety Defined

The World Health Organization (WHO) defines safety as "the prevention of errors and adverse effects to patients associated with health care" (WHO, 2017). The Agency for Healthcare Quality (AHRQ) (Mitchell, 2008) defines it as "freedom from accidental or preventable injuries produced by medical care" (Mitchell, Ch. 1, p. 2). A health-care organization focused on safety prevents errors, learns from errors when they do occur, and promotes a culture of safety, which is covered later in this chapter (Mitchell, 2008). Hospital and skilled nursing facility safety indicators are monitored and reported regularly to assess harm prevention (Box 11-1).

Quality Defined

The Institute of Medicine (IOM) defines quality as "the degree to which health services for individuals

---

box 11-1
Hospital Patient Safety Indicators (PSI)

- Pressure ulcer rate
- Iatrogenic pneumothorax rate
- In-hospital fall with hip fracture rate
- Perioperative hemorrhage or hematoma rate
- Postoperative acute kidney injury rate
- Postoperative respiratory failure rate
- Perioperative pulmonary embolism (PE) or deep vein thrombosis (DVT) rate
- Postoperative sepsis rate
- Postoperative wound dehiscence rate
- Unrecognized abdominopelvic accidental puncture or laceration rate

Source: Agency for Healthcare Quality. (2016a). PSI 90 fact sheet. AHRQ Quality Indicators. Retrieved from http://www.qualityindicators .ahrq.gov/downloads/modules/psi/v31/psi_guide_v31.pdf

and populations increase the likelihood of desired health outcomes and are consistent with current and professional knowledge" (IOM, 2001, p. 232).

The IOM (2001) also lists the characteristics of quality health care:

1. **Safe** Avoiding injuries to patients from the care that is intended to help them
2. **Effective** Providing services based on scientific knowledge to all who could benefit and refraining from providing services to those not likely to benefit (avoiding underuse and overuse)
3. **Patient-centered** Providing care that is respectful of and responsive to individual patient preferences, needs, and values and ensuring that patient values guide all clinical decisions
4. **Timely** Reducing waits and sometimes-harmful delays for those who receive and those who give care
5. **Efficient** Avoiding waste, in particular that of equipment, supplies, ideas, and energy
6. **Equitable** Providing care that does not vary in quality because of characteristics such as gender, ethnicity, geographic location, and socioeconomic status

Safety in the U.S. Health-Care System

Patient safety is the prevention of harm caused by errors. The IOM defines errors as "the failure of a planned action to be completed as intended (e.g., error of execution) or the use of a wrong plan to achieve an aim (e.g., error of planning)" (IOM, 2000, p. 57). It is important to note that errors are usually unintentional and that not all errors lead to an adverse event causing harm or death.

In the United States, medical errors account for approximately 250,000 deaths per year (Anderson & Abrahamson, 2017; Sternberg, 2016). It is estimated that this represents less than 10% of the total errors that actually occur (Anderson & Abrahamson, 2017). These are the result of poorly coordinated care, medication errors, falls, hand-off errors, diagnostic and surgical errors, and health care-acquired (nosocomial) infections (HAI) and conditions (HAC). The Centers for Disease Control and Prevention (CDC, 2020) approximates that one in 31 patients in the United States contracts at least one infection associated with their hospitalization. The most common HAIs and HACs include adverse drug events (ADEs), bacteremia, catheter-associated urinary tract infections (CAUTI), ventilator-associated pneumonia (VAE), and surgical site infections (SSI) (CDC, 2020; Pham et al, 2012). Falls, while not as frequent as other HACs, are associated with an increase in mortality, extended lengths of stay, and a decrease in the ability of individuals to return to their previous health status (Haines et al., 2011; Oliver et al., 2010). Most falls are the result of impaired balance and mobility, unrecognized cognitive impairment, and failure of health-care personnel to institute safety measures.

The AHRQ National Scorecard on hospital-acquired conditions (2019a) trended patient safety data from 2014 to 2017. This report showed that in 2014 the average number of HACs was 99 HACs per 1,000 discharges or roughly 2,940,000 HACs among hospitalized adults. In 2017, this rate had fallen to approximately 2,550,000 HACs, which means there were 910,000 fewer HACs as compared with 2014 data. The impact on patients and hospitals has been significant as AHRQ (2019b) estimates that over 20,700 deaths were averted and roughly $7.7 billion in costs were saved between 2015 and 2017 alone.

ADEs represent the largest number of HACs. The AHRQ (2017a) indicates that 1.2 million ADEs occur annually in the United States, and as many as 50% are preventable (AHRQ, 2017a). More recently, it is estimated that one in 20 hospitalized patients experienced an ADE (AHRQ, 2019b). Although there has been a notable decrease in the number of HAIs and ADEs over the past 8 years, their impact is still significant and may result in death, increased financial costs, and extended hospital stays.

Hand-off errors involve a break in continuity of care when different providers in one care area assume responsibility of the patient (change of shift, for example) or the patient moves from one care area or care facility to another (discharge to home health, for example). These are most commonly the result of communication errors. In order to take on responsibility for the patient, adequate and accurate information has to be clearly transferred to continue to provide safe, effective care decisions (Raduma-Tomas et al., 2012; Raduma-Tomas et al., 2011).

Another significant source of error is misdiagnosis. Approximately 80,000 to 160,000 people suffer significant permanent injury or death because of diagnosis-related errors each year (Johns Hopkins Medicine, 2013). They are also the greatest source of errors in emergency departments (EDs) (T. W. Brown et al., 2010). Diagnostic errors occur more often in certain specialties such as oncology, neurology, and cardiology.

Types of Errors

The IOM report *To Err Is Human* (2000) relied on the work of Leape, Bates, and Petrycki (1993) to categorize types of errors. After categorizing the errors, Leape and colleagues concluded that 70% of all errors were preventable. Studying errors and identifying how each occurred offers data that may be used to improve safety.

- **Near miss** A near miss, sometimes called a good catch, is an error or mishap that results in no harm or very minimal patient harm (IOM, 2000, p. 87). Near misses are useful in identifying and remedying vulnerabilities in a system before more serious harm can occur. An example of a near miss is catching a medication error before the medication is administered.
- **Adverse event** An adverse event is an injury to a patient caused by the care provider rather than an underlying condition of the patient (IOM, 2000). The IOM (2000) reports have highlighted the prevalence of errors, especially preventable adverse events. Adverse events have been classified into four types (p. 36) (Box 11-2).

Risk Management, Error Identification, and Error Reporting

Risk Management

Risk management is a process of identifying, analyzing, treating, and evaluating real and potential

Four Types of Adverse Events

Diagnostic
Error or delay in diagnosis
Failure to employ indicated tests
Use of outmoded tests or therapy
Failure to act on results of monitoring or testing

Treatment
Error in the performance of an operation, procedure,
  or test
Error in administering the treatment
Error in the dose or method of using a drug
Avoidable delay in treatment or in responding to an
  abnormal test
Inappropriate (not indicated) care

Preventive
Failure to provide prophylactic treatment
Inadequate monitoring or follow-up of treatment

Other
Failure of communication
Equipment failure
Other system failure

Source: Leape, L. L., Lawthers, A. G., Brennan, T. A., & Johnson, W.
(1993). Preventing medical injury. Quality Review Bulletin, 19(5),
144–149.

hazards. Health-care organizations usually have a risk manager who ensures that adverse events, errors, and safety issues are investigated and are reported to administration and, if needed, state and federal regulatory agencies such as the Centers for Medicare and Medicaid Services (CMS) or the state department of health. As a nurse, it is your responsibility to report adverse incidents to the risk manager, according to your organization's policies and procedures. In many states, this is a legal requirement.

Error Identification

Risk events are categorized according to severity. Although all untoward events are important, not all carry results with the same severity of outcomes (Benson-Flynn, 2001).

1. **Service occurrence** A service occurrence is an unexpected occurrence that does not result in a clinically significant interruption of services and that is without apparent patient or employee injury. Examples include minor property or equipment damage, unsatisfactory provision of service at any level, or inconsequential interruption of service. Most occurrences in this category are addressed as a patient complaint process.

2. **Minor injuries** These are usually defined as needing medical intervention outside of hospital admission or physical or psychological damage.

3. **Serious incident** A serious incident results in a clinically significant interruption of therapy or service, minor injury to a patient or employee, or significant loss or damage of equipment or property.

4. **Sentinel events** A sentinel event is an unexpected occurrence involving death or serious or permanent physical or psychological injury, or the risk thereof. The phrase "or the risk thereof" includes any process variation for which a recurrence would carry a significant chance of a serious adverse outcome. Such events are called sentinel because they signal the need for immediate investigation and response. Sentinel events require immediate notification of the organization's risk manager and senior leadership. The risk manager conducts an investigation to identify the cause of the event, and changes in the organization's systems and processes are made to reduce the probability of such an event in the future (The Joint Commission [TJC], 2017b).

5. **Never events** Never events are "shocking medical errors that should never occur" (AHRQ, 2017a). These events must be reported to a state licensing agency (e.g., the Department of Public Health [DPH]) and may be submitted to TJC. They include occurrences that meet at least one of the following criteria:
   ▪ The event has resulted in an unanticipated death or major permanent loss of function that is not related to the natural course of the patient's illness or underlying condition.
   ▪ Any of the following even if the outcome was not death or major permanent loss of function: suicide of a patient in a setting where the patient receives around-the-clock care (e.g., hospital, residential treatment center, crisis stabilization center), infant abduction or discharge to the wrong family, rape, hemolytic transfusion reaction involving administration of blood or blood products having major blood group incompatibilities, or surgery on the wrong patient or wrong body part (AHRQ, 2017a).

Adhering to standards of care and exercising the amount of care that a reasonable nurse would demonstrate under the same or similar circumstances can protect the nurse from litigation. Understanding what actions to take when something goes wrong is imperative. The main goal is patient safety. Reporting and remediation must occur quickly. Nursing standards of care as well as the policies and procedures of the institution greatly decrease the nurse's risk. Common risks for nursing error include:

■ Medication errors
■ Documentation errors or omissions
■ Failure to perform nursing care or treatments correctly, which includes timeliness of care that could result in or contribute to infection
■ Errors in patient safety that result in falls
■ Failure to rescue (e.g., recognize complications and relay significant data to patients and other providers) and failure to appropriately intervene in a timely manner (Burke et al., 2022; Delamont, 2016; Kalisch et al., 2009)

Risk management also includes attention to areas of employee wellness, safety, and injury prevention. Latex allergies, repetitive stress injuries, biohazardous exposure because of needlesticks or sharps injuries, carpal tunnel syndrome, barrier protection for tuberculosis, back injuries, the rise of antibiotic-resistant organisms, and workplace violence all fall under the area of risk management.

Incident and Error Reporting

Incidents are things that occur which would be considered unexpected or abnormal. It could be an actual event or an event that was averted. Once an incident has occurred, you must complete an incident report immediately. Depending on the severity of the incident, you should notify your immediate supervisor. When in doubt, include the supervisor as they may be able to assist you with the reporting process. The incident report is used to collect and analyze data for determination of future risk and more importantly the opportunities to improve workplace and patient safety. The report should be accurate, objective, complete, and factual. If there is future litigation (a lawsuit), the plaintiff's (person with the complaint) attorney can subpoena the report. Today, most organizations have computer-based incident reporting. In the event that this is not the case, the report should be prepared in only a single copy and never placed in the medical record (Swansburg & Swansburg, 2002). It is kept with internal hospital correspondence.

Incident reports should also be used to capture near misses, which are potentially harmful errors that were not realized either because of early detection or good fortune (AHRQ, 2017a). You might think that because you or a colleague caught an error before it occurred that it doesn't need to be reported. The benefit of reporting near misses is that it allows the organization to study the event and the activities leading up to it and make policy and procedure changes that can prevent it from happening again. By taking the time to report the error that almost occurred, you may be able to help your organization prevent future patient harm.

Nurses have a responsibility to be informed and to become active participants in understanding and identifying potential risks to their patients and to themselves. Ignorance of the law is no excuse. Maintaining a knowledgeable, professional, and caring nurse–patient relationship is the first step in decreasing your own risk. Hansten and Washburn (2001) recommend that you focus attention on six steps to ensure the delivery of safe, high-quality, patient-centered care (p. 24D):

1. **Think critically** Use your creative, intuitive, logical, and analytical processes continually in working with patients and their families.
2. **Plan and report outcomes** Emphasizing results is a necessary part of managing resources in today's cost-conscious environment. Focusing on outcomes moves the nurse and other members of the interprofessional team away from tasks.
3. **Make introductory rounds** Begin each shift with the interprofessional team members introducing themselves, describing their roles, and providing patient updates.
4. **Plan in partnership with the patient** In conjunction with the introductory rounds, spend a few minutes early in the shift with each patient, discussing care objectives and long-term goals. This event becomes the center of the nursing process for the shift and ensures that the patient, nurse, and other members of the interprofessional team are working toward the same outcomes.
5. **Communicate the plan** Avoid confusion among members of the interprofessional team by communicating the intended outcomes and

the important role that each member plays in the plan.

6. **Evaluate progress** Schedule time during the shift to quickly evaluate outcomes, assess the progress of the plan, and make revisions as necessary.

Nurses are on the front line in identifying and reporting errors. In the past, individuals involved in medical errors suffered punitive consequences; thus, many errors went unreported. Providers and organizations may fear blame or punishment for mistakes or errors. This culture of blame prevents or discourages individuals from coming forward, whereas a culture of safety encourages them to come forward.

Building a Culture of Safety

To achieve safe patient care, a *culture of safety* must exist. Organizations and senior leadership must drive change to create and maintain a culture of safety—a blame-free environment in which reporting of errors is promoted and rewarded. A culture of safety promotes trust, honesty, openness, and transparency. In general, hospitals that practice a culture of safety show fewer reported cases of adverse events (Mardon et al., 2010).

When a culture of safety exists, individual providers do not fear reprisal and are not blamed for identifying or reporting errors. Health systems that fully embrace the culture of safety are committed to a journey to high reliability. Some organizations acknowledge and celebrate the results of investigating the cause of errors because the data and information help the organization learn why or how the error occurred, thus improving care and preventing harm.

Event-reporting systems hold organizations accountable and lead to improved safety. Mandatory reporting systems are operated by regulatory agencies and have a strong focus on errors associated with serious harm or death. One example is the Food and Drug Administration (FDA), which mandates the reporting of serious harm or death (adverse events) related to drugs and medical devices. Failure to report mandatory requirements may lead to fines, withdrawal of participation in clinical trials, or loss of licensure to operate.

TJC recommends that *root cause analysis (RCA)* be conducted for each sentinel event. The RCA is the process of learning from consequences; although these can be positive consequences, most

RCA deal with adverse consequences. An example of an RCA is a review of a medication error, especially one resulting in a death or severe complications. Principles of RCA include:

1. Engage the people who played a role in the event to learn the context in which the incident occurred. These key stakeholders should be led by a facilitator.
2. Determine what influenced the consequences (i.e., determine the necessary and sufficient influences that explain the nature and the magnitude of the consequences).
3. Establish tightly linked chains of influence.
4. At every level of analysis, determine the necessary and sufficient influences.
5. Whenever feasible, drill down to root causes.
6. Know that there are always multiple root causes.

The International Center for Patient Safety, developed by TJC, establishes National Patient Safety Goals each year and publishes sentinel event strategies (TJC, 2017b). These tools offer health-care organizations goals and strategies to prevent harm and death based on what has been learned from other sentinel events. An example of an RCA is the following review of a sentinel event involving a medication error that could have resulted in a death or severe complications.

A nurse working in a pediatric intensive care unit administered an intravenous blood thinner to an infant to maintain the patency of the central venous catheter. The baby was doing well until the next day when it was realized that the baby had received an accidental overdose. Instead of receiving 10 units of the medication, he had received 10,000 units. The baby survived this life-threatening ordeal, but how did this error happen?

An RCA was initiated. Key stakeholders—nurses, physicians, and other members of the health-care team directly involved with the medical error—were gathered together with a facilitator, in this case the chief medical officer. The facilitator established ground rules for the fact finding that was about to begin, stressing the confidentiality and safety of the review. This is important so that staff feel safe enough to honestly share experiences, observations, and actions without judgment or recrimination. This allows the true cause of the error to be discovered. More often than not, the cause of medical error is usually a system failure rather than a caregiver's act.

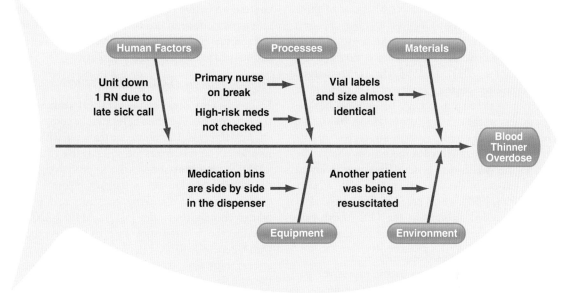

Figure 11.1 Fishbone diagram for cause-and-effect analyses.

During the RCA, the team, guided by the facilitator, listened to each team member recount personal experiences when caring for the baby. This allowed the entire team to hear the circumstances surrounding the medical error so that they might identify the true or root cause of the incident. RCA teams usually employ cause-and-effect tools to capture the relationships between variables. A fishbone diagram was used to identify the factors or causes that led to the sentinel event, which in this case was a medication overdose. Possible causes of the problem are sorted into five different categories (Fig. 11.1).

The findings from the RCA revealed that, although staffing issues may have contributed to the error, issues around medication storage and medication administration processes were root causes of the incident. The medication was stored in alphabetical order with the two different dose vials of the blood thinner stored next to each other in the medication dispenser, making it very easy to grab the wrong drug. In addition, the medication labels and packaging, except for the concentration, were almost identical.

The remedies from this analysis were far reaching. First, the hospital separated the two different vials from one another in medication dispensers hospital-wide and also notified the manufacturer about the labeling. Then, a preventative measure was put into action. Because of the life-threatening nature of this drug, the nursing staff instituted an independent double check of this medication. This practice change required two RNs to independently calculate the medication dose and compare their results; then one of them would draw up the medication, with the second nurse confirming the proper medication and dose were selected for administration to the patients. A decision was made to extend the use of this independent double check for all high-risk medications for this patient care unit, as well as across the hospital.

At no time during this process was a single person blamed for this incident. The occurrence was not caused by one person; in fact, it was caused by multiple factors that required systemic change to prevent such incidents. The staff's participation and candor allowed the organization to improve patient safety (Oz, 2009).

Quality in the Health-Care System

Issues of Safety and Quality

The drive to decrease costs and improve outcomes has increased attention to improved quality and safety. We look first at some important reports that have focused our attention on existing safety and quality concerns and suggested solutions.

The IOM, now the National Academy of Medicine (NAM), is a private, nonprofit organization chartered in 1970 by the U.S. government to provide unbiased, expert scientific advice for the purpose of improving health. Today, the NAM is one of three academies chartered by Congress to offer objective advice on matters of health, technology, and science (National Academies of Science, Engineering, and Medicine, 2021). In 1998, the IOM charged the Committee on the Quality of Health Care in America to develop a strategy to improve health-care quality in the coming decade (IOM, 2000). The committee completed a systematic review of the literature that highlighted some serious shortcomings in the health-care system. This was followed by the release of the *Statement on Quality of Care* (Donaldson, 1998), which urged health-care leaders to make needed changes in the U.S. health-care system. Consensus was reached on four areas:

1. Quality can be defined and measured.
2. Quality problems are serious and extensive.
3. Current approaches to quality improvement (QI) are inadequate.
4. There is an urgent need for rapid change.

This statement launched today's movement to improve quality and safety in the 21st century.

The IOM's work led to the series of reports that serve as the foundation for efforts to improve the quality of health care provided in the United States. Two in particular, *To Err Is Human: Building a Safer Health System* (IOM, 2000) and *Crossing the Quality Chasm: A New Health System for the 21st Century* (IOM, 2001), provide a framework upon which the 21st-century health-care system is being built.

Quality Improvement (QI)

QI has been part of nursing care since Florence Nightingale critically evaluated the care provided to wounded and ill soldiers during the Crimean War (Nightingale & Barnum, 1992). In the past, health-care organizations focused on quality assurance (QA), which is an inspection process meant to ensure that hospitals followed minimum standards of patient care quality. Activities focused on retrospective chart audits and fixing errors that are found. Little emphasis was placed on organization-wide change, system improvement, or taking a proactive approach to learn from errors; rather, it remained reactive and punitive in nature (AHRQ, 2013)

Today, QI has evolved into a framework designed to reduce variation in care by standardizing health care and medical processes and structures with the goal of improving patient, clinical, and operational outcomes (CMS, 2021). Given the continuous nature of QI and the complex and hazardous work done in health-care organizations, it is not unusual to find yourself working in an organization on a journey to high reliability.

High-Reliability Organizations (HRO)

High-reliability organizations (HRO) acknowledge the inherent risk of technologies and the complexities of care delivery and acknowledge that even with organizational controls, errors are still possible (Sutcliffe, 2011). These organizations strive to proactively identify possible weaknesses or failures before adverse events, effectively managing the risks and probabilities therein (Sutcliffe, 2011). AHRQ (2019b) describes the characteristics of a HRO as preoccupied with failure so as to avert it, reluctant to simplify processes before truly understanding them, sensitive to the complexity of systems and the importance of the context, seeking out those with the most knowledge about the work at hand, and vigilant in cross monitoring and assessment of potential threats to safety.

The goal of QI is that "All people should always experience the safest, highest quality, best value health care across all settings" (TJC, 2009). This improvement process is data-driven and dependent on teamwork. The success of teams is largely dependent on the unit's culture and the leader's ability to instill the importance of safe, high-quality care as an organizational key value. A unit-based QI team should be composed of key stakeholders who share a common purpose. This purpose may require a temporary team dedicated to solving a particular issue or a permanent team dedicated to the oversight and implementation of a quality plan for the unit (C. Brown et al., 2008).

QI involves (a) identifying areas of concern (indicators), (b) continuously collecting data on these indicators, (c) analyzing and evaluating the data, and (d) implementing needed changes. When one indicator is no longer a concern, another indicator is selected. Common safety indicators used to evaluate the quality of care include the number of falls with injuries, frequency of medication errors, incidence of skin breakdown, and infection rates. These indicators can be identified by the accrediting agency or by the facility itself. Regardless of the type of team, once an issue is identified, the structure and processes are the same (C. Brown et al., 2008):

- Identify key stakeholders.
- Collect, analyze, and evaluate data.

■ Determine the root cause or area of concern.

■ Compare and review findings with current evidence-supported best practice.

■ Design an improvement plan with an implementation timeline.

■ Monitor progress to ensure that the practice change is sustained.

The purpose of QI is to continuously improve the capability of everyone involved to provide high-quality, safe patient care. QI aims to act proactively and avoid a blaming environment, providing a path to improving the standard of care for the entire system.

Identifying opportunities for QI is everyone's responsibility. Once identified, collecting comprehensive, accurate, and representative data is the next step in the QI process. You may be asked to brainstorm your ideas with other nurses or members of the interprofessional team, complete surveys or checklists, or keep a log of your daily activities. How do you administer medications to groups of patients? What steps are involved? Are the medications always available at the right time and in the right dose, or do you have to wait for the pharmacy to bring them to the floor? Is the pharmacy technician delayed by emergency orders that must be processed? Looking

at the entire process and mapping it out on paper in the form of a flowchart may be part of the QI process for your organization (Fig. 11.2).

Health-care organizations are expected to have QI programs that promote QI strategies and an overarching plan that serves as a roadmap for high-quality care and service. This plan is typically part of an organization's multiyear strategic plan, which is shared across the system in the form of an annual quality program report, complete with goals and tactics to ensure safe, high-quality patient care. Successful strategies may address improving the culture and work environment of the organization, attracting and retaining the right staff, ensuring that QI processes are effective, and providing staff with the tools needed to do their jobs (Drewniak, 2014) (Box 11-3).

An organization's QI plan should include the following (Health Resources and Services Administration [HRSA], 2011; McLaughlin & Kaluzny, 2006):

■ QI goals linked to the organization's strategic plan
■ A quality council that includes the institution
■ Education about QI processes and tools for all levels of personnel
■ Process for identifying improvement opportunities

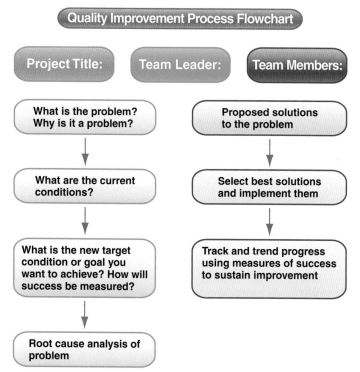

Figure 11.2 QI process.

Strategic Planning

A strategic plan is a short, visionary, conceptual document that:

- Serves as a framework for decisions or for securing support and approval
- Provides a basis for more detailed planning
- Explains the business to others in order to inform, motivate, and involve
- Assists benchmarking and performance monitoring
- Stimulates change and becomes the building block for the next plan

Source: Drewniak, R. (2014). White paper: 7 steps to healthcare strategic planning. Hayes Management Consulting. Retrieved from https://www.hayesmanagement.com/wp-content/uploads/2014/06/Whitepaper-Hayes-White-Paper_7-Steps-to-Healthcare-Strategic-Planning.pdf

- Formation of process improvement teams
- Policies that motivate and support staff participation in process improvement

Many health-care organizations use the FOCUS-PDCA model: **F**ind an opportunity to improve, **O**rganize a team, **C**larify the process, **U**nderstand the root cause, and **S**tart an improvement process (Taylor et al., 2013). The improvement process is a cyclical problem-solving process that consists of a **p**lan where the problem is identified, **d**oing or implementing the solution, **s**tudying or monitoring progress, and **a**cting on your results (Taylor et al., 2014). This creates a continuous QI process. The FOCUS-PDCA model is usually incorporated into an organization's QI plan as part of their Lean or Six Sigma performance improvement methodology. Regardless of the model used, QI provides a structured process for involving the health-care team in planning and executing a continuous flow of improvements to provide quality care (McLaughlin & Kaluzny, 2006, p. 3).

Using QI to Monitor and Evaluate Quality of Care

QI involves (a) identifying areas of concern (indicators), (b) continuously collecting data on these indicators, (c) analyzing and evaluating the data, and (d) implementing needed changes. Quality measures or indicators of quality are identified because they help us make good decisions that improve care and reduce the incidence of error or harm. QI is an ongoing activity and continues until the improvement goal has been sustained, When one indicator is no longer a concern, it is moved into a monitoring phase and another indicator is selected. Common indicators include the number of falls with injuries, frequency of medication errors, incidence of skin breakdown, and infection rates, especially those related to SSI, CAUTI, and central line-associated bloodstream (CLABSI) infections. These indicators may be selected because accrediting and licensing agencies such as TJC or the CMS have noted them as patient safety measures or they have been chosen by your organization as an patient care improvement opportunity. The purpose of QI is to continuously improve the capability of everyone involved to provide high-quality, safe patient care. QI aims to act proactively and avoid a blaming environment, providing a path to improving the entire system.

QI at the Organizational and Unit Levels

Structured Care Methodologies (SCMs)

Most agencies have tools for tracking outcomes. These tools, called structured care methodologies (SCMs), are interprofessional tools designed to "identify best practices, facilitate standardization of care, and provide a mechanism for variance tracking, quality enhancement, outcomes measurement, and outcomes research" (Cole & Houston, 1999, p. 53). SCMs include guidelines, protocols, algorithms, standards of care, and clinical pathways that identify core aspects of nursing performance and create a shared and stable set of performance indicators and benchmarks to measure outcomes (Dubois et al., 2013).

SCMs do not take the place of expert nursing judgment. The fundamental purpose of the SCM is to assist health-care providers in implementing practices identified with good clinical judgment, evidence-based interventions, and improved patient outcomes. Data from SCMs allow comparisons with outcomes, development of evidence-based decisions, identification of high-risk patients, and identification of issues and problems before they escalate into disasters. Although they sound complicated, they are actually very practical and straightforward.

- **Clinical practice guidelines** Guidelines first appeared in the 1980s as statements to assist health-care providers and patients in making appropriate health-care decisions. Guidelines are based on current research strategies and are often developed by experts in the field. The use of guidelines is seen as a way to decrease variations in practice.

- **Protocols** Protocols are specific, formal documents that outline how a procedure or intervention should be conducted. Protocols have been used for many years in research and specialty areas but have been introduced into general health care as a way to standardize approaches to achieve desired outcomes. Protocols are oftentimes tied to order sets in the electronic medical record (EMR). When a provider selects an orderset, it usually will autopopulate the protocol into the patient's record, which will initiate a prompt or nursing intervention. An example in use in many facilities is a chest pain protocol.
- **Algorithms** Algorithms are systematic procedures that follow a logical progression based on additional information or patient responses to treatment. They were originally developed in mathematics and are frequently seen in emergency medical services. Advanced cardiac life support algorithms are now widely used in health-care agencies.
- **Standards of care** Standards of care are often discipline-related and help to operationalize patient care processes and provide a baseline for quality care. Lawyers often refer to a discipline's standards of care in evaluating whether a patient has received appropriate services.

Standard work is the safest efficient and effective way to do a job. It is designed to reduce variation in care, which is a leading cause of medical error. Standard work helps people understand how care is to be delivered, which helps set clear expectations for the care team. Standard work, which comes from process improvement (PI) methods such as Lean and Six Sigma, is derived from defining best practice and should include creating the most effective way to carry out that work and then monitoring performance improvement outcomes to meet that standard (Quisenberry, 2021).

Aspects of Health Care to Evaluate

QI programs are designed to ensure the performance of safe, high-quality health care by evaluating three aspects of health care: the *structure* within which care is given, the *process* of delivering care, and the *outcomes* of that care. A comprehensive evaluation should include all three aspects (Brook et al., 1980; Donabedian, 1969, 1977, 1987). When evaluating nursing care, the independent, dependent, and interdependent functions of nurses should be added to the model (Irvine, 1998). Each of these dimensions is described here, and their interrelationship is illustrated in Table 11-1.

Structure

Structure refers to the setting in which the care is given and to the resources (human, financial, and material) that are available. The following structural aspects of a health-care organization can be evaluated:

- **Facilities** Comfort, convenience of layout, accessibility of support services, and physical safety (fire or disaster preparedness, for example)
- **Equipment** Adequate supplies, state-of-the-art equipment, and staff skilled in their use

table 11-1

Dimensions of QI in Nursing: Examples

	Independent Function	Dependent Function	Interdependent Function
Structure	Pressure ulcer risk assessment tool	Tablet access to patient puts nurse in touch with patient, who in turn texts physician.	Nursing case management model of care adopted on rehabilitation unit.
Process	Risk score and associated nursing interventions outlining preventative measures populate the EMR.	Physician immediately enters order to increase dosage of pain medication, and patient is medicated within the hour.	Nurse-led interdisciplinary team meeting engages physicians, therapists, social workers, and pharmacists to meet patient needs for discharge to home. Team determines the need for a customized wheelchair.
Patient outcome	Skin intact at discharge	Relief from pain	Patient ability to enter narrow doorway to bathroom unassisted.

Source: Adapted from Irvine, D. (1998). Finding value in nursing care: A framework for quality improvement and clinical evaluation. Nursing Economics, 16(3), 110–118.

- **Staff** Education, credentials, experience, absenteeism, turnover rate, and staff–patient ratios
- **Finances** Salaries, adequacy to operate the facility, and sources of funds

Although none of these structural factors alone can guarantee quality care, they make good care more likely. A larger number of nurses each shift and a higher proportion of RNs are associated with shorter lengths of stay; higher proportions of RNs are also related to fewer adverse patient outcomes (Lichtig et al., 1999; Rogers et al., 2004).

Process

Process refers to the activities carried out by the health-care providers and all the decisions made while a patient is interacting with the organization (Jones, 2016). Examples include:

- Scheduling an appointment
- Conducting a physical assessment
- Ordering an x-ray or magnetic resonance imaging (MRI) scan
- Administering a blood transfusion
- Completing a home environment assessment
- Preparing the patient for discharge
- Telephoning the patient postdischarge

Each of these processes can be evaluated in terms of timeliness, appropriateness, accuracy, and completeness (Irvine, 1998). Process variables include psychosocial interventions such as teaching and counseling, as well as physical care measures. Process also includes leadership activities such as interprofessional team conferences. When process data are collected, a set of objectives, procedures, or guidelines is needed to serve as a standard or gauge against which to compare the activities. This set can be highly specific, such as listing all the steps in a catheterization procedure, or it can be a list of objectives, such as offering information on breastfeeding to all expectant parents or conducting weekly staff meetings.

Outcome

An *outcome* is the result of all the health-care providers' activities. Outcome measures evaluate the effectiveness of nursing activities by answering such questions as: Did the patient recover? Is the family more independent now? Has team functioning improved? Outcome standards address indicators such as physical and mental health; social and physical function; health attitudes, knowledge, and behavior;

utilization of services; and customer satisfaction. Research on outcomes can guide the formation of the best strategies for the delivery of safe, effective, and quality patient care (Patient-Centered Outcomes Research Institute [PCORI], 2012).

The outcome questions asked during an evaluation should address observable behavior, such as the following:

- **Patient** Wound healed, blood pressure within normal limits, infection absent
- **Family** Increased time between visits to the ED, applied for food stamps
- **Team** Decisions reached by consensus, attendance at meetings by all team members

Some of these outcomes, such as blood pressure or time between ED visits, are easier to measure than other, equally important outcomes such as patient-reported outcomes; for example, increased patient or nurse satisfaction with care or changes in attitude. Although the latter cannot be measured as precisely, it is important to include the full spectrum of biological, psychological, and social aspects (Hostetter & Klein, 2012). For this reason, considerable effort has been put into identifying the patient outcomes that are affected by the quality of nursing care.

There is considerable evidence that patient care outcomes can be improved by employing a better-educated nursing workforce (Benner et al., 2010). The IOM *Future of Nursing* report (2011) recommended increasing "the proportion of nurses with a BSN to 80% by 2020" and challenges health-care organizations to encourage and support associate degree nurses (ADNs) in their pursuit of advancing their education (p. 3). This recommendation does not negate the value of the ADN. Instead, it promotes the concept of lifelong learning and the need to continue one's education. In 2021, the National Academies of Science, Engineering, and Medicine released the NAM *Future of Nursing 2020–2030* (2021), which furthers the importance of nurses "practicing to the full extent of their education and training" (p. 2). This report recommends that nurses expand their education and practice to include incorporating social determinants of health and taking steps to achieve health equity (National Academies of Science, Engineering, and Medicine, 2021).

A major challenge in using and interpreting outcome measures is that outcomes are influenced by many factors. For example, the outcome of patient teaching done by a nurse on a home visit is affected by the patient's interest and ability to learn, social determinants of health, the quality of the teaching materials, the presence or absence of family support, information from other caregivers (which may conflict), and the environment in which the teaching is done. If the teaching is successful, can the nurse be given full credit for the success? If it is not successful, who has failed?

In order to determine why an intervention such as patient teaching succeeds or fails, it is necessary to evaluate the factors contributing to the teaching moment, the actual teaching process, and the outcome of the nurse–patient interaction. A comprehensive evaluation includes all three aspects: structure, process, and outcome.

Organizations, Agencies, and Initiatives Supporting Quality and Safety in the Health-Care System

The ongoing movement to improve quality and safety has led to the development of several governmental and private organizations that monitor, evaluate, accredit, influence, research, finance, and advocate for quality in the health delivery system.

Government Agencies

Federal- and state-level government agencies provide tools and resources for improving quality and safety within the U.S. health-care system. They also oversee regulation, licensure, and both mandatory and voluntary reporting programs. The U.S. Department of Health and Human Services (HHS) is the principal agency for protecting the health of all Americans and providing essential human services, including health care (HHS, 2018). HHS works closely with state and local governments to meet the nation's health and human needs. HHS also administers the CMS and the Medicare Quality Improvement Organization (QIO) program. The QIO was created in 1982 to monitor the quality and efficiency of care and services delivered to its beneficiaries. Current initiatives include:

- **MedQIC** This initiative aims to ensure that each Medicare recipient receives the appropriate level of care. MedQIC is a community-based QI program that provides tools and resources to encourage changes in processes, structures, and behaviors within the health-care community.
- **Post-acute care reform plan** CMS is examining post-acute care transfers, to places such as skilled nursing facilities, rehabilitation centers, or long-term acute care hospitals with the aim of reducing care fragmentation and unsafe transitions of care.
- **Development of quality indicators for inpatient rehabilitation facilities (IRFs)** The goal of this initiative is to develop quality measures for inpatient rehabilitation services, including expected outcomes for Medicare beneficiaries in IRFs.
- **Hospital quality initiative** This is a major initiative aimed at improving the quality of care at the provider and organization level using a uniform set of quality measurements by which consumers can compare organizations and by which organizations can benchmark progress. Organizations provide data to CMS through public reporting of quality measures. These data feed the *Hospital Compare* Web site (www.hospitalcompare.hhs.gov). Organizations are incentivized to participate with an offering of increased reimbursement.

The AHRQ is the lead federal agency charged with improving the quality, safety, efficiency, and effectiveness of health care for all Americans (AHRQ, 2016b). Initiatives currently under way include:

Health IT (AHRQ, 2017b) A multifaceted initiative that includes (a) $260 million in grants and contracts to support and stimulate investment in health information technology (IT); (b) the newly created AHRQ National Resource Center, which provides technical assistance and research funding to aid technology implementation within communities; and (c) learning laboratories at more than 100 hospitals nationwide to develop and test health IT applications.

National Quality Measures Clearinghouse (NQMC) A Web-accessible database providing access to evidence-based quality measures and measure sets. NQMC provides access for obtaining detailed information on quality measures and to further their dissemination, implementation, and use in order to inform health-care decisions.

AHRQ quality indicators Set of quality indicators used by organizations to highlight potential quality concerns, identify areas that need further study and investigation, and track changes in these indicators through time.

Health-Care Provider Professional Organizations

Professional organizations directly address concerns regarding the quality and safety of the professionals they represent. Each organization offers programs, access to evidence-based practices, toolkits, and newsletters to aid their members in driving quality within their own practice and organization. Key organizations for nursing include the American Nurses Association (ANA) and specialty nursing associations such as the American Association of Critical-Care Nurses (AACN) and the Emergency Nurses Association (ENA).

One of the most significant quality initiatives evolved from 10 quality indicators identified by the ANA that relate to the availability and quality of professional nursing services in hospitals, which evolved into the National Database of Nursing Quality Indicators (NDNQI). This database is comprised of unit-specific nurse-sensitive information collected at hospitals. The indicators reflect the structure, process, and outcomes of nursing care, lead to improved quality and safety at the bedside, and are continually updated at www.nursingworld .org, the official ANA Web site. The ANA also has a strong focus on safe nurse staffing levels to promote safe, high-quality patient care.

Specialty nursing associations have also placed safe, high-quality patient care on their agendas. They have been instrumental in developing, establishing, and implementing standards of care; many health-care institutions promote and require implementation of these specialized standards within their own patient care units. Examples of these specialty associations include the AACN (www.aacn .org) and the American Association of Neurosciences Nurses (www.aann.org).

Nonprofit Organizations and Foundations

Nonprofit organizations and foundations generally focus on consumer education, policy development, and research to improve quality and safety within the health-care system. Many serve multiple missions. The Kaiser Family Foundation (2018) has a strong emphasis on U.S. and international nonpartisan health policy and health policy research.

The Robert Wood Johnson Foundation (RWJF) seeks to improve health for all Americans in four focus areas—healthy communities; healthy children, healthy weight; health leadership; and health systems (RWJF, 2017). RWJF's success comes from leveraging partnerships and its commitment to "building evidence and producing, synthesizing and distributing knowledge, new ideas and expertise" (RWJF, 2017).

The Leapfrog Group is a nonprofit organization interested in improving the safety, quality, and affordability of health care through incentives and rewards to those who use and pay for health care (Leapfrog Group, 2011). This group focuses on reducing preventable medical mistakes and is committed to improving safety and quality through improving transparency by (a) reporting hospital safety and quality survey results, (b) incentivizing better quality and safety performance, and (c) collaborating with other organizations to improve quality and safety. The Leapfrog letter grade continues to be an important quality standard for many hospitals (Galvin et al., 2005). For example, the Leapfrog calculator is designed to measure lives and dollars lost by hospitals based on their Leapfrog letter grade. Austin and Derk (2016) found that organizations with letter grades of D or F had a 50% greater risk of mortality or more than 33,000 lives lost than hospitals with an A letter grade.

Quality Organizations

Quality organizations strive to improve system-wide quality for Americans through a variety of programs and methods. One of the best known is TJC. TJC was established in 1951 by the American College of Physicians, the American Hospital Association, and the Canadian Medical Association as an independent, not-for-profit organization dedicated to accrediting hospitals using the American College of Surgeons' Minimum Standard for Hospitals (TJC, 2017a). Today, hospitals, health-care networks, long-term care facilities, ambulatory care centers, home health agencies, behavioral health-care facilities, and clinical laboratories are among the organizations seeking TJC accreditation. Although accreditation by TJC is voluntary, it is necessary for Medicare and Medicaid reimbursement.

TJC evaluates and accredits more than 21,000 health-care organizations and programs using structural and process measures of quality, assessment of the physical plant, life safety, staffing plans, credentialing of service providers, and other department-specific standards. The accreditation survey is a dynamic QI model focused on both the structures and processes necessary to achieve clinical outcomes. Evaluation of nursing services and the delivery of patient care are important parts of the accreditation. Professional nurses' ability to describe and demonstrate the planning and delivery of patient care are key factors during the survey process. Understanding your organization's policies and procedures regarding the coordination of care and care planning will prepare you for the TJC survey process.

Integrating Initiatives and Evidence-Based Practices Into Patient Care

As you familiarize yourself with each of these organizations and their respective initiatives, consider how they will affect the management of patient care. Your responsibility as a professional RN is to be aware of their presence, understand their importance, and participate in your facility's safety and quality initiatives. As a leader and manager, you will be expected to drive changes based upon their recommendations, ensuring that quality and safety continue to improve.

Nurses are key to improving patient safety (RWJF, 2011). The IOM report proposed five core competencies (Box 11-4) that health-care professionals need to be effective as providers and leaders

---

box 11-4

Core Competencies for Health Professionals

Provide patient-centered care. Identify, respect, and care about patients' differences, values, preferences, and expressed needs; relieve pain and suffering; coordinate continuous care; listen to, clearly inform, communicate with, and educate patients; share decision making and management; and continuously advocate disease prevention, wellness, and promotion of healthy lifestyles, including a focus on population health.

Work in interprofessional teams. Cooperate, collaborate, communicate, and integrate care teams to ensure that care is continuous and reliable.

Employ evidence-based practice. Integrate best research with clinical expertise and patient values for optimum care, and participate in learning and research activities to the extent feasible.

Apply QI. Identify errors and hazards in care; understand and implement basic safety design principles, such as standardization and simplification; continually understand and measure quality of care in terms of structure, process, and outcomes in relation to patient and community needs; and design and test interventions to change processes and systems of care with the objective of improving quality.

Utilize informatics. Communicate, manage knowledge, mitigate error, and support decision making using information technology.

Source: Institute of Medicine. (2003). Core competencies for health professionals. National Academies Press.

---

in the 21st century health-care system. The IOM's report *The Future of Nursing: Leading Change, Advancing Health* (2011) and *The Future of Nursing 2020–2030: Charting a Path to Achieve Health Equity* (National Academies of Science, Engineering, and Medicine, 2021) focus on nursing education, research, and leadership that include mechanisms and technology that help nurses address the impacts of social determinants of health and help achieve health equity as ways to improve patient safety. Nurses need to be full partners with physicians and other members of the interprofessional team in the delivery of health care.

By integrating these competencies into 21st-century health profession education, you can support safe and effective patient care. As a practicing professional, you can use the competencies to guide future professional development and ensure a positive impact on health-care reform while improving quality and safety.

Influence of Nursing

Nurses are empowered through self-determination, meaning, competence, and impact. They play vital roles in decision making within their organizations and their communities. Your role as a staff nurse and a member of the community offers you the opportunity to make a difference to your patients. Your attention to detail in the course of your everyday practice offers you regular opportunities to correct processes to reduce the risk of harm to patients and your colleagues.

Bedside change-of-shift huddles and hand-offs foster frequent review of care planning and interventions, which can result in good catches. Whether it is an averted medication error, the prevention of a fall, or sepsis detection, early recognition of impending complications offers you and your colleagues the opportunity to prevent harm to a patient and even initiate the QI process. Working within organizations and health-care institutions, nurses can create guidelines for safe staffing, develop systems that measure patient acuity by nursing time and expertise, encourage shared decision making, and promote safe practice (Aiken et al., 2012; CDC, 2020; Pham et al., 2012).

A nurse's influence extends beyond the bedside; your knowledge of challenges at the bedside and in your health-care organization make you an excellent addition to community boards as well as your organization's interprofessional committees.

Community boards, hospital committees, and memberships in professional organizations give nurses the opportunity to promote safety and quality in nursing practice and care delivery as well as community health.

Nurses are respected and trusted health-care professionals. To influence change in their organizations, professional nurses must first acknowledge the power within their profession and recognize their central role in health care. Nurses can leverage their professional expertise and the trust and respect they have garnered, but they need to act, not stand on the sidelines. Bottom line, get involved!

Conclusion

Focusing on quality of care reduces cost, increases patient and nurse satisfaction, and improves patient outcomes. As the people who are often closest to the patient, nurses are in a unique position to affect both the patient experience and clinical outcomes by ensuring that delivery of care is patient-centered, safe, and of the highest quality. Start by learning about your organization's QI plan and initiatives. Familiarize yourself with the causes of medical errors. Participate on committees to affect positive change by creating policies that promote safe, high-quality care.

Study Questions

1. How have historical, social, political, and economic trends affected nursing practice? Give specific examples and their implications.

2. What problems have you identified during your clinical experiences that could be opportunities for QI?

3. How does your organization ensure patient safety?

4. What is a high-reliability organization (HRO)?

5. Discuss the role of the nurse in QI, PI, and risk management.

6. Describe the FOCUS-PDCA process and how it is used by organizations to improve safety and quality.

7. Based on TJC patient safety goals, what will you do to ensure adherence to these goals?

8. Describe how regulatory agencies and accrediting agencies affect patient care and outcomes at the bedside.

9. Review the nonprofit organizations and government agencies that influence and advocate for quality and safety in the health-care system.
   a. What have been the results of their efforts for patients, facilities, the health-care delivery system, and the nursing profession?
   b. How have these organizations or agencies affected your facility and professional practice?

10. How would you begin a discussion on safety and quality issues with your nurse manager or a colleague?

11. What issues may arise when the care delivery system is changed? What does the RN need to consider when implementing these changes?

12. How can you, as a nurse, get involved to effect change at work or in your community?

Case Study to Promote Clinical Judgment

Your manager has called a meeting with the entire interprofessional team on your floor and included the director of QI. Based on the past 6 months, the readmission rate of patients who have infections after hip replacements for osteoarthritis is twice that of the national average. The director has requested that the staff identify members who wish to be QI team members investigating this problem. You have volunteered to be a member of the team. The team will consist of an orthopedic surgeon, the physical therapist on the unit, a physician's assistant who works with the hospital's orthopedic surgeons, the clinical nurse educator, the case manager, and you.

1. Why were these people selected for the team?

2. What data needs to be collected to evaluate this situation?

3. What are the potential outcomes for patients who have had hip replacements?

4. Develop a flowchart of a typical hospital discharge and readmission rate for patients who have had hip replacements.

NCLEX®-Style Review Questions

1. You are a new nurse. The hospital where you work is committed to providing safe, high-quality care. Which of the following activities would let you know that your organization is committed to improving patient safety?
   1. The hospital has a good catch program for staff who recognize errors and near misses.
   2. The hospital subscribes to TJC safety publications.
   3. The hospital measures performance every month, monitors quality indicators, and regularly reports on quality.
   4. All of the above

2. Your new organization is committed to quality patient care. Which of these are considered characteristics of quality health care?
   1. The nurses use evidence-based research to guide care delivery.
   2. The nurses are respectful and responsive to their clients' individual preferences.
   3. The nurses perform an independent double check when administering chemotherapy medication.
   4. All of the above

3. Medical errors account for 250,000 deaths per year. It is estimated that as many as 50% of these errors may be preventable. What steps would you take to avoid a medication error?
   1. Review the patient's medication administration record during bedside shift report.
   2. Ask your colleagues to get your medication so that you can give it on time.
   3. Call the pharmacist.
   4. Review the medication administration policy.

4. Studying errors and identifying how they occur helps organizations improve patient safety. Which category of errors is the most useful in identifying and remedying vulnerabilities in an organization?
   1. Sentinel event
   2. Adverse event
   3. Near miss event
   4. Wrong procedure event

5. Nursing standards of care and the organization's policies and procedures greatly decrease risk to patient safety. Which of the following steps can a nurse take to further reduce risk?
   1. Submit event or incident reports for near misses.
   2. Follow medication administration policies and procedures.
   3. Always report significant data on care to patients and providers in a timely manner.
   4. All of the above

6. To achieve safe patient care, a culture of safety must exist. What are characteristics of an organization with a culture of safety?
   1. Transparency, openness, reporting of errors is rewarded, blame-free environment
   2. Honesty, studying of serious events
   3. Privacy, reporting of errors appreciated
   4. Blame-free environment, openness, error reporting is encouraged

7. The purpose of QI is to continuously improve the capability of everyone involved to provide safe, high-quality patient care. What is important to know about the QI process?
   1. It is independent of teamwork.
   2. It is a data-driven approach to improving process.
   3. Common safety indicators are not used to evaluate quality of care.
   4. Opportunities for QI are selected by organization leadership.

8. Structured care methodologies (SCM) are
   1. Nursing tools designed to identify best practices and facilitate standards of care
   2. Used to create a stable set of performance indicators to measure outcomes
   3. Used to assist employees with wellness and injury prevention
   4. Helpful when making staffing assignments

9. When evaluating the quality of care, a health-care organization must consider structures, processes, and outcomes of care delivery. Which of the following is a good example of an organizational process?
   1. Budgeting adequate money for nursing salaries
   2. Preparing a patient for discharge
   3. Monitoring for infections
   4. Increasing time between clinic visits

10. The HHS is charged with protecting the health of all Americans and providing essential health services. Which of the following HHS quality initiatives is currently under way?
    1. Post-acute care reform initiative
    2. National health-care research and quality indicators aimed at helping improve access to care
    3. NDNQI
    4. Health IT

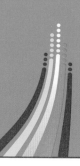

chapter 12

Maintaining a Safe Work Environment

OBJECTIVES

After reading this chapter, the student should be able to:

- Recognize threats to employees' safety in the health-care environment.
- Identify agencies responsible for overseeing workplace safety.
- Describe methods for dealing with threats to employees' safety in the workplace.
- Discuss the role of the nurse in dealing with threats to employee and workplace safety.

OUTLINE

Most people spend the majority of their waking hours in the workplace, which makes it easy to take the safety and security of the work environment for granted. Although committed to providing safe, high-quality care to patients, health-care organizations and hospitals are just as susceptible to overlooking hazardous conditions and unsafe practices as other industries. Hospitals and health-care organizations employ hundreds of people in multiple buildings, across multiple campuses, and even across state lines. National and state safety standards ensure that organizations reduce the risk of injury to employees and protect them from environmental harm.

Although the bulk of responsibility for maintaining a safe work environment rests with organizational leaders who have the authority and resources to initiate improvements, employees are essential in identifying issues and reporting incidents to ensure prompt action. Nurses play a key role in identifying safety issues and advocating for improvements, especially in patient care settings. This chapter focuses on these issues.

Workplace Safety

Threats to Safety

A health-care facility may be one of the most dangerous work environments in the United States. Health and safety threats include infectious diseases, physical violence, ergonomic injuries related to the movement and repositioning of patients, exposure to hazardous chemicals and radiation, and sharps injuries (American Nurses Association [ANA], 2022a). Although many of these risks can be managed by following guidelines and standards, others are less predictable. Injury caused by physical violence is one example.

Wey (2016) cited 40 incidents of violence in one large New York hospital in only 2 months. The worst incidents involved a nurse who was knocked to the floor by a patient and repeatedly kicked in the head, suffering a severe brain injury. The Occupational Safety and Health Organization (OSHA) cited this hospital for its ineffective violence prevention program (Wey, 2016). In 2017, a Massachusetts nurse was cornered by a patient and stabbed multiple

times (Go Local Worcester News Team, 2017). In June of 2022, a doctor and two nurses were stabbed by a patient demanding treatment for anxiety in a Los Angeles hospital emergency department (ED) (National Public Radio [NPR], 2022). Fortunately, these nurses survived; however, these reports represent a growing number of assaults on health-care workers across the country. Today, health-care workers are five times more likely to suffer injury because of workplace violence than in any other industry. In 2018, over 70% of nonfatal injuries and illnesses in health-care environments were caused by workplace violence (U.S. Bureau of Labor Statistics, 2020).

Not all violence occurs in hospitals. Clinic and home health employees are also vulnerable:

A social services coordinator regularly visited potentially violent clients at home and drove them to facilities for mental and physical evaluations. A mentally ill client with a history of violence stabbed her to death in front of his home. Again, OSHA cited her employer for failing to have a comprehensive violence prevention program or assisting employees who express concern about their safety (Wey, 2016).

The ANA surveyed 4,614 nurses in 2011 to learn about their primary concerns related to workplace safety. Their top concerns were stress and overwork (74%) and ergonomic (musculoskeletal) injuries (62%). Shift lengths have increased, but mandatory overtime requirements have declined slightly, reported by 53% in 2011 compared with 68% in 2001 (ANA, 2011). An encouraging finding is that nurses reported the greater availability of effective devices to assist them in patient transfers and reduced sharps injuries, fewer assaults, and less illness because of the work environment (ANA, 2011). When surveyed about factors considered essential to a healthy workplace environment, employees listed collaborative work relationships, good communication, empowerment, recognition, opportunities for growth, effective leadership, adequate staffing, and workplace safety (Dempsey & Reilly, 2016; Lindberg & Vingård, 2012; Sherman & Blum, 2019).

Workplace safety threats vary from one setting to another and from one individual to another. For example, a pregnant staff member may be more vulnerable to risks from radiation. Likewise, staff members working in the ED are at more risk for exposure to infectious diseases such as SARS-CoV-2 (COVID-19), tuberculosis, and HIV than staff who work in the newborn nursery. All staff members have the right to be made aware of potential risks and provided with as much protection as possible. No worker should feel uncomfortable or unsafe in the workplace.

Agencies Addressing Threats to Safety

The modern movement for safety in the workplace began near the end of the Industrial Revolution. The National Council for Industrial Safety (now the National Safety Council [NSC]) was formed in 1913. The Occupational Safety and Health Act of 1970 created the National Institute of Occupational Safety and Health (NIOSH) and OSHA. As part of the U.S. Department of Labor, OSHA is responsible for developing and enforcing workplace safety and health regulations. NIOSH supports research, education, and training, whereas the NSC partners with OSHA to provide training. The NSC maintains that safety in the workplace is the responsibility of both the employer and the employee. Employers must ensure a safe, healthy work environment, and employees are accountable for knowing and following safety guidelines and standards (Hagen et al., 2015).

OSHA

The goal of OSHA is to prevent injuries and illness and save the lives of employees across the United States (OSHA, 2020). Employers must comply with OSHA regulations to provide a safe, healthful work environment. They are also required to keep records of all occupational (job-related) illnesses and accidents such as chemical exposures, lacerations, hearing loss, respiratory exposure, musculoskeletal injuries, and exposure to infectious diseases. A workplace may be inspected with or without prior notification to the employer. Catastrophic or fatal accidents and employee complaints may trigger an OSHA inspection. OSHA promotes collaboration between employers and employees to identify and remove workplace hazards before contacting OSHA. If the employer cannot or will not resolve the issue, the employee may file a complaint with OSHA, and an inspection will be ordered (OSHA, 2020; U.S. Department of Labor, 1995). Notice of any violations is posted where all employees can view them. However, the employer has the right to contest the OSHA decision. The law also states that the employer cannot punish or discriminate against employees for exercising their rights related to job safety and health hazards or participating in OSHA inspections (OSHA, 2020; U.S. Department of Labor, 1995).

OSHA inspections of health-care facilities have focused mainly on blood-borne pathogens, exposure to infectious diseases, lifting and ergonomic (proper body alignment) guidelines, confined-space regulations, respiratory guidelines, and workplace violence. OSHA added protecting the work site against terrorism after the September 11, 2001 terrorist attacks.

Centers for Disease Control and Prevention (CDC)

The CDC partners with other agencies to investigate health problems, conduct research, implement prevention strategies, and promote safe and healthy environments. The CDC publishes continuous updates of recommendations for workplace HIV transmission prevention and universal precautions related to blood-borne pathogens and other infectious diseases such as coronavirus, commonly referred to as COVID-19 (CDC, 2019). The CDC also targets public health emergency preparedness and response related to biological and chemical agents and threats (CDC, 2019). CDC recommendations can be found in the *Morbidity and Mortality Weekly Report* (MMWR) on the Internet (www.cdc.gov/health/diseases) or at its toll-free phone number (800-311-3435).

American Nurses Association (ANA)

The ANA Web site (www.nursingworld.org) provides up-to-date information on workplace advocacy and safety for all nurses. In 1999, the ANA established its Commission on Workplace Advocacy, which addresses issues such as collective bargaining, workplace violence, mandatory overtime, staffing ratios, conflict management, delegation, ethical issues, compensation, needlestick safety, latex allergies, pollution prevention, and ergonomics.

The Joint Commission (TJC)

The Joint Commission (TJC) accredits hospitals and health-care organizations on behalf of the

box 12-1

Federal Laws Enacted to Protect the Worker in the Workplace

- **Equal Pay Act of 1963** Employers must provide equal pay for equal work, regardless of gender.
- **Title VII of Civil Rights Act of 1964** Employees may not be discriminated against on the basis of race, color, religion, sex, or national origin.
- **Age Discrimination in Employment Act of 1967** Private and public employers may not discriminate against persons 40 years of age or older except when a certain age group is a bona fide occupational qualification.
- **Pregnancy Discrimination Act of 1968** Pregnant women cannot be discriminated against in employment benefits if they are able to perform job responsibilities.
- **Fair Credit Reporting Act of 1970** Job applicants and employees have the right to know of the existence and content of any credit files maintained on them.
- **Vocational Rehabilitation Act of 1973** An employer receiving financial assistance from the federal government may not discriminate against individuals with disabilities and must develop affirmative action plans to hire and promote individuals with disabilities.
- **Family Education Rights and Privacy Act—Buckley Amendment of 1974** Educational institutions may not supply information about students without their consent.
- **Immigration Reform and Control Act of 1986** Employers must screen employees for the right to work in the United States without discriminating on the basis of national origin.
- **Americans With Disabilities Act of 1990** Persons with physical or mental disabilities or who are chronically ill cannot be discriminated against in the workplace. Employers must make "reasonable accommodations" to meet the needs of the disabled employee. These include such provisions as installing foot or hand controls; readjusting light switches, telephones, desks, tables, and computer equipment; providing access ramps and elevators; offering flexible work hours; and providing readers for blind employees.
- **Family Medical Leave Act of 1993** Employers with 50 or more employees must provide up to 13 weeks of unpaid leave for family medical emergencies, childbirth, or adoption.
- **Needlestick Safety and Prevention Act of 2001** This act directed OSHA to revise the blood-borne pathogens standard to establish in greater detail requirements that employers identify and make use of effective and safer medical devices.
- **Lilly Ledbetter Fair Pay Act of 2009** This act supports fair pay and provides protection against discrimination in compensation based upon race, color, religion, sex, or national origin.

Source: Adapted from Strader, M., & Decker, P. (1995). Role transition to patient care management. Appleton and Lange; Pub L. 111-2. Retrieved from eeoc.gov/eeoc/history/50th/thelaw/ledbetter.cfm; Lilly Ledbetter Fair Pay Act of 2009, S.181, 123 Stat. 5; and General Industry Regulations Book. (2018). Subpart Z Occupational Safety and Health Standards, Title 29 Code of Federal Regulations, Part 1910.

U.S. Department of Health and Human Services (HHS) Center for Medicare and Medicaid (CMS). This triennial accreditation includes an on-site survey of up to 4 days. During this review, the TJC team, made up of health-care professionals, ensures that workplace safety policies are in practice. This is done by policy review and validated by the team's inspection of the work environment and interviews with staff.

National Academy of Medicine (NAM)

The National Academy of Medicine (NAM), originally named the Institute of Medicine (IOM), was founded in 1970. It is a private, nongovernmental organization whose mission is to improve people's health everywhere; thus, the topics it studies are extensive. In 1996, the NAM began a quality initiative to assess the nation's health-care system. One result was the 2004 report, *Keeping Patients Safe: Transforming the Work Environment of Nurses.* The report identified concerns related to organizational management, workforce deployment practices, work design, and organizational culture (Beyea, 2004). Funded by the Agency for Healthcare Research and Quality (AHRQ), it has served as an action plan for organizations that depend on nurses (AHRQ, 2005). Box 12-1 lists the most important federal laws enacted to protect individuals in the workplace.

Developing Workplace Safety Programs

Today, health-care organizations strive to build healthy, safe work environments by becoming high-reliability organizations through creating a culture of safety (American College of Healthcare Executives [ACHE], 2017; AHRQ, 2019). High-reliability organizations seek to minimize the incidence of adverse events by maintaining a commitment to safety at every level of their organization. This includes frontline workers, managers, senior executives, and the governing board (AHRQ, 2019). Their commitment to safety is foundational to beginning the journey to high reliability. The culture of safety has four tenets:

- Everyone recognizes that the work the organization does consists of high-risk activities and rugged determination to maintain consistently safe operations.

- Errors and near misses are reported without reprisal. Sometimes called a blame-free environment, everyone should feel compelled to report errors and near misses for continuous quality and safety improvements.
- Interdepartmental and interprofessional collaboration are used to find solutions to safety problems.
- The organization prioritizes and commits resources to address safety issues (AHRQ, 2019).

Workplace safety programs should protect staff members from harm and the organization from any liability.

1. The first step in developing a workplace safety program is to recognize a potential hazard. OSHA (2020; U.S. Department of Labor, 1995) requires employers to inform employees of any potential health hazards and provide as much protection as possible. Initial warnings often come from the CDC, NIOSH, and other federal, state, and local agencies. Employers must provide tuberculosis testing and the hepatitis B vaccine; personal protective equipment (PPE) such as face shields, gloves, gowns, and masks or respirators; and immediate treatment after exposure for all staff members who may have contact with bloodborne pathogens or other contagions such as coronavirus disease. They are expected to remove hazards, educate employees, and establish institution-wide policies and procedures to protect their employees (Herring, 1994; Roche, 1993). If not provided with appropriate PPE, employees may refuse to participate in activities involving patients requiring isolation or exposure to blood or blood products. Reasonable accommodations must also be made. For example, a nurse with latex allergies should have access to non-latex materials if not already provided.
2. The second step in a workplace safety program is a thorough assessment of the amount of risk entailed. For example:

Tracey Wu is the nurse manager on a busy geriatric unit. Most patients require total care: bathing, feeding, and positioning. She observed that several staff members working on the unit have not been using the new lift equipment and are using body mechanics when lifting and moving the patients. Several had gone to the employee health department complaining of back and shoulder pain. This past week, she noticed that patients seemed to remain in the same position for long periods and were rarely out of bed or were left in a chair for the entire day. When she confronted the staff, the response was the same from all of them: "I have to work for a living. I cannot afford to risk a back injury for someone who may not live past the end of the week." Tracey was concerned about the quality of patient care and her staff's lack of information about back safety. She decided to seek assistance from the nurse practitioner in the employee health department to develop a back injury prevention program.

Assessment of the workplace may require considerable data gathering. Formal committees are often formed to assess these risks. Staff from various levels and departments should be included.

3. The third step is to create a plan to provide optimal protection for staff members without interfering with quality patient care. For example, some devices worn to prevent tuberculosis transmission interfere with communication with the patient. Some attempts have been made to limit visits or withdraw home health-care nurses from high-crime areas, thus leaving homebound patients without care. This can result in an increased reliance on EDs and overcrowding (McElwee, 2019; Nadwairski, 1992), which merely shifts rather than mitigates employee risk. Developing a safety plan includes the following:
   - Distinguish real from imagined risks.
   - Consult federal, state, and local regulations and experts on work safety.
   - Seek evidence-based practices related to the problem.
   - Develop a plan to reduce risks.
   - Calculate the costs of the program or plan.
   - Seek administrative support for the plan.
4. The fourth and final stage in developing a workplace safety program is implementing the plan. Educating the staff, providing the necessary safety supplies and equipment, and modifying the environment may be necessary.

Violence

NIOSH defines *workplace violence* as "an act of violence or threat of violence, without regard to intent, that occurs at a covered facility or while a covered employee performs a covered service" (Alexander et al., 2022). Nurses' frequent and close contact with individuals in distress makes them a potential target (Magnavita & Heponiemi, 2011; McElwee, 2019). The overall private-sector rate for assault resulting in injury is 2 per 10,000 full-time workers; compare this with the rate for health service workers at 10.4, with the incidence rate for nurses at 13.9 (U.S. Bureau of Labor Statistics, 2020). Most of the incidents involve patients (McElwee, 2019; McPhaul & Lipscomb, 2004). Although a relatively rare occurrence, there is also the threat of an active shooter in the facility. Most of these incidents have occurred in EDs or patient rooms (Hodge & Nelson, 2014; McElwee, 2019). Some of the circumstances surrounding health-care work contribute to workers' susceptibility (Edwards, 1999; NIOSH, 2002), such as the following:

■ Units for treating violent individuals
■ Patients needing seclusion or restraint
■ Increased numbers of acute and chronic mentally ill patients being released without effective follow-up
■ Working late or until very early morning hours
■ Working in high-crime areas
■ Working in buildings with poor security
■ Treating weapons-carrying patients and families
■ Inexperienced staff who have not been trained to manage crises or handle volatile situations
■ Long wait times for service
■ Overcrowded, uncomfortable waiting areas

To assess the risk of violence, nurses must know their workplace (Public Services Health and Safety Association [PSHSA], 2018). Ask the following:

■ How frequently do assaultive incidents, threats, and verbal abuse occur in your facility? Where? Who is involved? Are incidents reported?
■ Are current emergency response systems effective?
■ Are staffing patterns sufficient? Is the staff experienced in handling these situations (Iennaco et al., 2013; PSHSA, 2018)?
■ Are post-assaultive treatment and support available to staff?

---

box 12-2

Behaviors Indicating a Potential for Violence

• History of violent behavior
• Delusional, paranoid, or suspicious speech
• Aggressive, threatening statements
• Rapid speech, angry tone of voice
• Pacing, tense posture, clenched fists, tightening jaw
• Alcohol or drug use
• Policies that set unrealistic limits

Source: Adapted from Kinkle, S. (1993). Violence in the ED: How to stop it before it starts. American Journal of Nursing, 93(7), 22–24; Kansas State Nurses Association (corporate author). (1996). Violence assessment in hospitals provides basis for action. The Kansas Nurse, 71(3), 18–20.

Although assaults that result in severe injury or death receive media coverage, most assaults on nurses by patients or coworkers go unreported by the nurse.

Be aware of clues that may indicate a potential for violence (Box 12-2). These behaviors may occur in patients, family members, visitors, or other staff members.

Not only are episodes of violence underreported, but there are persistent misperceptions that assaults are part of the job and that the victim somehow caused the assault. A lack of institutional reporting policies may also cause underreporting or employee fears that the assault was because of negligence or poor job performance (Arnetz et al., 2015; U.S. Department of Labor, 1995). Box 12-3 lists some faulty reasoning that leads to placing blame on the victim of the assault.

Actions to address violence in the workplace include (a) identifying the factors that contribute to violence and controlling as many as possible and

---

box 12-3

When an Assault Occurs: Placing Blame on Victims

• **Victim gender** Women receive more blame than men.
• **Subject gender** Female victims receive more blame from women than men.
• **Severity** The more severe the assault, the more often the victim is blamed.
• **Beliefs** The world is a just place, and therefore the person deserves the misfortune.
• **Age of victim** The older the victim, the more the victim is held to blame.

Source: Adapted from Lanza, M. L., & Carifio, J. (1991). Blaming the victim: Complex (nonlinear) patterns of causal attribution by nurses in response to vignettes of a patient assaulting a nurse. Journal of Emergency Nursing, 17(5), 299–309.

(b) preparing staff to prevent and manage violence (Mahoney, 1991; McElwee, 2019).

Preventing Violent Behavior

Preventing an incident is better than having to intervene after violence has occurred. The following are suggestions to nurses about how to participate in workplace safety related to the prevention of violence (ANA, 2015b).

- Participate in or initiate regular workplace assessments. Identify unsafe areas and factors within the organization that contribute to assaultive behavior, such as inadequate staffing, high-activity times of day, invasion of personal space, seclusion or restraint activities, and lack of experienced staff. Work with management to make and monitor changes. Consider using metal detectors, video surveillance, and increased use of security personnel, but remain aware of the need to maintain patient privacy (Hodge & Nelson, 2014).
- Be alert for behaviors that precede violence, such as verbal expressions of anger and frustration, threatening body language, signs of drug or alcohol use, or the presence of a weapon. Evaluate each situation for potential violence.
- Know your patients. Be aware of any history of violent behaviors, diagnoses suggesting potential for violent behavior, and alcohol or drug intoxication. Monitor those with a history of violence and alert staff members to take precautionary measures. This type of surveillance has been reported to reduce violent attacks by 92% (Hodge & Nelson, 2014).
- Maintain behavior that helps to defuse anger. Present a calm, caring attitude. Do not match threats, give orders, or present with behaviors that may be interpreted as aggressive. Acknowledge the person's feelings.
- If you cannot defuse the situation, then remove yourself from it quickly, call security, and report the situation to management.

Box 12-4 lists some additional actions that can be taken to protect staff members and patients from violence in the workplace.

If Violent Behavior Occurs

What if, despite all precautions, violence occurs? What should you do? You should:

- Report the incident to your supervisor, whether it is a threat or actual violence. Include a

---

box 12-4

Steps Toward Increasing Protection From Workplace Violence

- Security personnel and escorts
- Panic buttons in medication rooms, stairwells, activity rooms, and nursing stations
- Bulletproof glass in reception, triage, and admitting areas
- Locked or key-coded access doors
- Closed-circuit television
- Metal detectors
- Use of beepers or cellular phones
- Handheld alarms or noise devices
- Lighted parking lots
- Escort or buddy system
- Enforce wearing of photo identification badges

Source: Adapted from Simonowitz, J. (1994). Violence in the workplace: You're entitled to protection. RN, 57(11), 61–63. www.nursingworld .org/practice-policy/advocacy/state/workplace-violence2/

---

description of the situation; names of victims, witnesses, and perpetrators; and other pertinent information.
- Call security. Nurses are entitled to the same protections as anyone else who has been assaulted.
- Get medical attention. This includes medical care, counseling, and evaluation.
- Contact your collective bargaining unit, your state nurses association, or OSHA if the problems persist.
- Be proactive. Get involved in policy making (ANA, 2015b; Gilmore-Hall, 2001).

Natural Disasters and Terrorism Threats

From the 2001 anthrax outbreak and attacks on the World Trade Center to the Las Vegas shooting that killed 58 and injured 851 in 2017, concern related to terrorism has heightened. The ANA provides nurses with valuable information on how they can better care for their patients, protect themselves, and prepare their hospitals and communities to respond to acts of bioterrorism and natural disasters (ANA, 2022a).

Nurses are often called upon when a disaster occurs. For example, many worked with the ANA to provide support for the victims of Hurricane Katrina. A nurse holding a newborn rescued from the severely damaged NYU Langone Medical Center became a symbol of the rescue efforts following the destruction caused by Super Storm Sandy (2012) in New York.

Disasters can be natural or man-made, either accidental or an act of terrorism. They may be:

- Natural or environmental (e.g., tornados, floods, hurricanes)
- Biological (e.g., a flu pandemic)
- Chemical (e.g., a chemical spill)
- Radiological (e.g., a nuclear event)
- Explosive (e.g., a terrorist bombing)

Special considerations during these disasters include attention to mental health needs of victims and responders, addressing special needs populations (elderly or patients dependent on mechanical support), and the surges in the volume of patients presenting to hospitals and clinics (ANA, 2011).

Following are some steps that can be implemented in the workplace to better prepare for these threats (Altman, 2002; AWHONN, 2001):

- Know the evacuation procedures and routes for your facility.
- Monitor your patient caseload for any unusual disease patterns and notify appropriate authorities.
- Know the backup systems available for communication and staffing in the event of emergencies.

Become familiar with the disaster policies in your facility.

Needlestick (Sharps) Injuries

Between 600,000 and 800,000 needlestick injuries occur annually in the United States, and approximately 75% are preventable (ANA, 2010). Why is this a concern? Percutaneous exposure is the principal route for human immunodeficiency virus (HIV) infection and hepatitis B and C, as well as other blood-borne pathogens.

In 1997, a 27-year-old nurse, Lisa Black, attended an in-service session on post-exposure prophylaxis for needlesticks. A short time later, she attempted to aspirate blood from a patient's intravenous line when the patient moved, and the needle went into Lisa's hand. Nine months later, she tested positive for HIV and 3 months later for hepatitis C (Trossman, 1999).

There are several legal sources of protection from sharps injuries. For example, the Needlestick Safety and Prevention Act was enacted on April 18, 2001. The revised OSHA Blood Borne Pathogens Standard obligates employers to consider safer needle devices when conducting their annual reviews (Foley, 2012). TJC surveyors routinely ask if health-care organization leaders are familiar with the Needlestick Safety Prevention Act and what action has been taken to comply (OSHA, 2018b). Although much progress has been made in preventing sharps injuries, a recent consensus statement from the ANA and other groups calls for more attention to (Daley, 2012):

- Greater safety in surgical settings
- Sharps safety outside the hospital
- Including nurses in the selection of safety devices
- Encouraging product design and development to fill existing gaps (e.g., in dentistry, use of longer needles)
- Increased staff training

Your Employer's Responsibility

All health-care facilities should have a written plan to prevent sharps injuries that is updated annually. Staff should receive annual training during work hours and have a right to be involved in selecting safety devices. Additional control measures include (Foley, 2012):

- The employee must be evaluated and treated within 2 hours of a sharps injury, including a free hepatitis B vaccine.
- The safety and efficacy of sharps purchased must be evaluated.
- Recapping of needles and related practices should be prohibited.
- Contaminated work surfaces must be cleaned according to established guidelines.
- Employers must provide good-quality PPE, including gloves, gowns, eye protection, respirators, and masks in all needed sizes.

The surgical setting presents unique challenges in preventing sharps injuries. Sharps such as scalpels must be transferred from person to person safely, but the urgency and the number of staff at the surgical table increase the risk of harm. Of note, 30% of sharps injuries are sustained by those other than the primary user (ANA, 2010). Some recommendations for addressing this risk include (Dugdale, 2021; Guglielmi & Ogg, 2012):

- Use blunt-tip suture needles where possible.
- Use safety scalpels, either sheathed or retractable.
- Initiate the hands-free technique (HFT) or neutral passing zone (a container or sterile towel) instead of passing instruments hand-to-hand.
- Double glove to increase protection from punctures.
- Share information (educate) with staff about sharps injury prevention.

Employee Responsibilities

What are your responsibilities related to preventing sharps injuries? You will need to learn how to use new devices and ensure that the current safety requirements are enforced. Also (ANA, 1993; Brooke, 2001; Dugdale, 2021):

- Always use universal precautions.
- Use and dispose of sharps properly.
- Obtain immunization against hepatitis B.
- Get involved in sharps selection.
- Keep your training up to date.
- Report all exposures immediately following your facility's protocol.
- Comply with post-exposure follow-up procedures and policies.

If you have questions about treatment for a needlestick, you can call the National Clinician's Post-Exposure Prophylaxis (PEPLine) number, 1-888-448-4911 (CDC, 2022; Handelman et al., 2012).

Latex Allergy

Since the 1987 CDC recommendations for universal precautions, the use of gloves has increased the exposure of health-care workers to natural rubber latex (NRL). Allergic reactions to latex include contact dermatitis to generalized urticaria, rhinitis, wheezing, swelling, shortness of breath, and anaphylaxis.

Latex allergy should be suspected if an employee develops symptoms after latex exposures. A complete medical history can reveal latex sensitivity, and blood tests approved by the U.S. Food and Drug Administration (FDA) are available to detect latex antibodies. Skin testing and glove-use tests are also available.

Given the increased need for PPE and associated sensitivities, hospitals have converted to non-latex products. Before this conversion, the incidence of illness, anaphylaxis, and death have been reported (Bauer et al., 1993; Rosen et al., 1993).

Complete latex avoidance is the most effective approach. Medications may reduce allergic symptoms, and special precautions are needed to prevent exposure during medical and dental care. Employees with a latex allergy should consider wearing a medical alert bracelet.

Although the use of products containing latex has been dramatically reduced and, in some cases, eliminated in the acute care and clinical settings, it is important to note that there are specialty products that contain latex. Check with your supervisor and read labels to ensure safety.

The following will help to decrease the potential for latex allergy problems (CDC, 1998):

- Evaluate any cases of hand dermatitis or other signs of latex allergy.
- Use latex-free procedure trays and crash carts.
- Use non-latex gloves for activities that do not involve contact with infectious materials.
- Avoid using oil-based creams or lotions, which can cause glove deterioration.
- Seek ongoing training and the latest information related to latex allergy.
- Wash, rinse, and dry hands thoroughly after removing or changing gloves.
- Use powder-free gloves.

If you develop a latex allergy, be aware of the following precautions (CDC, 1998):

- Avoid all types of latex exposure.
- Wear a medical alert bracelet.
- Carry an EpiPen with auto-injectable epinephrine.
- Alert your employer and colleagues to your latex sensitivity.
- Carry non-latex gloves.

The number of new cases of latex allergy has decreased because of improved diagnostic methods, education, accurate labeling, and powder-free gloves. Although current research does not demonstrate whether the amount of allergen released during shipping and storage of medications from vials with rubber closures is sufficient to induce a systemic allergic reaction, nurses should take special precautions when patients are identified as high risk for latex allergies. Nursing staff should work closely with the pharmacy staff to follow universal one-stick-rule precautions, which assume that every pharmaceutical vial may contain a natural rubber latex closure. In addition, the nurse should remain with any patient at the start of medication administration and keep frequent observations and vital signs for 2 hours (Hamilton et al., 2005).

Ergonomic Injuries

Around 42% of nurses report they are at risk of an ergonomic injury, and 13% have had a serious injury. For some, the injury means they can no longer practice their profession. In addition, 75% have access to safe patient handling technology, yet only half use it regularly (Francis & Dawson, 2016). Why don't they use the equipment? There are several possible reasons:

> It may not be easily accessible.
> It may be too heavy or clumsy to use.
> Staff may not have been trained in its use.

Francis and Dawson (2016) note that appropriate safe patient handling equipment must be selected and made readily available to staff, staff have to be well trained, and leaders have to monitor actual use.

Back Injuries

Occupation-related back injuries affect more than 75% of nurses during their careers. Every year, 12% of nurses leave the profession because of back injury, and 52% complain of chronic back pain. In 2010, nursing aides, orderlies, and attendants had the highest rates of musculoskeletal disorders, seven times the average across all workplaces, higher even than construction workers (OSHA, 2018c). The problem with lifting a patient is not just one of overcoming heavy weight but also of overcoming improper lifting techniques. Size, shape, and deformities of the patient, as well as the patient's balance, combativeness, uncooperativeness, and contractures, must be considered. Any unexpected movement or resistance from the patient can throw the nurse off balance and result in a back injury. Limited space, equipment, beds, chairs, and commodes also contribute to back injury risk (Edlich et al., 2001).

OSHA has issued several safe patient handling publications and presentations, which can be found on its Web site (OSHA, 2018c).

For example, the *Back Facts,* a training workbook to prevent back injuries in nursing homes (OSHA, 2003), and the OSHA guidelines for nursing homes (OSHA, 2009) are comprehensive resources. Employers must keep their workplaces free from recognized hazards, including ergonomic hazards.

The ANA has conducted a Handle With Care campaign and developed safe patient handling and mobility programs to prevent back and other musculoskeletal injuries. Health-care facilities that have invested in recommended assistive patient handling programs report cost savings in the thousands of dollars for direct costs of back injuries and lost workdays (OSHA, 2018b). "All it takes," notes the ANA on its Web site, "is one bad lift to change a nurse's life. Just one fast-paced decision has the potential to end a nursing career." Your responsibility is to learn safe patient handling in school and at work. Your employer's responsibility is to provide safe patient handling education and assistive patient handling equipment that can improve the quality care of patients, improving patients' comfort, dignity, and safety during transfers.

Repetitive Stress Injuries

The use of computers continues to increase exponentially for all health-care personnel. Repetitive stress injuries (RSIs) affect people who spend long hours at computers, switchboards, and other occupations where repetitive motions are performed. The most common RSIs are carpal tunnel syndrome and mouse elbow. Poorly designed computer workstations present the highest risk of RSIs. Preventive measures include the following (Feiler & Stichler, 2011; Krucoff, 2001; OSHA, 2018c):

■ Keep the monitor screen straight ahead, about an arm's length away. The top of the screen should be at eye level.
■ Align the keyboard so that your forearms, wrists, and hands are parallel to the floor. Tilt if needed to keep wrists in a neutral position.
■ Position the mouse (if used) directly next to you and on the same level as the keyboard.
■ Keep thighs parallel to the floor as you sit on the chair. The feet should touch the floor, and the chair back should be ergonomically sound. Alternatively, use a stand-up desk to vary position further.
■ Vary tasks. Avoid long sessions of sitting. Do not use excessive force when typing or clicking the mouse.

Finally, those employees who have been injured at work need support and guidance when they return to work. They may also need modifications to their work-related activities, an explanation of policies related to their situation, and access to continued care for their injury (OSHA, 2018c; Spector & Reul, 2017).

Indoor Air Pollution and Exposure to Hazardous Chemicals

The list of potentially hazardous chemicals found in a health-care setting is a long one: hazardous drugs, disinfectants and sterilizing agents, pesticides, and an array of cleaning products. Patients and staff need to be protected from unnecessary exposure to these chemicals (ANA, 2018). OSHA (2018a) classifies hazardous chemicals as carcinogenic, corrosive, toxic, irritant, sensitizer, or target organ effector. OSHA requires employers to label all their hazardous materials clearly and provide them with Material Safety Data Sheets (MSDSs). Employers must also train their employees to prevent hazards and provide PPE and immediate emergency treatment for potentially injurious exposure.

Inside air pollution is a more recently identified problem. Dioxin emissions, mercury, and battery waste are often not handled properly in the hospital environment. Disinfectants, chemicals, waste anesthesia gases, and laser plumes that float in the air are other sources of pollution exposure for nurses. Rethinking product choices, such as avoiding polyvinyl chloride or mercury products, providing convenient collection sites for battery and mercury waste, and making waste management education mandatory for employees, is a way to a more pollution-free environment (Romjue, 2020; Slattery, 1998). Better ventilation and air filtration can keep the air cleaner (Feiler & Stichler, 2011; Romjue, 2020). Recycled paper and products, minimized use of toxic disinfectants, and waste disposal choices that reduce incineration to a minimum are needed. Nurses as professionals need to be aware of the consequences of the medical waste produced by the health sector, which supports continued education for both nurses and patients as well as specific policy statements and advocacy efforts of our professional organizations, such as reduction of medical waste incinerator emissions and use of mercury-free and PVC-free products (ANA, 2007; Romjue, 2020).

Disabled Employees

The Americans With Disabilities Act, enacted in 1990, makes it unlawful to discriminate against a qualified individual with a disability. Employers are required to provide reasonable accommodations for a person with a disability. A reasonable accommodation is a modification or adjustment to the job, work environment, work schedule, or work procedures that enables a qualified person with a disability to perform the job. Both you and your employer may seek information from the Equal Employment Opportunity Commission (EEOC) for information (EEOC, 2018).

Shift Work Disorders

Although nurses who work nights permanently often can readjust their sleep–wake cycle from night to day, even permanent night workers may be subject to continuous sleep deprivation. Those who continuously rotate shifts may seriously disturb their circadian rhythms: A typical night shift worker's scenario is to feel sleepy during work and travel home but have difficulty falling asleep during the day. Symptoms that continue for more than a month indicate the presence of shift work disorder. Up to 40% of shift workers may suffer from this disorder and have a higher risk of ulcers, heart disease, depression, chronic fatigue, poor work performance, and accidents on and off work (Cleveland Clinic, 2021; O'Malley, 2011). Suggestions for nurses who rotate shifts (Cleveland Clinic, 2021; O'Malley, 2011; Shandor, 2012) include the following:

■ Shorter (8-hour) shifts allow you to get at least 7 hours' sleep before returning to work.
■ Try to schedule the same shifts for an entire scheduling period instead of rotating different shifts within one scheduling period.
■ Try to schedule the same days off consistently.
■ If you become sleepy during the shift, try exercise (take a walk or climb stairs), bright light, a brief nap if possible, and a cup of coffee (not near the end of your shift).
■ If you work evenings or nights, do not eat a big meal or take caffeine or alcohol at the end of the shift as this interferes with sleep. Try to avoid using sleep medications.
■ If driving home in bright morning light, put on sunglasses.

- Try to sleep for a continuous block of time at regularly scheduled times instead of catching a few hours here and there.
- Make sure the room you are sleeping in is a comfortable temperature and as dark and noise-free as possible.
- Find time to maintain good nutrition and daily exercise.
- Self-scheduling increases perceived control and may reduce the stress of shift work.

It is evident from this list that there are several ways an employer can help reduce the stress of shift work. Making healthy food available around the clock and providing nap facilities can help employees stay healthy and alert during their shifts (Shandor, 2012). The ANA's position on reducing the risks of nurse fatigue is that both nurses and their employers are responsible for considering the nurse's need for adequate sleep in allowing on-call status, as well as voluntary or mandatory overtime (ANA, 2011).

Mandatory Overtime

The ANA calls mandatory overtime a "dangerous staffing practice" that can have a negative impact on patient care (ANA, 2022b). When nurses are routinely forced to work beyond their scheduled hours, they can suffer emotional and physical effects. As patient acuity and workloads increase, overtime puts patients and nurses at greater risk. Working overtime should be a choice, not a requirement; however, nurses have been threatened with dismissal or a charge of patient abandonment if they refuse to participate in mandatory overtime.

The ANA opposes mandatory overtime, stating that nurses should be allowed to refuse overtime if they believe that they are too fatigued to provide quality care. In a 2006 position statement regarding nurses working when fatigued, the ANA (2022b) maintains the position that, regardless of the number of hours worked, each registered nurse has an ethical responsibility to carefully consider their level of fatigue when accepting an assignment extending beyond the regularly scheduled workday or week. This includes a mandatory or voluntary overtime assignment (ANA, 2006, 2022b). Rogers et al. (2004) found that nurses' error rates increase significantly during overtime, after 12 hours, or after working more than 60 hours per week. Currently, half of staff nurses are routinely scheduled to work 12-hour shifts, whereas 85% of staff nurses routinely work longer than scheduled hours (Caruso et al., 2015).

Staffing Ratios

Findings from 12 key studies cite specific effects of low nurse staffing on patient outcomes: incidences of failure to rescue, inpatient mortality, pneumonia, urinary tract infections, and pressure ulcers. Effects on the nurses include needlestick injuries and eventual burnout (Aiken et al., 2002). Hospital length of stay and finances are affected as well. Aiken and colleagues further identified a relationship between staffing, patient mortality, nurse burnout, and job dissatisfaction (Aiken et al., 2002). With each additional patient assigned to a nurse, the following occurred:

- A 30-day mortality increase of 7%
- Failure-to-rescue rate increase of 7%
- Nursing job dissatisfaction increase of 15%
- Burnout rate increase of 23%
- A reported 43% of nurses surveyed suffer from burnout

Staffing ratios are setting dependent with intensive care unit patients requiring a higher nurse-to-patient ratio (one nurse to two patients) than an acute care unit where there may be one nurse to four to five patients (AHRQ, 2021). The ANA recommends moving staffing decisions from the industrial model of measuring time and motion to a professional model that examines the factors needed to provide quality care. The effect of changes in staffing levels should be evaluated using nursing-sensitive indicators, the patient care complexity or acuity, the number of admissions and discharges from a unit in a workday, the number of professional staff and ancillary staff, the size and layout of the unit, and availability of technical support and other resources (ANA, 2022b).

A survey of 820 nurses and 621 patients in 20 hospitals across the United States (Vahey et al., 2004) showed that units characterized by nurses as having adequate staff, adequate administrative support for nursing care, and good relations between physicians and nurses were twice as likely as other units to report high satisfaction with nursing care. Nursing shortages can make staffing ratios challenging to maintain, as seen with the recent shortages caused by the COVID-19 pandemic as hospitals and health systems struggle to recruit, retain, and supplement nursing staff to ensure safe, quality patient care (Hausman et al., 2022).

Reporting Questionable Practices

The Code for Nurses (ANA, 2015a) is very specific about nurses' responsibility to report questionable behavior that may affect a patient's welfare. Suppose you become aware of inappropriate or questionable practices in the provision of health care. In that case, the concern should be addressed directly with the person with the questionable practice and attention called to the possible detrimental effect on the patient's welfare. Use official channels if it becomes necessary to report these practices. ANA's Code of Ethics further states that:

When nurses become aware of the inappropriate or questionable practice, the concern must be expressed to the person involved, focusing on the patient's best interests and the integrity of nursing practice. When practices in the healthcare delivery system or organization threaten the patient's welfare, nurses should express their concern to the responsible manager or administrator or, if indicated, to an appropriate higher authority within the institution or agency or an appropriate external authority.

When an incompetent, unethical, illegal, or impaired practice is not corrected, it continues to jeopardize patient well-being and safety. Nurses must report the problem to appropriate external authorities such as practice committees of professional organizations, licensing boards, and regulatory or quality assurance agencies. Some situations are sufficiently egregious to warrant the notification and involvement of all such groups and/or law enforcement. (p. 28)

Most employers have policies that encourage the reporting of behavior that may adversely affect the workplace environment, including but not limited to (ANA, 1994, 2015a):

1. Endangering a patient's health or safety
2. Abusing one's authority
3. Violating laws, rules, regulations, or standards of professional ethics
4. Grossly wasting funds

Protection should be afforded to both the accused and the person doing the reporting, but this is not always the case:

Two Texas nurses not only lost their jobs but also were charged with misuse of official information when they reported a physician to the medical board for patient safety concerns. The charges against one were dropped eventually, and the other was found not guilty in court. The Texas Nurses Association (TNA) Legal Defense Fund helped pay their legal expenses, and the nurses won a civil judgment of $750,000 against the county. The physician was placed on 4 years' probation. "Nurses need to be able to advocate for patient safety," said Cindy Zolnierek, TNA director of practice, "and anything that stands in the way is not good for patients or nurses" (Trossman, 2011, p. 11).

Staff willingness to identify and report problems is essential to ensuring patient safety and improving outcomes. A study of nursing home nurses found they were frustrated by the lack of feedback on submitted incident reports, the limited culture of safety (some noted that reporting a problem could affect their social life and relationships with colleagues), and that lack of time also hindered reporting problems (Praug & Jelsness-Jorgensen, 2014). Another study done in Australia found that nurses who had been whistleblowers not only experienced retaliation at work but it also sometimes disrupted their family life (Wilkes et al., 2011). Whistleblowers are sometimes ostracized (isolated or cast out), which is a painful experience for those who enjoy the comradery of nursing colleagues (Watson & O'Connor, 2017).

Whistleblower is the term used for an employee who reports employer violations to an outside agency. You cannot assume that doing the right thing will protect you: Speaking up could actually get you fired unless you are protected by a union contract or other formal employment agreement. Your state professional organization may also be able to support you. It is important that you know reporting a quality or safety issue sometimes results in reprisals from one's employer. Does this mean that you should never speak up? Not necessarily. Case law, federal and state statutes, and the federal False Claims Act may afford a certain level of protection. Some states have whistleblower laws, but they often apply only to state employees or to certain types of workers. Although these laws may offer some protection, the most important point is to work through the employer's chain of command and internal procedures.

You may also (a) make sure that whistleblowing is addressed at your facility, either through a collective bargaining contract or workplace advocacy program; (b) contact your state nurses association to find out if your state offers whistleblower protection or has such legislation pending; (c) be politically active by contacting your state legislators and urging them to support a pending bill or by educating your elected state officials on the need for such protection for all health-care workers; and (d) contact your U.S. congressional representatives and urge them to support the Patient Safety Act.

Conclusion

Workplace safety is an area of increasing concern for employers and employees alike. Staff members have a right to be informed of any potential risks in the workplace. Employers have a responsibility to provide adequate equipment and systems to protect employees and to create programs and policies to inform employees about minimizing risks as much as possible. Issues of workplace violence, sexual harassment, impaired workers, ergonomics and workplace injuries, and terrorism should be addressed to protect both employees and patients.

There are also work issues related to fatigue and sleepiness because of overlong workdays, mandatory overtime, and inadequate staffing. All these concerns affect not only the staff but also the quality of care and the outcomes of that care. For these reasons, professional organizations, government agencies, and legislative bodies have taken action to encourage employers to provide a safe work environment.

Study Questions

1. Why is it important for nurses to understand the major federal laws and agencies responsible for protecting the individual in the workplace?

2. What actions can nurses take if they believe that OSHA guidelines are not being followed in the workplace?

3. What are nurses' responsibilities in dealing with the following workplace issues: transmission of blood-borne pathogens, violence, sexual harassment, and impaired coworkers?

4. What information do you need to obtain from your employer related to disasters or a terrorist threat?

5. What factors will you look for in the work environment that make it a safe place to work?

Case Studies to Promote Clinical Judgment

Whistleblower

Selena Suriaga noticed that one of the surgeons whose patients were brought to her unit after their time in the recovery area had more difficulty regaining full consciousness than did the other postsurgical patients. When she mentioned it at lunch one day, a recovery area nurse said, "Sure, he insists on deep anesthesia and wants us to keep his patients sedated. He believes that this will improve his satisfaction ratings."

"That's no reason to overmedicate," said Selena.

"Of course not," said the recovery nurse, "but he gets very angry if we don't give his patients the full amount ordered."

"I think we should tell someone," suggested Selena.

1. If you were Selena, would you leave this concern to the recovery nurses or would you try to resolve it? Why?

2. What are some of the concerns Selena might have about bringing this problem to the attention of hospital management?

3. Describe the steps Selena should take if she decides to follow up on this problem.

4. After speaking with her unit nurse manager and the nursing director of her service, Selena realizes that they do not intend to take any action to resolve this problem. What are her next steps in advocating for patient safety? To whom can she turn? What are the potential consequences for Selena if she talks about this concern to authorities outside the hospital?

5. Selena finally concludes that she will be the whistleblower who reports this problem to the state licensure agency and TJC. What are the personal consequences she might face as a whistleblower? To whom can she turn for support?

Incidence of Violence

Robert Jones works on the evening shift in the ED at a large urban hospital that frequently receives victims of gunshot wounds, stabbings, and other gang-related incidents. Many are high on alcohol or drugs. Robert has just interviewed a 21-year-old male patient awaiting treatment for injuries resulting from a fight after an evening of heavy drinking. Because his injuries were determined not to be life-threatening, he had to wait to see a physician. "I'm tired of waiting. Let's get this show on the road!" he screamed as Robert walked by. "I'm sorry you have to wait, Mr. P., but the doctor is busy with another patient and will get to you as soon as possible." He handed him a cup of juice he had been bringing to another patient. The patient grabbed the cup, threw it in Robert's face, and then grabbed his arm. Slamming him against the wall, the patient jumped off the stretcher and yelled obscenities at him. He continued to scream until a security guard intervened.

1. Critically evaluate the incident: What was done correctly? What was done incorrectly?

2. What could have been done by staff of the ED to prevent this incident?

3. What should be done by the organization to prevent other incidents similar to this one?

4. Rewrite the incident to illustrate an effective response to this situation.

NCLEX®-Style Review Questions

1. OSHA, a federal government agency, is responsible for
   1. Providing training to handle difficult clients and their families
   2. Providing research and education training
   3. Upholding the standards of nursing practice
   4. Developing and enforcing workplace safety and health regulations

2. A *surprisingly* dangerous job in the United States is working
   1. In a coal mine
   2. As a window cleaner in New York City
   3. In a health-care facility
   4. As a police officer

3. A federal agency that partners with other agencies throughout the nation to investigate health problems, conduct research, implement prevention strategies, and promote safe and healthy environments is known as the
   1. FDA
   2. IOM
   3. ANA
   4. CDC

4. Actions to address violence in the health-care workplace include: **Select all that apply**.
   1. Identifying the factors that contribute to violence and controlling as many as possible
   2. Allowing the violence to escalate
   3. Assessing staff attitudes and knowledge regarding responses to violence
   4. Providing weapons training to those identified as having a potential for physical violence

5. According to NIOSH, a common reaction to latex allergy is
   1. Increased appetite
   2. Allergic contact dermatitis
   3. Increased falls
   4. An increase in violent outbursts

6. A common ergonomic occupational-related risk in the health-care environment is
   1. Indoor air pollution
   2. Active shooters
   3. Nosocomial infection
   4. Back injuries

7. A suburban hospital recently announced that staff nurses could no longer choose their shift. Instead, they would be assigned to either a 12-hour day shift or a 12-hour night shift on an as-needed basis. An informal group of staff nurses met to discuss this new policy. They came up with several arguments against it. Which of the following suggestions would help to alleviate the deleterious effects of this new policy?
   1. Allow self-scheduling by staff nurses in each unit.
   2. Provide free dinner for nursing staff at the end of the night shift.
   3. Allow staff members to request consistent days off.
   4. End visiting hours before the day shift ends so that the night shift nurses do not have to deal with visitors.

8. Which of the following are considered reasonable accommodations for an employee with a disability? **Select all that apply**.
   1. Modification of the work schedule
   2. Salary reduction to reflect lower output
   3. Additional days off and extended vacations
   4. Adjustment of work procedures

9. Which of the following procedures and modifications contributes to reducing indoor air pollution?
   1. Windows that may be opened by staff as needed
   2. More powerful ventilation systems and air filtration
   3. Selection of products with more polyvinyl chloride (PVC)
   4. Increased use of medical waste incinerators

10. Stephanie Beals was a little nervous during her first week of work as a licensed nurse. Distracted by a lead nurse behind her, her hand slipped, and she was stuck by the needle she had just used. What is most important for Stephanie to do?
    1. Disinfect the site of the needlestick.
    2. Apologize to the patient, clean the site, and properly dispose of the needle.
    3. Update her hepatitis B immunization.
    4. Report the incident and obtain post exposure prophylaxis (PEP) within 2 hours.

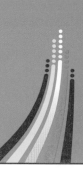

chapter 13

Promoting a Healthy
Work Environment

Social Environment

Many aspects of the social environment of the workplace received attention in earlier chapters. Team building, communicating effectively, and developing leadership skills are essential to developing working relationships.

The day-to-day interactions with one's peers and supervisors have a significant impact on the quality of the workplace environment. Most employees feel the difference between a supportive and a nonsupportive environment keenly. For example:

> Ms. B came to work already tired. Her baby was sick and had been awake most of the night. Her team expressed concern about the baby when she told them she had a difficult night. Each team member voluntarily took an extra patient so that Ms. B could have a lighter assignment that day. When Ms. B expressed her appreciation, her team leader said, "We know you would do the same for us." Ms. B worked in a supportive environment.
>
> Ms. G came to work after a sleepless night. Her young son had been diagnosed with leukemia, and she was apprehensive about him. When she mentioned her concerns, her team leader interrupted her, saying, "Please leave your personal problems at home. We have a lot of work to do, and we expect you to do your share." Ms. G worked in a nonsupportive environment.

In a supportive environment, people are willing to make difficult decisions, take risks, and "go the extra mile" for team members and the organization. In a nonsupportive environment, members are afraid to take risks, avoid making decisions, and limit their commitment to their coworkers and the individuals in their care. Incivility, discussed later in this chapter, contributes to a nonsupportive environment.

Involvement in Decision Making

Having a voice in the decisions made about one's work and patients is very important to health-care professionals. There are many actions that leaders can take to empower nurses. They include removing barriers to nurse participation in decision making, providing regular coaching on each nurse's professional development, publicly recognizing nurses for their contributions, valuing their initiative and assertiveness, and serving as role models who demonstrate confidence and competence (Gallup, 2022). The following illustrates the difference between empowerment and powerlessness:

> Soon after completing orientation, Nurse A heard a new nurse aide scolding a patient for soiling the bed. Nurse A did not know how incidents of possible verbal abuse were handled in this institution, so she reported it to the nurse manager. The nurse manager asked Nurse A several questions and thanked her for the information. The new aide was counseled immediately after their meeting. Nurse A noticed a positive change in the aide's manner with patients after this incident. Nurse A felt good about contributing to a more effective patient care team. Nurse A felt empowered and will take action when another occasion arises.
>
> A colleague of Nurse B was an instructor at a community college. This colleague asked Nurse B if students would be welcome on her unit. "Of course," replied Nurse B. "I'll speak with my nurse manager about it." However, when Nurse B did so, the response was that the unit was too busy to accommodate students. In addition, Nurse B received a verbal reprimand from the supervisor for overstepping her authority by discussing the placement of students. "All requests for student placement must be directed to the education department," she said. The supervisor directed Nurse B to write a letter of apology for having made an unauthorized commitment to the community college. Nurse B was afraid to make any decisions or public statements after this incident. Nurse B felt alienated and powerless.

Professional Growth and Innovation

The difference between a climate that encourages staff growth and creativity and one that does not can be very subtle. Many people are only partly aware of whether or not they work in an environment that fosters professional growth and learning. Yet the effect on the quality of the work done is pervasive, and it is an essential factor in distinguishing a good health-care organization from an excellent one.

The rapidly increasing accumulation of knowledge in medical science and its impact on health-care organizations mandates continuous learning for safe practice. Much of the responsibility for staff development and promotion of innovation lies with upper-level management. First-line managers can develop and support a climate of professional growth that encourages critical thinking and innovation, provides opportunities to take advantage of educational programs, supports new ideas and projects, and rewards professional development.

Encouraging Innovation, New Ideas, and Critical Thinking

Intellectual curiosity is a hallmark of the professional, but a curious frame of mind is relatively easy to suppress in a work environment. Patients and staff will quickly sense a nurse's impatience or defensiveness when they raise questions and may simply stop asking. However, if you are a critical thinker and support other critical thinkers, you can contribute to an open-minded work environment.

Participating in brainstorming sessions, group conferences, and discussions encourages the generation of new ideas. More recently, many organizations have strengthened their efforts to cultivate new nursing knowledge and innovation. This was especially true during the COVID-19 pandemic when frontline nurses collaborated with their leaders and found safer alternatives when caring for COVID-19 patients. The use of nurses as safety monitors who offered physical and emotional support to their peers, IV tubing extensions to migrate the pumps out of the isolation rooms in ICUs to ensure timely titration of life-saving medication, and even the redesign of the care delivery model were beneficial. These ideas resulted from blending novel concepts from novice nurses with senior, more experienced nurses' knowledge.

Although new nurses may think they have nothing to offer, remember that this rarely the case. They need to participate in activities that encourage them to contribute fresh, new ideas.

Rewarding Professional Growth

A primary source of discontent in the workplace is a lack of recognition by leaders for individual and group accomplishments (Ellrich & Nelson, 2020). Everyone enjoys praise and recognition, and there is no monetary cost to providing it. An acknowledgment for a job well done in a card, a verbal thank you, or a public announcement at a staff meeting goes a long way with coworkers recognizing a job well done. Recognition is praise for accomplishment and, more importantly, colleague or leader appreciation for that achievement. Nurse leaders also consider it a top priority because of its ties to nursing engagement in their work, making nurses feel valued, improving morale, and enhancing teamwork (Peterson, 2016; Zwickel et al., 2016).

Many leaders underestimate the powerful effect of meaningful recognition on a nurse. Meaningful recognition can improve nurse retention and indirectly affect nurse recruitment as those recognized nurses tell others of their experiences (Peterson, 2016). In addition to the work of individual leaders, many health-care organizations have staff recognition programs that serve as another means of increasing self-esteem, social gratification, morale, and job satisfaction (Hurst et al., 1994).

Horizontal Violence

Horizontal violence may occur among employees in a health-care environment. This phenomenon is defined as "hostile, aggressive, and harmful behavior by a nurse or a group of nurses toward a co-worker or group of nurses via attitudes, actions, words, and other behaviors" (Thobaben, 2007, p. 83). Terms to describe horizontal violence, which are often used interchangeably, include *lateral violence, incivility, bullying,* and *disruptive behavior* (Taylor, 2016). Horizontal violence behaviors include verbal abuse, punishment, humiliating comments, intimidation, malicious gossip, and sabotage or interference with work (Grant et al., 2020). Bullies in the workplace may be coworkers, superiors, or subordinates. Regardless of their place on the organizational chart, they can cause a great deal of distress to others in the workplace. The Joint Commission (TJC) characterizes horizontal violence as a sentinel event because it may threaten patient safety (Kear, 2012; TJC, 2022).

How common is bullying in the workplace? Unfortunately, it is not a rare event. Before the COVID-19 pandemic, in a sample of 2,659 registered nurses (RNs) from 19 facilities in New York State, 22% reported they were expected to do others' work, 9% had been reprimanded in front of others, 9.8% said attempts were made to destroy their credibility, 9.2% reported being constantly criticized, and 6% had been threatened with negative consequences (Sellers & Millenbach, 2012).

Trépanier and colleagues (2016) estimate that almost 40% of nurses are exposed to bullying. Their research found that workgroup cohesion, social support from the supervisor and mentor, communication and trust within the teams, and value congruence were protective.

In 2017, the American Nurses Association (ANA) initiated a campaign, #endnurseabuse, to raise public and professional awareness of violence in nursing (Ross et al., 2019; ANA, 2017). Despite this and other industry efforts, findings from American Hospital Association research shows over 44% of nurses surveyed reported physical violence, and close to 68% experienced verbal abuse during the pandemic (American Hospital Association, 2022)). The presence of cliques, lack of trust, poor communication, and a lack of support are related to the occurrence of bullying.

Australian and United Kingdom (UK) nursing students were asked if they had experienced bullying during their clinical placements. Among the students, 50% of the 833 Australian nursing students and 35% of the 561 UK students reported they had experienced bullying, primarily from other nurses (Birks et al., 2017). Similarly, a study of new graduates in Canada found that most had observed some incivility in their workplace, primarily by coworkers rather than supervisors (Smith et al., 2010). On a positive note, nursing managers in Canada have noticed an increase in the reporting of horizontal violence as the staff has become more aware of their rights and protections as employees (Rocker, 2012). Although lower in intensity than physical violence, the long-term effects of incivility are far from benign and need to be addressed. The following are a few ways in which these behaviors can be addressed (Kear, 2012; Lewis & Malecha, 2011; Ross et al., 2019):

- Establish a zero-tolerance policy for these behaviors.
- Develop a code of conduct that explicitly addresses these behaviors.
- Ensure administrators, supervisors, and managers model appropriate behavior.
- Discuss strategies for handling such behavior in meetings with staff.
- Report bullying behavior to your nurse manager.
- Confront bullying and belittling behavior; express your concerns objectively.

Kear (2012) suggests an objective response to this behavior: "When you call me incompetent, I feel angry. Instead, I would like you to teach me what I may not know . . ." (p. 1). It requires courage to confront these behaviors directly; however, failing to do so allows them to continue and even increase.

Similar to some of the other workplace problems (discrimination, for example), bullying creates a toxic environment that hurts the individual targeted, interferes with the smooth functioning of a health-care facility, and reduces the quality of the care provided.

Sexual Harassment

After months of interviewing, a new supervisor was hired, a young male nurse whom the staff members jokingly described as "a blond Tom Cruise." The new supervisor was an instant hit with the predominantly female executives and staff members. However, he soon found himself on the receiving end of sexual jokes and innuendoes. He had been trying to prove himself a competent supervisor with hopes of eventually moving up to a higher management position. He viewed the female staff members and supervisor's behavior as undermining his credibility and being embarrassing and annoying. He attempted to stop the unwelcome conduct by discussing it with his boss, a female nurse administrator. She told him jokingly that it was nothing more than "good-natured fun" and that "men can't be harassed by women" (Outwater, 1994).

Sexual harassment is a persistent problem in the workplace and is considered violence or aggression toward another person or persons (AAUW, 2018). The Equal Employment Opportunity Commission (EEOC) list of industries with the most sexual harassment claims ranks health care as number 4 (Ross et al., 2019). In a multihospital study (Cogin & Fish, 2009), findings revealed that 60% of female nurses and 34% of male nurses reported being victims of sexual harassment. Internationally, the percentage of nurses experiencing sexual harassment is approximately 20% (Ross et al., 2019).

Significant contributors to the high percentage of sexual harassment experienced by nurses include sex-role stereotypes, persistent societal tolerance of sexual harassment, and the unequal balance of power between men and women. Findings from studies on sexual violence show that female nurses are prone to sexual harassment because attributes such as caring attitudes, gentleness, and compassion are wrongly perceived as sexual signals (Ross et al., 2019). Nurses frequently dismiss and seldom report verbal sexual harassment or inappropriate, nonsexual touching by patients as unintentional because of medication or illness despite how uncomfortable it made them feel. Underreporting sexual harassment is common, even though the emotional costs of anger, humiliation, and fear are high (McClendon & Farbman, 2018).

In 1980, the EEOC issued a statement prohibiting sexual harassment. Then, in 1993, the ANA issued a statement calling for the elimination of sexual harassment in all work settings (Ross et al., 2019). Title VII of the Civil Rights Act of 1964 prohibits discrimination based on sex, race, color, national origin, and religion (AAUW, 2018). Two forms of unwelcomed sexual conduct are

1. **Quid pro quo** This involves sexual favors solicited in exchange for favorable job benefits or continuation of employment. In these cases, the employee must demonstrate that they were required to endure unwelcome sexual advances to keep the job or job benefits, and that rejection of these behaviors would have resulted in deprivation of a job or benefits. Example: An administrator approaches a nurse for a date in exchange for a promotion.
2. **Hostile work environment (HWE)** HWE is the most common sexual harassment claim and the most difficult to prove. The employee making a claim must prove that gender is the basis for the harassment. They must show that it has affected conditions of employment or created an offensive environment where the employee could not effectively discharge their job responsibilities (Outwater, 1994; Ross et al., 2019). If an environment is determined to be hostile or abusive, there is no further need to establish that it was also psychologically damaging. Although sexual harassment against women is more common, men can also be victims (Box 13-1).

Do not ignore the issue of sexual harassment in the workplace. If you supervise other employees, it is essential to review your agency's policies and procedures and seek appropriate guidance from the human resources department if needed. Initiating

---

box 13-1

Behaviors That Could Be Defined as Sexual Harassment

- Pressure to participate in sexual activities
- Asking about another person's sexual activities, fantasies, or preferences
- Making sexual innuendoes, jokes, or comments; showing sexual graffiti or visuals
- Continuing to ask for a date after the other person has expressed disinterest
- Making suggestive facial expressions or gestures with hands or body movements
- Making remarks about a person's gender or body

---

a confidential investigation of the allegation is required when an employee approaches you with a complaint. Do not dismiss any incidents or accounts of sexual harassment involving yourself or others as "just having fun" or respond, "There is nothing anyone can do." Responses such as this can have serious consequences in the workplace (Outwater, 1994).

If you do experience sexual harassment, you should do the following:

Consult your employee handbook or online published policies You may find guidance on responding to the harassment, including recording the incidents and reporting them in these documents.

Confront Indicate immediately and clearly to the harasser that the attention is unwanted. In a unionized facility, ask the nursing representative to accompany you.

Report Immediately inform your supervisor of the incident. If the harasser is your supervisor, report the incident to a higher authority and file a formal complaint.

Document Record the incident immediately while it is fresh in your mind—what happened, when and where it occurred, and how you responded. Name any witnesses. Keep thorough records in a safe place away from work.

Support Seek support from friends, relatives, and organizations such as your state nurses association. If you are a student, seek help from a trusted faculty member or advisor.

Contact the EEOC The EEOC must be contacted within 180 days of the incident, so don't delay if you think this is the route you will have to take to resolve the problem. Its Web site has contact details (AAUW, 2018).

If you are a student, your employer (or the director of your program) is responsible for maintaining a harassment-free workplace. You should expect your employer to demonstrate commitment to creating a safe, healthy work environment; provide written solid policies prohibiting sexual harassment; describe how employees will be protected; and educate all employees verbally and in writing. For a list of other important federal laws to protect workers, please see Chapter 12, Box 12-1.

Implicit Bias

Ms. V is beginning orientation as a new staff nurse, and as part of her orientation she must attend a class on diversity, equity, and inclusion (DEI). She tells the human resources orientation coordinator, "I don't think I need to attend that class. I treat all people as equal. Besides, anyone living in our country should learn the language and how we do things, not the other way around."

Examples of implicit bias (IB) that can lead to false assumptions include perceptions that obese people are lazy, those who attend state schools are less intelligent than people admitted to private colleges and universities, or that patients who ask for pain medication are drug-seeking.

All cultures, races, and ethnic groups need to examine their assumptions and possible biases concerning people of different gender, ages, culture, race, ethnic group, or abilities. Edgoose, Quiogue, and Sidhar (2019) describe IB as the "unconscious collection of stereotypes and attitudes that we develop toward certain groups of people, which can affect our patient relationships and care decisions" (p. 30). IB develops with an individual's experience and usually lines up with their cultural and social hierarchies. IB is created by the mental shortcuts that help recognize patterns and sum up situations using approaches that worked in the past (Narayan, 2019). Triggered by a new situation, the brain formulates quick assessments and judgments based on prior, similar experiences. Unfortunately, these automatic responses, or stereotyping, can result in subtle, discriminatory behaviors (Narayan, 2019).

The report *Unequal Treatment: Confronting Racial and Ethnic Disparities in Health Care* concluded that IB-associated stereotyping and health-care provider clinical uncertainty contribute to racial and ethnic disparities in health care (u Long, 2003). Health-care disparities refer to minority population clinical outcomes compared with the dominant or majority populations. Health inequities can also be based on gender, age, sexual orientation, religion, socio-economic status, gender identity, disability, and stigmatizing diagnoses such as mental illness or substance use.

A lack of awareness of your IBs can directly and possibly negatively impact patient outcomes, especially regarding patient assessment, treatment decisions, time with patients, and effective care planning and discharge teaching (Narayan, 2019). IB, although not preventable, is manageable. Edgoose and colleagues (2019) recommend three strategies with associated tactics to mitigate IB and enhance situational awareness: educating yourself and others about IB to be able to confront our own biases using techniques such as mindfulness and periods of introspection; embracing diversity by learning about the other person's perspective and acknowledging differences; and, slowing down to recognize your own IB. Addressing IB requires vigilance. In addition to an individual's attempts to understand and manage IB, hospitals and health-care systems need to promote equity, diversity, and inclusion by providing ongoing education and continuous process improvement (Edgoose et al., 2019).

Equity, Diversity, and Inclusion

Equity and Health Equity

Equity is "the state, quality or ideal of being just, impartial and fair" (Annie E. Casey Foundation [AECF], 2021, p. 5). It is different from equality because people may have the same opportunities, but there are barriers to helping them take advantage of them. Creating an equitable solution may require policies or programs to improve access to ensure access for all. Equality assumes that everyone starts from the same place and receives the same opportunities. Policies and laws at a national and local level improve social equity.

Similar to social equity, health equity ensures that everyone has the same access to care and the opportunity to be as healthy as possible. Both social and health equity acknowledge that care disparities exist and work to eliminate them.

Diversity and Inclusion

Diversity in health-care organizations includes ethnicity, race, culture, gender, sexual orientation, lifestyle, primary language, age, physical capabilities, and career stages of employees and patients. Working with and caring for people with different customs, traditions, communication styles, and beliefs can be rewarding and challenging. An organization that fosters diversity encourages respect and understanding of human characteristics and accepts the similarities and differences that make us human.

Inclusion has been defined as a commitment from leadership, colleagues, and coworkers to provide space and create a sense of belonging where individuals feel valued and respected for who they are (Schmidt et al., 2016). This creates an environment where people do their best work collectively and individually.

Fostering inclusion requires cultivating diversity, being culturally humble, and continually assessing personal and organizational biases (Campinha-Bacote, 2002; Davidhizar et al., 1999; Stubbe, 2020). Consider several factors that enhance understanding diversity and fostering inclusion:

1. **Communication** Communication and culture are closely bound. Culture is transmitted through communication and influences how people express themselves. Vocabulary, voice qualities, intonation, rhythm, speed, silence, touch, body posture, eye movements, and pronunciation differ among cultural groups and vary among persons from similar cultures. Maintaining respect is central to building relationships (Davidhizar et al., 1999). Active listening or focusing all of your attention on your audience to ensure a shared understanding of a topic is essential when setting expectations and goals (Gelinas, 2018). Everyone needs to assess the communication preferences of others in the workplace.
2. **Space** Personal space is the area that surrounds a person's body. The amount of personal space individuals prefer varies from person to person and from situation to situation. Understanding coworkers' comfort related to personal space is essential in the workplace. Individuals relay discomfort using nonverbal rather than verbal communication, such as pulling back or a change in facial expression.
3. **Social organization** A person's social organization can be focused on family, friends, work, or some combination of the three and influences their choices (Davidhizar et al., 1999). For some people, the importance of family supersedes that of other personal, work, or national issues. For example, caring for a sick child may override the importance of being on time or even coming to work, regardless of staffing needs or policies.
4. **Time** Time orientation can be culturally related (Davidhizar et al., 1999). Some cultures are more past-oriented, emphasizing traditions. People from cultures with a future orientation may be more likely to forego current pleasure for later rewards, returning to school for a higher degree or earning certification. Working with people who have different time orientations may cause difficulty managing rotating shifts, planning schedules, setting deadlines, and even defining what "on time" means.
5. **Internal or external control** Individuals with an external locus of control believe in the importance of fate or chance. People with an internal locus of control believe they can influence, and even determine, outcomes (Davidhizar et al., 1999). Thus, nurses influence patient outcomes when delivering care. Depending on personal or cultural beliefs, a nurse might dismiss an outcome as fateful or lucky rather than a result of care provided.

Indications of an organization's commitment to building a diverse and inclusive workplace include the following (Carter et al., 2020; Mitchell, 1995):

■ Minorities are represented at all levels of personnel, and an organization's demographic should mirror that of its consumer or client base.
■ Individual preferences about issues of social distance, touching, voice volume and inflection, silence, and gestures are respected.
■ Recognition of and respect for cultural and religious holidays is displayed.

Ways that you can model cultural humility (Campinha-Bacote, 2002):

■ Awareness of your IB, values, and personal preferences when addressing others
■ Recognition of opportunities to be more inclusive of diverse groups, opinions, and ideas
■ Knowledgeable about other cultures and people who are different from you

- Respectful of and sensitive to diversity among individuals
- Skilled in using culturally sensitive intervention strategies

Discrimination

Discrimination is the unjust treatment of people and groups based on characteristics they possess, or groups or classes to which they belong (APA, 2019). It is harmful to all and is not in keeping with the nursing profession's Code of Ethics to "respect the inherent dignity, worth, unique attributes, and human rights of all individuals" (ANA, 2015, p. 17). ANA position statements support eliminating all forms of discrimination and call for equality and justice at both the individual and population levels (ANA Ethics Advisory Board, 2019). Discrimination is linked to health inequity or disparity, leading to poor clinical outcomes (ANA Ethics Advisory Board, 2019). The ANA Code of Ethics (2019) calls for nurses to treat all patients equally with civility and respect.

Times of crisis, such as a pandemic, amplify societal issues and disparities and create stress and uncertainty. The coming together to advocate for the rights of Black individuals and people of color (BPOC) during the Black Lives Matter rallies heightened our awareness of social inequities, especially as they relate to health disparities and systemic racism.

Discrimination, in any form, is intolerable. Most health-care organizations and agencies have zero-tolerance policies and practices to ensure a safe and healthy work environment. In addition, there are laws that prohibit discrimination in the workplace based on the 5th and 14th Amendments to the Constitution and mandate due process and equal protection under the law. The federal EEOC oversees the administration and enforcement of issues related to workplace equality. The Civil Rights Act of 1964 applies to employers of 15 or more people, including federal, state, and local government employers (AAUW, 2018). Although there may be exemptions from any law, nurses must recognize that significant legislation prohibits employers from making workplace decisions based on race, color, sex, age, disability, religion, or national origin. The employer may ask questions about these issues but cannot make employment decisions based on them.

Cultural Humility and Culturally Competent Care

More than one in three Americans are members of a racial or ethnic minority. However, more importantly, the members of these minorities, and society in general, are unique individuals (U.S. Census Bureau, 2020). This noted growth in cultural diversity requires nurses to practice with cultural humility. *Cultural humility* is defined as "having traits of respect, empathy, and a critical self-reflection at both interpersonal and interprofessional levels" (Hughes et al., 2020, p. 28). It ensures that a nurse knows the importance of knowing each patient and incorporating their needs and preferences into care delivery. This individualized approach to care planning reduces the incidence of bias. It stresses using evidence-based data to ensure that the patient's unique culture, ethnicity, beliefs, and values are blended into care. The nurse's ability to take a situation or person, professionally or personally, at face value in cultural and social contexts shows genuine interest and can foster better understanding and collaboration. Assumptions about an individual's preferences based on race, ethnicity, gender, age, or gender orientation are biased because they are based on one's perspective, not fact. It is important to continually expand your knowledge of different cultures and ethnic groups to expand your worldview, which can reduce IB and stereotyping (Campinha-Bacote, 2002; Leininger, 1999; Schmidt et al., 2016).

Culturally Competent Care

Cultural competence is an "ongoing process in which the healthcare provider [nurse] continuously strives to achieve the ability to effectively work within the cultural context of the client [patient, community]" (Campinha-Bacote, 2002, p. 181). It is a process wherein someone is continually and sincerely learning and acknowledging the needs and concerns of the patient by getting to know every patient as an individual with unique needs, goals, and attributes. It takes cultural awareness and the desire to be with and learn from the patient (Campinha-Bacote, 2002).

Nurses are somewhat similar to anthropologists as they seek to learn about being human, one patient at a time. This holistic approach blends the subjective data from the patient with the objective data or evidence to form an assessment of the patient's condition that is then used to make a plan of care.

Campinha-Bacote (2002) notes that culturally competent care is built on five constructs:

Cultural awareness This involves the exploration and understanding of one's background to identify personal biases, prejudice, and stereotypes.

Cultural knowledge This involves finding and learning facts about different cultures and ethnic groups to understand a patient's interpretation of their illness and population-specific prevalence and incidence of disease.

Cultural skill The ability of the nurse to collect pertinent information about a patient's presenting problem and physical assessment. It is important to understand body structure and skin color related to normal and abnormal presentation. This knowledge can give the nurse more confidence and prove reassuring to the patient.

Cultural encounters Putting oneself in different situations to experience new and diverse groups can broaden understanding of other cultures and ethnic groups. It refines one's beliefs and can help identify and reduce personal biases.

Cultural desires This means being motivated or caring enough to want to become culturally knowledgeable and skilled in cultural encounters. Campinha-Bacote (2002) notes that "cultural desire involves the concept of caring" (p. 182).

Cultural humility gives nurses the insight, ability, and vigilance necessary to provide culturally competent care. The constructs of culturally competent care are interwoven, and when addressing one, it strengthens nursing care. Nurses must respect a patient's beliefs and practices and show real motivation to provide genuine, responsive, and meaningful care to the patient.

Addressing Job Stress and Burnout to Create a Healthy Work Environment

Workplace Stress

Workplace stress is a mismatch between an individual's perception of their demands and their ability to meet them, compounded by predisposing factors and the general nature of clinical work (Grant et al., 2020). Tully and Tao (2019) note that although some stress can be beneficial, prolonged stress can negatively affect physical and psychological health. Understanding the cause of stress is critical to maintaining optimal health and well-being. More than 50% of Americans experience stress, with 61% attributing that stress to work-related pressures (Tully & Tao, 2019). Other factors contributing to a person's threshold for stress are personal characteristics and experiences, coping mechanisms, and the circumstances of the event (Grant et al., 2020; McVicar, 2003, 2016; Tully & Tao, 2019).

Sources of Workplace Stress

Before the COVID-19 pandemic, nurses reported higher levels of work-related stress than other health-care workers (ANA, 2011; Roberts & Grubb, 2014; Tully & Tao, 2019). The nature of nurses' work creates the potential for experiencing stress (Grant et al., 2020; McGibbon et al., 2010; Roberts & Grubb, 2014; Tully & Tao, 2019), especially for younger, less experienced nurses (Africa & Trépanier, 2021; Purcell et al., 2011). Five themes describing barriers to reducing work-related stress are:

- Inadequate or "short" staffing, high nurse–patient ratios, time constraints, and shift
- Government regulations and hospital requirements that create barriers to care which can cause moral distress
- Bullying, incivility, and other disrespectful behaviors and unrealistic expectations by patients and their families
- Lack of authentic leadership within practice environments
- Hostile workplace culture, including workplace violence and interpersonal conflict (Grant et al., 2020; Healy & Tyrrell, 2011; Purcell et al., 2011; Tully & Tao, 2019)

Nurses in a pediatric intensive care unit reported some additional sources:

- When caring requires inflicting pain on a child
- Being tied to their patients continuously for 12 hours
- Dealing with inexperienced medical residents
- Taking on others' work (e.g., therapy on the weekend, double-checking doctors' orders, discharge planning) without credit for it

- Malfunctioning equipment and a lack of supplies and equipment to provide care (McGibbon et al., 2010; McVicar, 2016)

Outside demands such as family caregiving can also be a source of stress (Tucker et al., 2012). Over time, minor stressors can accumulate, with adverse effects on one's health, such as cardiovascular disease or psychological disorders (Evans et al., 2011; Grant et al., 2020; Roberts & Grubb, 2014; Tully & Tao, 2019).

Although most discussions emphasize the stressful nature of nurses' work, it is essential to keep in mind that there are many sources of satisfaction in the work of nurses as well. For example, a study of more than 2,000 staff nurses from a midwestern medical center found that the nurses reported an average level of perceived stress (Tucker et al., 2012), suggesting most nurses learn how to manage these stresses. Additional information about managing stress and capturing job satisfaction will be discussed later.

Why Is Health Care a Stressful Occupation?

The National Institute for Occupational Safety and Health (NIOSH, 1999) broadly defines *work-related stress* as the "harmful physical and emotional responses that occur when the job requirements do not match the capabilities, resources, or needs of the worker" (p. 6). Stress experienced by nurses is related to the nature of their work: continued intensive, intimate contact with people who often have serious physical, mental, emotional, or social problems and terminal conditions (Grant et al., 2020). Efforts to save patients or help them achieve a peaceful ending to their lives are not always successful. Crises such as the COVID-19 pandemic can exponentiate workplace stressors such as inadequate staffing, urgent changes in government regulations or hospital policy, unrealistic expectations, workplace violence, and insufficient resources to care for patients (Grant et al., 2020; Tully & Tao, 2019). The continued loss of patients alone can lead to burnout. Coupled with these additional stressors, the chance of work-related stress grows.

In some instances, human service professionals also experience lower pay, longer hours, and more extensive regulation than professionals in other fields. Inadequate advancement opportunities for women and minorities in lower-status, lower-paid positions may also contribute to job dissatisfaction.

Signs of and Responses to Stress

Whether the stress you experience results from significant life changes or the cumulative effect of minor everyday hassles, how you respond to these experiences determines how stress will affect your life (Davis et al., 2000). Those daily hassles include heavy workloads, time constraints, and a lack of resources which individually are manageable but may cause stress if these hassles are general working conditions (Roberts & Grubb, 2014; Tully & Tao, 2019). Chronic exposure to stressors such as these can lead to burnout, compassion fatigue, and even physical illness (Grant et al., 2020; Tully & Tao, 2019).

Occupational exposure to stressful situations mounts up and can cause anxiety and depression (Grant et al., 2020; Roberts & Grubb, 2014). This, coupled with conflict and workplace violence, adds a complexity that exacerbates stress. People cope with stress differently. Some people effectively manage stressful events, whereas others, in the same situation, may feel anxious or afraid (Crawford, 1993; Teague, 1992; Tully & Tao, 2019). Also, a patient care situation that one nurse considers stressful may not seem stressful to a coworker. The following is an example:

A new graduate nurse working on a busy telemetry unit experienced physical discomfort when admitting patients. Patients were often in acute distress, with shortness of breath, diaphoresis, agitation, and chest pain. Family members were troubled, anxious, and sometimes angry.

Each time the nurse had to admit a patient, she experienced a "sick-to-the-stomach" feeling, tightness in the chest, and difficulty concentrating. She was afraid that she would miss something essential and that the patient would die during admission. In contrast, the more experienced nurses seemed to handle each admission with ease, even when the patients exhibited life-threatening symptoms.

Compassion Fatigue and Burnout

Compassion Fatigue

Compassion is a required professional nursing value according to the International Council of Nurses' Code of Ethics (Gustafsson & Hemberg, 2022). Compassion is an attribute of caring (Roach, 2002). When caring for patients, nurses are intimately involved in patient experiences and feelings, witness human suffering, and may experience moral distress, emotional trauma, and loss daily (Gustafsson & Hemberg, 2022; Upton, 2018). Nurses experience satisfaction in positive feelings of caring for patients. Constant exposure to job stress such as working short-staffed or not having the right supplies when caring for patients can be physically, emotionally, and mentally taxing. Inability to cope with the long-term exposure to the demands of caring can result in an emotional and physical disconnection or desensitization from patients, families, and even colleagues or compassion fatigue (Gustafsson & Hemberg, 2022; Henson, 2020; Upton, 2018). Symptoms of compassion fatigue manifest in physical, psychological, and social symptoms ranging from cardiovascular disease, diabetes, and obesity to cynicism, boredom, isolation, and, in some instances, substance use, anxiety, and depression (Gustafsson & Hemberg, 2022; Upton, 2018). An essential attribute of compassion fatigue is sudden onset with immediate behavioral changes noted such as apathy, a loss of connection with their patients, and even physical symptoms such as nightmares and anxiety (Henson, 2020). Unlike compassion fatigue, burnout is the result of constant job-related stress over time (Henson, 2020; U.S. Department of Health and Human Services (NIOSH, 2022).

Burnout

The ultimate result of unmediated, unresolved job-related stress is burnout. The term *burnout* was a favorite buzzword of the 1980s and continues to be part of today's vocabulary. Burnout is considered an occupational hazard for service industries such as health care (Maslach & Leiter, 2016). Herbert Freudenberger formally identified it as a leadership concern in 1974. The literature on job stress and burnout grows as new books, articles, workshops, and videos regularly appear. Signs of burnout include emotional exhaustion, cynicism, a perceived loss of control, and depersonalization (Henson, 2020; Maslach & Leiter, 2016). It is also considered a precursor to compassion fatigue (Sabo, 2011).

Moreover, burnout is the "progressive deterioration in work and other performance resulting from increasing difficulties in coping with high and continuing levels of job-related stress and professional frustration" (Paine, 1984, p. 1).

Frustration created by challenges that prevent nurses from delivering their idea of perfect patient care contributes to burnout. Anything that interferes with providing the highest-quality care causes work-related stress and feelings of failure for nurses who take their greatest satisfaction from caring for patients. Nurses routinely put the needs of their patients, colleagues, and others ahead of theirs, sometimes to the nurse's detriment. Job demands that occasionally result in a skipped meal break, working overtime last minute, or taking a heavier assignment are qualities of a team player. However, nurses may begin to experience burnout when it becomes a regular occurrence. Things such as a heavy workload, a lack of recognition, poor interpersonal relationships, perceived inequities, and misaligned values can preempt care delivery and cause job-related stress and burnout (Maslach & Leiter, 2016).

The number of nurses and health-care workers experiencing burnout has escalated during the COVID-19 pandemic, which threatens both the individual worker and public health (HHS, 2022). The National Academy of Medicine (NAM, 2019) estimated that up to 54% of nurses and physicians suffer from burnout and more than 50% of health-care workers reported mental health symptoms (HHS, 2022).

"People who expect to derive a sense of significance and meaning from their work enter their professions with high hopes and motivation and relate to their work as a calling. When they feel that they have failed, that their work is meaningless and makes no difference in the world, they may feel helpless and hopeless and eventually burn out" (Pines, 2004, p. 67). Goliszek (1992) identified four stages of burnout. Building on this description, Maslach and Leiter (2016) described burnout as a three-dimensional syndrome consisting of extreme exhaustion, cynicism, negative behaviors, disengagement from work, and a lack of personal accomplishment (Maslach & Leiter, 2016). Maslach and Leiter's work closely aligns with attributes and behaviors found in Goliszek's stages of burnout:

1. **High expectations and idealism** At the first stage, the individual is enthusiastic, dedicated, and committed to the job and exhibits a high energy level and a positive attitude despite job-related stressors (Goliszek, 1992). An inability to cope with prolonged stress contributes to emotional exhaustion (Maslach & Leiter, 2016).

2. **Pessimism and early job dissatisfaction** In the second stage, frustration, disillusionment, or boredom with the job develops (Goliszek, 1992). This stage can result in individual strain, manifesting in physical and psychological symptoms such as anxiety and exhaustion (Maslach & Leiter, 2016).

3. **Withdrawal and isolation** As the individual moves into the third stage, anger, hostility, negativism, and cynicism are exhibited (Maslach & Leiter, 2016). At this stage, the physical and psychological stress symptoms worsen. During these first three stages, simple changes in job goals, attitudes, self-care, and behaviors may reverse the burnout process (ANF, 2022; Goleszik, 1992).

4. **Detachment and loss of interest** As the physical and emotional stress symptoms become severe, the individual exhibits low self-esteem, chronic absenteeism, reduced productivity, low morale, and an inability to cope

(Goleszik, 1992; Maslach & Leiter, 2016). Once the individual has moved into this stage and remains there for any length of time, burnout is inevitable.

Sharon had wanted to be a nurse for as long as she could remember. However, she married early, had three children, and put her dreams of being a nurse on hold. Now that her children are grown, Sharon has finally realized her dream by graduating from the local community college last year with a nursing degree. She has been working in an acute care oncology unit, and there have been many changes. Sharon has difficulty adapting to the restructuring changes at her hospital and goes home angry and frustrated every day. Her colleagues have noticed that she has become sarcastic, frequently overwhelmed, and argumentative. Recently Sharon mentioned having trouble sleeping and had stopped playing tennis with her league. Sharon's husband lost his job during the pandemic, making her the primary breadwinner; however, she is seriously considering changing her career. "I am tired of dealing with people. Maybe machines will be more friendly and predictable." Sharon is experiencing burnout. Box 13-2 lists factors to consider to determine whether you may be experiencing stress or burnout.

box 13-2

Assessing Your Risk for Stress and Burnout

- Do you feel more exhausted than energetic?
- Do you work harder but accomplish less?
- Do you feel cynical or disenchanted most of the time?
- Do you often feel sad or cry for no apparent reason?
- Do you feel hostile, negative, or angry at work?
- Are you short-tempered? Do you withdraw from friends or coworkers?
- Do you forget appointments or deadlines? Do you frequently misplace personal items?
- Are you becoming insensitive, irritable, and short-tempered?
- Do you experience physical symptoms such as headaches or stomachaches?
- Do you feel as if you want to avoid people?
- Do you laugh less? Feel less joy often?
- Are you interested in sex?
- Do you crave junk food more often?
- Do you skip meals?
- Have your sleep patterns changed?
- Do you take more medication than usual? Do you use alcohol or other substances to alter your mood?
- Do you feel guilty when your work is not perfect?
- Are you questioning whether the job is right for you?
- Do you feel as if no one cares what kind of work you do?
- Do you constantly push yourself to do better yet feel frustrated that there is no time to do what you want?
- Do you feel as if you are on a treadmill all day?
- Do you use holidays, weekends, or vacation time to catch up?
- Do you feel you are "burning the candle at both ends"?

Source: Adapted from Golin, M., Buchlin, M., & Diamond, D. (1991). Secrets of executive success. Rodale Press; and Goliszek, A. (1992). Sixty-six second stress management: The quickest way to relax and ease anxiety. New Horizon.

Managing Stress and Building Resilience

Managing Stress

Psychologists noted more than 100 years ago (1908) that too little stress can cause a lackadaisical attitude, whereas too much hurts performance and eventually one's health. However, a moderate amount can stimulate high performance without deleterious effects (Beck, 2012; Tully & Tao, 2019) (see Box 13-3 for signs that your work-related stress level is too high).

You can take action to manage your stress at work while your employer undertakes others. The use of coping strategies such as proactively planning your workday, setting goals, and seeking help reduce work-related stress (Tully & Tao, 2019). A healthy lifestyle, including attention to exercise, adequate sleep, and spiritual concerns, is fundamental to caring for oneself (ANA, 2017; Johnson,

Signs That Your Stress Level Is Too High

- Dreading going to work
- Thinking frequently about mistakes or failures
- Avoiding patients, colleagues, and assignments
- Using alcohol or drugs to relax after work
- Worrying about all of the above

Source: Adapted from Beck, M. (2012, June 19). Anxiety can bring out the best. Wall Street Journal, D1.

2011; Tucker et al., 2012). Riahi (2011) suggests maintaining a healthy work–life balance: self-reflect on your perceived role, develop hardiness through positive coping styles, and embrace various prevention and stress-reduction actions. The ANA (2017) Healthy Nurse, Healthy Nation (HNHN) campaign echoes this sentiment.

Building Resilience and Buffering Against Stress

Building Resilience

Resilience is the ability to thrive (rather than experience stress) in adverse situations (Meyer et al., 2020). Resilience characteristics include equanimity, grit, and self-reliance (Meyer et al., 2020). Grit is simply the passion, perseverance, and personal commitment to reach a goal despite obstacles (Duckworth et al., 2007). Building resilience requires self-awareness to identify situations and triggers that evoke feelings of stress. Early identification of these events can result in proactive interventions and reduce or eliminate work-related stress. In order to create this level of surveillance, both the work environment and the nurse need to be healthy.

In 2017, the ANA launched the HNHN campaign to help nurses improve their health. Research findings revealed that Americans are healthier than nurses. Nurses were "more likely to be overweight, have higher stress levels, and get less sleep" (ANA, 2017, 2022). HNHN stresses the importance of nurses focusing on their physical exercise, getting enough sleep, eating right, improving their quality of life, and being safe (ANA, 2017).

Your self-awareness, your ability to identify stressors, and your response or coping mechanisms are excellent ways to gain control of the external stressors or your emotions next time (Tully & Tao, 2019). Research suggests mindfulness-based stress reduction (e.g., noting your physical response to stress), cognitive-behavioral training (screening out

negative thoughts) (Shellenbarger, 2012), conflict resolution, and crisis intervention (Grant et al., 2020) are more helpful than earlier relaxation approaches. Still, they require a substantial investment of time.

Self-compassion and realistic expectations of yourself and your new profession will also reduce stress related to unrealistic goals:

Jane, a new graduate nurse taking her first independent clinical assignment on a busy acute care unit, was asked to admit a patient due to arrive from the emergency department (ED). She was very excited about the opportunity and prepared the room. As the stretcher wheeled into the room, she noticed the patient was very pale, diaphoretic, and agitated. She could feel her stomach churn, and her palms were sweaty. Her body wanted to run, but she knew she had to care for the patient. Jane gathered her thoughts, assessed her patient, and quickly called for the rapid response team, who helped her stabilize and transfer the patient to the ICU. Once the patient had gone, she noticed she was anxious and almost in tears.

The lead nurse approached Jane and complimented her on a job well done. Then, the lead nurse noticed Jane looked shaken and took her to her office to debrief the situation. Jane spent several minutes blaming herself for not recognizing the patient's deteriorating symptoms. While discussing how she felt about her patients' physical and emotional stress, Jane found that her colleague had a different perspective. "Jane, you are new, and the fact that he decompensated was not your fault. You handled the situation beautifully. You should be proud rather than beating yourself up; you probably saved his life. Indeed, we don't save every patient admitted to our unit," the lead nurse said, "but our patients get great care, and most go home feeling better. Very few would have survived if we weren't here to take care of them."

The lead nurse described her first days as a new nurse hoping to help Jane understand the unpredictable nature of patient conditions. Jane asked how she could better prepare for her next patient admission. The lead nurse recommended Jane take advantage of education modules and classes on stress management and mindfulness training offered at the hospital.

Nursing demands a lot of physical and emotional stamina. Practicing good self-care and self-compassion are excellent ways to meet job demands, and equally important is the work environment. Learning about your employer's support and the resources available will further your ability to manage stress and build resilience. Steps taken to mitigate and reduce workplace stress and its effects include

- Providing well-prepared preceptors and mentors for newly hired nurses
- Maintaining sufficient staffing so that employees can take breaks and vacation time
- Offering peer support groups
- Debriefing after critical events have occurred
- Creating well-developed employee-assistance programs (EAPs) for professional counseling
- Offering stress reduction training and workshops
- Utilizing smartphone apps and other technology that promote things such as mindfulness and physical fitness
- Offering on-site exercise rooms
- Providing on-site relaxation rooms, sometimes called serenity or meditation rooms

Hoolahan and Greenhouse (2012) describe a restoration or serenity room created from a conference room and separate from break rooms for use by nursing staff as a safe place to step away and collect their thoughts. Staff called this calming "chair time" and occasionally used it for family members after critical incidents. Regardless of their names, both the break rooms and serenity rooms offer respite in stressful work environments. They are places where nurses can get away from the constant stimulation of alarms, monitors, and call lights to rest and talk with coworkers away from patients, families, visitors, and other providers. Break rooms should be close to care areas for two reasons: Nurses will not use the break room if it is too far away. They need to know that they are close enough to their care area and can respond if a crisis arises (Nejati & colleagues, 2016; Salmela et al., 2020).

Ultimately, you are in control. Every day you have choices. By gaining power regarding your options and the stress they cause, you empower yourself. Focus on the present moment rather than being preoccupied with that past or future, and say the following to yourself (Davidson, 1999):

- I choose to relish my days.
- I choose to enjoy this moment.
- I choose to be fully present to others.
- I choose to engage in the activity at hand fully.
- I choose to proceed at a measured, effective pace.
- I choose to acknowledge all I have achieved so far.
- I choose to focus on where I am and what I am doing.
- I choose to recognize that this is the only moment I can take action.

Managing and reducing work-related stress requires vigilant self-awareness (ANA, 2022; Baclig, 2015). Techniques for managing personal, professional, and organizational things include

- Make time for things that you enjoy and do them with some regularity.
- Know what is meaningful for you and consistently honor it by setting boundaries.
- Recognize when you feel stressed. Situational and self-awareness will help identify and manage triggers.
- Surround yourself with positive people who are supportive and collaborative.
- Know what resources are available such as counseling and employer-offered education. Explore resources available through professional associations and your community
- Participate and advocate for a healthy work environment. Recognize colleagues and peers for their contributions, and be inclusive of leadership when discussing issues and challenges such as communication breakdown and acuity-based staffing (Adapted from Baclig, 2015).

People cannot live in a problem-free world, but they can learn to handle stress. Putting yourself in the best possible condition physically and mentally enhances coping strategies and can reduce the incidence of compassion fatigue and burnout. Using the suggestions in this chapter, you will be able to adopt a healthier personal and professional lifestyle. The self-assessment questions in Box 13-4 can help you manage stress and help you understand your responses better. Boxes 13-5, 13-6, and 13-7 offer some guidelines for dealing with stress in the workplace.

Buffers Against Stress

Hardiness, stress resistance, and grit are attributes found in nurses that help them deal with work-related issues that can contribute to stress, compassion fatigue, and the possibility of burnout (Lambert & Lambert, 1987; Meyer et al., 2020). Research continues on the concept and

Questions for Self-Assessment

- What does the term *health* mean to me?
- What prevents me from living this definition of health?
- Is health important to me?
- Where do I find support?
- Which coping methods work best for me?
- What tasks cause me to feel pressured?
- Can I reorganize, reduce, or eliminate these tasks?
- Can I delegate or rearrange any of my family responsibilities?
- Can I say no to less important demands?
- What are my hopes for the future in terms of (a) career, (b) finances, (c) spiritual life and physical needs, (d) family relationships, and (e) social relationships?
- What do I think others expect of me?
- How do I feel about these expectations?
- What is important to me?
- Can I prioritize to have balance in my life?

Useful Relaxation Techniques

- Guided imagery
- Yoga
- Tai chi
- Meditation
- Relaxation tapes or music
- Exercise
- Favorite sports or hobbies
- Quiet corners or favorite places

Coping With Daily Work Stress

- Spend time on outside interests and take time for yourself.
- Increase your professional knowledge.
- Identify problem-solving resources.
- Identify realistic expectations for your position. Make sure you understand what is expected of you; ask questions if anything is unclear.
- Assess the rewards your work can realistically deliver.
- Develop good communication skills and treat coworkers with respect.
- Join rap sessions with coworkers. Be part of the solution, not part of the problem.
- Do not exceed your limits—you do not always have to say yes.
- Deal with other people's anger by asking yourself, "Whose problem is this?"
- Recognize that you can teach other people how to treat you.

Ten Daily De-Stressors

1. Express yourself! Communicate your feelings and emotions to friends and colleagues to avoid isolation and share perspectives. Sometimes, another opinion helps you see the situation in a different light.
2. Take time off. Taking breaks, or doing something unrelated to work, will help you feel refreshed as you begin work again.
3. Understand your energy patterns. Are you a morning or an afternoon person? Schedule stressful duties during times when you are most energetic.
4. Do one stressful activity at a time. Although this may take advanced planning, avoiding more than one stressful situation at a time will make you feel more in control and satisfied with your accomplishments.
5. Exercise! Physical exercise builds physical and emotional resilience. Do not put physical activities "on the back burner" as you become busy.
6. Tackle big projects one piece at a time. Having control of one part of a project at a time will help you avoid feeling overwhelmed and out of control.
7. Delegate if possible. If you can delegate and share in problem-solving, do so. Not only will your load be lighter, but others will be able to participate in decision making.
8. It's okay to say no. Do not take on every extra assignment or special project offered to you.
9. Be work-smart. Improve your work skills with new technologies and ideas. Take advantage of additional job training.
10. Relax. Find time each day to consciously relax and reflect on the positive energies you need to cope with stressful situations more readily.

Source: Adapted from Bowers, R. (1993). Stress and your health. *National Women's Health Report, 15(3),* 6.

- Commitment to work and life's activities rather than alienation
- Seeing life's demands and changes as challenges rather than as threats

The hardiness that comes from having this perspective leads to adaptive coping responses, such as optimism, effective use of support systems, and healthy lifestyle habits (Duquette et al., 1994; Lambert & Lambert, 1987; Nowak & Pentkowski, 1994). In addition, letting go of guilt, fear of change, and the self-blaming, "wallowing-in-the-problem" syndrome will help you buffer yourself against burnout (Lenson, 2001).

Job Satisfaction and the Joy of Work

Job satisfaction encompasses the feelings or attitudes, positive or negative, that an individual has about their work. Nurse work is often complex

impact of personal hardiness and grit on tempering job-related stress and building resilience. Hardiness includes the following:

- Feeling a sense of personal control over a situation rather than powerlessness

and unpredictable. In addition, mounting financial pressures have reduced the value of nursing care to meeting efficiency and productivity measures rather than helping nurses fulfill their passion to deliver excellent relationship-based care to their patients. In a study of 1,091 medical–surgical nurses, Amendolair (2012) found a positive relationship between perceived ability to express caring behaviors and job satisfaction. However, a nurse's inability to provide the care the patient needs because of organizational barriers can lead to moral distress, disengagement, and compassion fatigue.

Helping nurses maintain their passion and purpose contributes to their ability to do meaningful work, contributing to job satisfaction and better engagement with colleagues and patients (Sherman & Blum, 2019). Traditional job satisfaction surveys and nurse engagement surveys identify benefits and barriers to optimal nursing practice and care delivery. High nurse satisfaction and engagement correlate to reduced mortality, improved patient experience, and better clinical outcomes (Dempsey & Reilly, 2016).

The Health-Care Team

The health-care team and the employing organization are also important to the work. Nurses work with and interact with many different people in a day: patients, families, nursing assistants, many kinds of therapists, housekeeping and transport staff, social workers, and physicians, to name a few. How well everyone on a team works together affects job satisfaction. In a study of 3,675 nursing staff from five hospitals, Kalisch and colleagues (2010) found that higher levels of teamwork (trust, cohesiveness, mutual help and understanding, and leadership) and adequate staffing lead to greater job satisfaction.

The Employing Organization

An organization that supports its most valuable asset, its staff members, keeps its experienced nurses. The effect of the pandemic has resulted in a significantly higher number of resignations nationally, with health-care ranking in the top three industries affected (Boston-Fleischhauer, 2022). This year, the number of RNs intending to leave the bedside has risen to 32%, an increase of 10% over the prior year (Boston-Fleischhauer, 2022). Effective nurse leaders are key to accomplishing the goal of a healthy work environment (Blake, 2012; Wei et al., 2018). Higher pay, better benefits, and the means to turn

sources of dissatisfaction into actual improvements in the work environment (one could call this empowerment) are elements contributing to the retention of experienced nurses (Seago et al., 2011).

Burke, Ng, and Wolpin (2011) studied the effects of six "antidotes" to burnout: workload, autonomy, reward, communication, respect and civility, and constructive values. Findings revealed that restructuring, budget cuts, high workload, and low reward, control, or value incongruence were related to more significant distress for nurse participants (Burke et al., 2011). In 2015, the American Association of Critical Care Nurses (AACN) held public forums to identify things hampering optimal patient care in care environments. Barriers that further illustrated the need for implementing the antidotes recommended by Burke and colleagues included heavy workloads and staffing shortages, disrespectful behavior and hostile work environments, regulations, and a lack of leadership (Grant et al., 2020). Another study done in skilled nursing facilities found that nurse aides' attention to resident safety (rated by their supervisors) was affected by their level of empathy. Still, higher workloads, extended workdays, and financial hardships reduced this positive relationship (Leana et al., 2018). Employee physical and psychological wellness programs have proliferated in the workplace (Terry, 2018).

Before the COVID-19 pandemic, the Institute for Healthcare Improvement's (IHI) position paper on improving joy in work called burnout in health-care workers an epidemic (Feeley & Swensen, 2016; Perlo et al., 2017). Today, it has reached a critical level (Murthy, 2022). Burnout affects not only productivity but also the quality of the care provided. A few of the statistics the IHI report quotes are as follows:

- More than 50% of physicians reported burnout symptoms in a 2015 study.
- Within 1 year, 33% of nurses report looking for another job, according to 2013 study results.

"Turnover is up, and morale is down," they conclude (Perlo et al., 2017, p. 5). On the other hand, they also point out that health-care professions provide opportunities to "profoundly improve lives" and that "caring and healing should be naturally joyful activities" (p. 6), an effort full of meaning and purpose. Although published in 2017, the Get Ready phase with a four-step action plan remains relevant to help leaders create and maintain a healthy work environment capable of reducing the incidence of compassion fatigue and burnout (Boston-Fleischhauer, 2022; Sherman & Blum, 2019). To Get Ready (Perlo et al., 2017), leaders of a health-care organization should do the following:

- Listen and learn from the facility's employees regarding what matters most to them.
- Provide leaders with enough time to engage in the "what matters?" conversations and the follow-through needed to resolve problems. Failure to follow through on issues can increase employee frustration.
- Appoint a senior-level leader who can lead the effort and make needed changes at the organizational level.

Once ready, the action steps are to:

1. Have conversations with staff about what makes a bad day for them and what is needed to increase the number of good days.
2. Identify the main barriers (impediments) to experiencing joy in work in your organization.
3. Identify leaders at each level (unit to top administration) responsible for making the changes that will improve joy in work.
4. Select and use an improvement method to try out the changes identified: set an aim, select measures that indicate progress, decide on the change, and test it (Perlo et al., 2017). See Figure 13.1.

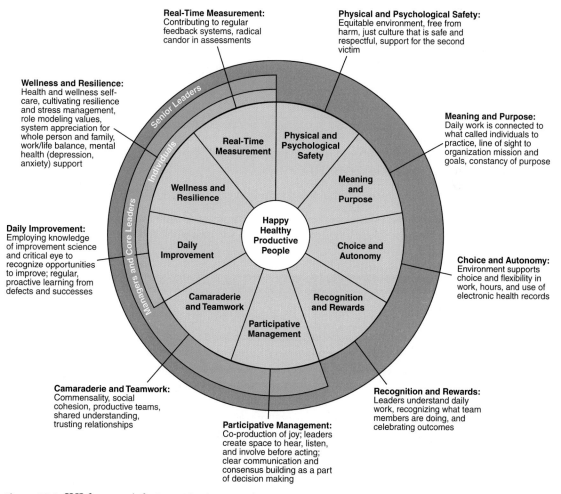

Figure 13.1 IHI framework for improving joy at work. *Source: Perlo, J., Balik, B., Swensen, S., Kabcenell, A., Landsman, J., & Feeley, D. (2017). IHI framework for improving joy in work. IHI White Paper. Institute for Healthcare Improvement.*

Conclusion

Nursing is a profession filled with a great deal of personal and professional meaning, resulting in a high degree of job satisfaction. Work consumes many hours in a person's life and the work can be stressful. Yet, the rewards and risks in nursing come from providing compassionate care to patients. Nursing can offer opportunities for professional growth, excitement, and satisfaction or create moments of frustration, dissatisfaction, and stress.

A work environment that promotes professional growth, engagement, and creativity is essential in improving the quality of work life. Cultural awareness, inclusion, respect for differences and diversity, professional growth, and involvement in decision making should be encouraged. Everyone plays a role in maintaining a healthy work environment and, as such, must confront incivility, bullying, harassment, and discrimination head-on.

Periodically ask yourself the questions shared in this chapter to help assess your stress level. Remember to review the stress management techniques described in this chapter to reduce the risk of burnout.

Study Questions

1. What characteristics would you look for in a workplace that will support a healthy work environment?

2. Consider experiences you have had in your clinical rotations: Were the environments supportive or nonsupportive? What recommendations would you make for improvement?

3. How would you respond if you experienced incivility or bullying at work?

4. Discuss the characteristics of health-care organizations that may lead to burnout among nurses. How could they be changed or eliminated?

5. What are the signs of work-related stress and burnout?

6. How is sexual harassment defined? If a colleague confides that she is a victim of sexual harassment, what would you recommend she do about it?

7. How can a nurse leader increase the cultural sensitivity of a unit staff?

8. Identify the physical and psychological signs and symptoms you exhibit during stress. What sources of stress are most likely to affect you? How do you deal with these signs and symptoms?

Case Studies to Promote Clinical Judgment

Diversity

You are a new nurse manager on a busy pediatric unit in a large metropolitan hospital. The hospital provides services for a culturally diverse population, including BPOC. Family members often practice alternative healing practices specific to their culture, for example, bringing special foods from home to entice a sick child to eat. One of the more experienced nurses said to you, "We need to discourage these people from fooling with all this hocus-pocus. We are trying to get their sick kid well in the time allowed under their managed care insurance plans, and all this medicine-man stuff is only keeping the kid sick longer. Besides, all this food stinks up the rooms and brings in bugs." You have observed how important these healing rituals and foods are to the patients and families and believe that both the families and the children have benefited from this nontraditional approach to healing.

1. How would you respond to the experienced nurse?

2. How can you be a patient advocate without alienating the staff?

3. What can you do to assist your staff in becoming more culturally sensitive to their patients and families?

4. How can health-care facilities incorporate Western, complementary, and alternative treatment and traditional medicine into patient care? Should they do this? Why or why not?

Burnout

Shawna Jefferson, a new staff member, has been working from 7 a.m. to 3 p.m. in an infectious disease unit since obtaining her RN license 6 months ago. Most of the staff members she works with have been there since the unit opened 5 years ago. The nursing staff includes a nurse manager, two RNs, a licensed practical nurse (LPN), and two technicians for approximately 40 patients on a typical day. Most patients are HIV-positive with multisystem failure. Many are severely debilitated and need help with their activities of daily living. Although staff members encourage family members and loved ones to help, most are unavailable because they work during the day. Several days a week, the nursing students from Shawna's community college program are assigned to the floor.

Tina Brown, the nurse manager, does not participate in any direct patient care, saying that she is "too busy at the desk." Laverne Sayed, the other RN, says the unit depresses her and that she has requested a transfer to pediatrics. Lynn Alvarez, the LPN, wants to "give meds" because she is "sick of the patients' constant whining," and Sheila, one of the technicians, is "just plain exhausted." Lately, Shawna has noticed that the other staff members seem to avoid the nursing students and reply to their questions with short answers in an annoyed tone. Shawna feels isolated and overwhelmed. She goes home at night worrying about the patients; she believes they need more care than they are receiving. She is afraid to tell Tina because she does not want to be considered a complainer. When she confided in Lynn about her concerns, Lynn replied, "Get real—no one here cares about the patients or us. All they care about is the bottom line! Why did a smart girl such as you choose nursing anyway?"

1. How would you feel if you were Shawna?

2. What is happening on this unit in leadership terms?

3. Identify the major problems on this unit.

4. What factors might have contributed to the harmful behaviors exhibited by Tina, Lynn, and Sheila?

5. Is there anything Shawna can do for herself, the patients, and the staff members?

6. How are the patients affected by the behaviors exhibited by all staff members?

7. How is the nurse manager reacting to the changes in her staff members?

8. If you were a new nurse manager brought in to intervene with this unit, what would you do?

9. What is the responsibility of the administration to create a healthier work environment on this unit?

NCLEX®-Style Review Questions

1. An incident of sexual harassment as identified by the EEOC is: **Select all that apply**.
   1. Telling jokes about sexual identity issues
   2. Offering separate restrooms
   3. Providing coffee and doughnuts to the nursing staff
   4. Demanding a daily kiss for writing a favorable evaluation

2. Factors found to increase nurses' joy at work include: **Select all that apply**.
    1. Ability to provide quality care
    2. Consistently high workload
    3. A pattern of continuous conflict and disagreement
    4. Civility and respect

3. Enhancing the quality of work–life can be achieved by
    1. Encouraging critical thinking and new ideas
    2. Discouraging a working relationship with one's peers
    3. Being negative
    4. Endangering a client's health or safety

4. The occurrence of sexual harassment may be reported to
    1. IHI
    2. ANA
    3. EEOC
    4. CDC

5. Burnout at work can be identified best by
    1. Expressions of frustration and powerlessness
    2. Fatigue and refusal to work double shifts
    3. Allergic reactions
    4. A preference for efficiency

6. New graduates usually experience a "honeymoon" period at their first job, which is characterized by
    1. Extreme criticism from colleagues
    2. Long hours and low pay
    3. Feeling undervalued
    4. Excitement about the new position

7. An effective way to help a diverse group of staff work together is to
    1. Provide equal opportunities for advancement
    2. Pretend there are no cultural differences
    3. Promote uniformity in communication styles
    4. Establish an English-only policy institution-wide

8. Which of the following events should be reported? **Select all that apply**.
    1. A patient is placed in a broken wheelchair that tips over.
    2. A staff member tells a neighbor about a famous athlete who is a patient.
    3. An employee reports to work under the influence of alcohol.
    4. A patient spills her supplemental protein drink on the floor; the certified nursing assistant (CNA; aide) mops it up.

9. A new nurse manager has observed several instances of horizontal violence between staff members on her unit, primarily verbal abuse and malicious gossip. What should she do?
    1. Ignore it because it is not physical violence and will not hurt anyone.
    2. Model this bullying behavior so that staff can see how it affects people.
    3. Keep a log of observed bullying behavior to discuss during the employees' annual evaluation.
    4. Confront the bullying behavior and discuss strategies for responding to it.

10. A colleague tells you, "I'm so burned out, I think it's time for me to resign." What can you tell your colleague?
    1. "You probably need a break from work. Why don't you ask for a 6-month leave of absence?"
    2. "Why don't you apply for a position at our rival hospital?"
    3. "Tell me how you take care of yourself and what you like about your work."
    4. "We're all burned out. Welcome to the club."

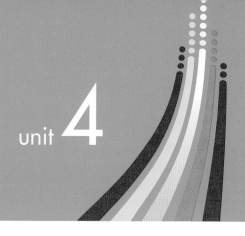

Your Nursing Career

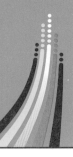

chapter 14

Launching Your Career

OBJECTIVES

After reading this chapter, the student should be able to:

- Evaluate personal strengths, weaknesses, opportunities, and threats using a SWOT analysis.
- Develop a résumé including objectives, qualifications, skills, experience, work history, education, and training.
- Compose job search letters including a cover letter, a thank-you letter, and acceptance and rejection letters.
- Discuss components of the interview process.
- Discuss the factors involved in selecting the right position.
- Explain why the first year is critical to planning a career.

Recently the U.S. Bureau of Labor Statistics (BLS) updated its projections regarding the nursing shortage. In the *Employment Projections 2018–2028,* the BLS listed registered nursing among the top careers in terms of job growth through 2028. The registered nurse (RN) workforce is now expected to grow to 3.4 million by 2028, an increase of 371,500 or 12% from the 2018 projections. The BLS also projects the need for 225,000 replacement nurses in the workforce (BLS, 2022).

This continued shortage of RNs permits those entering the profession many choices and opportunities as professional nurses. By now you have invested considerable time, expense, and emotion into preparing for your new career. Your educational preparation, technical and clinical expertise, interpersonal and management skills, personal interests and needs, and commitment to the nursing profession will contribute to meeting your career goals. Successful nurses view nursing as a profession and a lifetime pursuit, not as an occupational stepping stone.

This chapter deals with the most important endeavor: finding and keeping your first nursing position. The chapter starts with planning your initial search; developing a strengths, weaknesses, opportunities, and threats (SWOT) analysis; searching for available positions; and researching organizations. Also included is a section on writing a résumé and employment-related information about the interview process and selecting the first position.

Getting Started

By now at least one person has said to you, "Good career choice. Nurses are always needed and will never be out of a job." This statement is only one of several career myths. These myths include the following:

1. **"Good workers do not get fired."** They may not get fired, but many good workers have lost their positions during restructuring and downsizing.
2. **"Well-paying jobs are available without a college degree."** Even if entrance into a career path does not require a college education, the potential for career advancement is minimal without that degree. In many health-care agencies, a baccalaureate degree in nursing is required for an initial management position. The Institute of Medicine (IOM) reports

(2001, 2011) indicated that nurses with higher degrees promote better patient outcomes. For this reason, many health-care institutions are encouraging nurses to return for their BSN and MSN degrees in order to maintain employment.
3. **"Go to work for a good company, and move up the career ladder."** This statement assumes that people move up the career ladder because of longevity in the organization. In reality, the responsibility for career advancement rests on the employee, not the employer.
4. **"Find the 'hot' industry, and you will always be in demand."** Nursing is projected to continue to be one of the "hottest" industries well into the next decade. However, a nurse who performs poorly will never be successful, no matter what the demand.

Many students attending college today are adults with family, work, and personal responsibilities. On graduating with an associate degree in nursing, you may still have student loans and continued responsibilities for supporting a family. Your focus may be on job security and a steady source of income. The idea of career planning might not be a thought at this time; however, this is a strategic process and requires some thought and personal self-assessment (Borgatti, 2010; Gaines, 2020). The correct goal is to find a job that fits *you.* It is also not too early to begin formal planning of your career. In today's dynamic health-care environment, nursing managers and health-care organizations want nurses who consider nursing as a profession, not just a job. They look for individuals who express a commitment to forming partnerships with the health-care team and institution (Arvidsson et al., 2008; Papandrea, 2018).

SWOT Analysis

New graduates often secure their first position as a staff nurse on a medical–surgical floor. These individuals see themselves as "putting in their year" and then moving on to their dream position as a critical care or mother–baby nurse. However, as the health-care system continues to evolve and reallocate resources, this may no longer be the automatic first step for new graduates. Instead, new graduates should focus on long-term career goals and the different avenues by which they can be reached. Some of you may already have determined your career path knowing that you will need to pursue advanced nursing degrees to achieve your goal. If you are considering a graduate degree at some point in your future, now is the time to determine which of your early nursing experiences will help you achieve this goal. For example, if you envision yourself becoming an acute care nurse practitioner, securing a position in a critical care unit or emergency department (ED) will provide you with the experience needed to move in this direction. In contrast, those considering midwifery should consider working in a mother–baby or labor and delivery setting.

Consider your past experiences as they may be an asset in presenting your abilities for a particular position. A SWOT analysis, created in the 1960s and borrowed from the corporate world, guides you in discovering your internal strengths and weaknesses as well as external opportunities and threats that may help or hinder your job search and career planning. The SWOT analysis helps identify the activities and accomplishments that show how you best meet the requirements of the job or promotion you are seeking. By reviewing your strengths and weaknesses and comparing them with the position requirements, you can identify gaps. This helps prepare you to be the ideal candidate for the position you seek (Martin, 2019; Quast, 2013). Although you have already made the decision to pursue nursing, knowing your strengths and weaknesses can help you select the work setting that will be satisfying personally (Martin, 2019; Quast, 2013). Your SWOT analysis may include the following factors.

Strengths

- Relevant work experience
- Advanced education
- Product knowledge
- Good communication and people skills
- Computer skills
- Self-managed learning skills
- Flexibility

Weaknesses

- Ineffective communication and people skills
- Inflexibility
- Lack of interest in further education
- Difficulty adapting to change
- Inability to see health care as a business

Opportunities

- Expanding markets in health care
- New applications of technology
- New products and diversification

- Increasing at-risk populations
- Nursing shortage

Threats

- Increased competition among health-care facilities
- Changes in government regulation

(Box 14-1)

Take some time to strategically plan your career and personalize the preceding SWOT analysis. What are *your* strengths? What skills do *you* need to improve? What weaknesses do *you* need to minimize, or what strengths do *you* need to develop as you begin your job search? What opportunities and threats exist in the health-care community *you* are considering? Doing a SWOT analysis will help you make an initial assessment of the job market. It can be used again after you narrow your search for that first nursing position.

Many graduates find using the SMART acronym helpful to determine career goals. SMART represents specific (S), measurable (M), achievable (A), realistic (R), and timely (T) (Allnurses, 2018). SMART helps you specify what you want to accomplish during your career. For example, perhaps you desire to work as a perinatal nurse. Many health-care institutions promote certification as part of a clinical ladder. You would thus include obtaining certification as part of your plan https://www.nursingworld.org/ancc/.

In addition to completing a SWOT analysis, there are several other tools that can help you learn more about yourself. Two of the most common are the Strong Interest Inventory (SII) and the Myers–Briggs Type Indicator (MBTI). The SII compares

box 14-1

SWOT Analysis Diagram

Strengths	Weaknesses
Opportunities	Threats

the individual's interests with the interests of those who are successful in a large number of occupational fields in the areas of (a) work styles, (b) learning environment, (c) leadership style, and (d) risk-taking or adventure. Completing this inventory can help you discover what work environment might be best suited to your interests.

The MBTI is a widely used indicator of personality patterns. This self-report inventory provides information about individual psychological-type preferences on four dimensions:

1. Extroversion (E) or Introversion (I)
2. Sensing (S) or Intuition (N)
3. Thinking (T) or Feeling (F)
4. Judging (J) or Perceiving (P)

Although many factors influence behaviors and attitudes, the MBTI summarizes underlying patterns and behaviors common to most people. Both tools should be administered and interpreted by a qualified practitioner. Most university and career counseling centers are able to administer them. If you are unsure of where you fit in the workplace, consider exploring these tests with your college or university or take the MBTI online at www.myersbriggs.org.

Beginning the Search

Even with a nationwide nursing shortage, hospital mergers, emphasis on increased staff productivity, budget crises, staffing shifts, and changes in job market availability affect the numbers and types of nurses employed in various facilities and agencies. Instead of focusing on long-term job security, the career-secure employee focuses on becoming a career survivalist or developing resilience. Resilience requires that an individual develop the ability to recover or adapt to changes (Gray, 2012; Rees et al., 2016). A career survivalist or resilient individual focuses on the person, not the position. Consider the following career survivalist strategies (Morgan, 2013):

▪ **Be engaged** Your career belongs to you. Define your values and determine what motivates you. Be on the lookout for opportunities to break from the status quo. Opportunities for nurses are growing every day.
▪ **Stay informed** Health care is dynamic and changing daily. Go out there, stay informed, and start thinking about your options for riding the waves of change (Yilmaz, 2017).

▪ **Learn for employability** Take personal responsibility for your career success. Continue to be a "work in progress." Employability in health care today means learning technology tools, job-specific technical skills, and people skills such as the ability to negotiate, coach, work in interprofessional teams, and make presentations (Rees et al., 2016).
▪ **Plan for your financial future** Ask yourself, "How can I spend less, earn more, and manage better?" Often, people make job decisions based on financial decisions, which makes them feel trapped instead of secure.
▪ **Develop multiple options** The career survivalist looks at multiple options constantly. Moving up is only one option. Being aware of emerging trends in nursing, adjacent fields, lateral moves, and special projects presents other options.
▪ **Build a safety net** Networking is extremely important to the career survivalist. Joining professional organizations, taking time to build long-term nursing relationships, and getting to know other career survivalists will make your career path more enjoyable and successful.

What do employers think you need to be ready to work for them? In addition to passing the National Council Licensure Examination (NCLEX), employers cite the following skills as desirable in job candidates (Cazacu, 2010):

▪ Oral and written communication skills
▪ Responsibility and accountability
▪ Integrity
▪ Interpersonal skills
▪ Proficiency in field of study and technical competence
▪ Teamwork ability
▪ Willingness to work hard
▪ Leadership abilities
▪ Motivation, initiative, and flexibility
▪ Critical thinking and analytical skills
▪ Self-discipline
▪ Organizational skills

In today's world, there are multiple approaches to looking for a nursing position. The traditional approaches included looking through newspapers, professional magazines, and school career placement offices. Today, job seekers look to online job boards (Carlson, 2017; Papandrea, 2018; Williamson, 2021). Contacting specific health-care institutions and organizations and filling out a job application lets employers know that you are interested in working with them. Also think "outside the box." Although the acute care setting provides excellent experience with skill development and delegation concepts, good nursing positions exist outside the hospital setting (Williamson, 2021). Examples of alternative settings include community medical clinics, free-standing infusion centers, urgent care centers, and long-term care facilities.

Some Internet sites that post nursing opportunities are:

- www.careerbuilder.com
- www.nurse.com
- https://www.nurserecruiter.com
- www.Indeed.com

In recent years, three trends have emerged related to recruiting. First, employers are being more creative by using alternative sources to increase the diversity of employees. They commonly place advertisements in minority newspapers, Web sites, and magazines and recruit nurses at minority organizations. Second, some employers use temporary staff as a way to evaluate potential employees. Nursing staffing agencies are common in most areas of the country. Third, the Internet has become the major source for employers to advertise along with other media used by today's potential workforce.

Regardless of where you begin your search, explore the market vigorously and thoroughly. Speak to everyone you know about your job search. Encourage classmates and colleagues to share contacts with you, and do the same for them. Also, when possible, try to speak directly with the person who is looking for a nurse when you hear of a possible opening. The people in human resources offices may reject a candidate on a technicality that a nurse manager would realize does not affect that person's ability to handle the job if they are otherwise a good match for the position. For example, experience in day surgery prepares a person to work in other surgery-related settings, but a human resources interviewer may not know this.

Try to obtain as much information as you can about the available position. Is there a match between your skills and interests and the position? Ask yourself whether you are applying for this position because you really want it or just to gain interview experience. Be careful about going through the interview process and receiving job offers only to turn them down. Employers may share information with one another, and you could end up being denied the position you really want. Regardless of where you explore potential opportunities, use these "pearls of wisdom" from career nurses:

- Know yourself.
- Seek out mentors and wise people.
- Be a risk taker.
- Never, ever stop learning.
- Understand the business of health care.
- Involve yourself in community and professional organizations.
- Network.
- Understand diversity.
- Be an effective communicator.
- Set short- and long-term goals, and strive continually to achieve them.

Researching Your Potential Employer

After spending time looking at yourself and the climate of the health-care job market, you have narrowed your choices to the organizations that really interest you. Now is the time to find out as much as possible about these organizations.

It is important to evaluate your values and goals when researching an organization. Ownership of the company may be public or private, foreign or American. The company may be local or regional, a small corporation or a division of a much larger corporation. Depending on the size and ownership of the company, information may be obtained from the public library, chamber of commerce, government offices, or company Web site.

Has the organization recently gone through a merger, a reorganization, or downsizing? Information from current and past employees is valuable and may provide you with more details about whether the organization might be suitable for you. Be wary of gossip and half-truths that may emerge, however, because they may discourage you from applying to an excellent health-care facility. In other words, if you hear something negative about an organization, investigate it for yourself. Often, individuals jump at work opportunities before doing a complete assessment of the culture and politics of the institution.

The first step in assessing the culture is to review a copy of the company's mission statement. The mission statement reflects what the institution considers important to its public image. What are the core values of the institution? How do they compare with yours?

The department of nursing's philosophy and objectives indicate how the department defines nursing; they identify what the department's important goals are for nursing. The nursing philosophy and goals should reflect the mission of the organization. Where is nursing administration on the organizational chart of the institution? To whom does the chief nursing officer report? Does the organization value and promote nursing (Hu et al., 2022; Kuokkanen et al., 2014)? Although much of this information may not be obtained until an interview, a preview of how the institution views itself and the value it places on nursing will help you decide if your philosophy of health care and nursing is compatible with that of a particular organization. To find out more about a specific health-care facility, you can (Zedlitz, 2003):

- Talk to nurses currently employed at the facility.
- Access the facility's Web site for information on its mission, philosophy, and services.
- Visit an online chat room with other new nursing graduates.
- Join a local professional nursing organization while completing school.
- Check the library or complete an online search for newspaper and magazine articles related to the facility.

Writing a Résumé

Your résumé is your personal data sheet and a way of marketing yourself. It is the first impression the recruiter or your potential employer has about you. Consider your résumé your time to shine. The résumé highlights your skills, talents, and abilities. You may decide to write your own résumé or have it constructed by a professional service. Regardless of who prepares it, the purpose of a résumé is to get a job interview.

However, many people dislike the idea of writing a résumé. How can you sum up your entire career in a single page? How can you grab the employer's attention so they want to meet you and see what you have to offer? This one-page summary needs to work well enough to get you the position you want. Chestnut (1999) summarized résumé writing by stating, "Lighten up. Although a very important piece to the puzzle in your job search, a résumé is

box 14-2
Reasons for Preparing a Résumé

Assists in completing an employment application quickly and accurately.
Demonstrates your potential.
Focuses on your strongest points.
Gives you credit for all your achievements.
Identifies you as organized, prepared, and serious about the job search.
Serves as a reminder and adds to your self-confidence during the interview.
Provides initial introduction to potential employers in seeking the interview.
Serves as a guide for the interviewer.
Functions as a tool to distribute to others who are willing to assist you in a job search.

Source: Adapted from Marino, K. (2000). Résumés for the health care professional. John Wiley & Sons; and Zedlitz, R. (2003). How to get a job in health care. Delmar Learning.

not the only ammunition. What's between your ears is what will ultimately lead you to your next career" (p. 28). Box 14-2 summarizes reasons for preparing a well-considered, up-to-date résumé.

Although you might labor intensively over creating your résumé, most job applications live or die within 10 to 30 seconds as the receptionist or applications examiner decides whether your résumé should be forwarded to the next step or rejected. In many places, non-nursing personnel first screen your résumé. Some beginning helpful tips include the following (Gibson, 2018; Papandrea, 2017, 2018).

- Keep the résumé to one or two pages. Do not use smaller fonts to force more information on the page. Proofread, proofread, proofread. Typing errors, misspelled words, and poor grammar act as red flags. Use action verbs when possible. Do not substitute quantity of words for quality.
- Itemize your educational experiences on your résumé. Also include any certifications you may have. As a new graduate, it may be helpful to highlight specific clinical experiences as they relate to the position you wish to obtain.
- State your objective. Although you know very well what position you are seeking, the individual conducting the initial screening does not want to take the time to determine this. Tailor your résumé to the institution and position to which you are applying.
- Employers care about what you can do for them and your potential for future success with

their company. Your résumé must answer those questions.

- If sending electronically, choose a simple font and layout.
- Include pertinent keywords from the employer's job description. This helps your résumé get through any software filtering programs.

Essentials of a Résumé

Most résumés follow one of four formats: standard, chronological, functional, or a combination. There are several Web sites on résumé writing that offer free templates to assist you with this skill. Regardless of the type of résumé, basic elements of personal information, education, work experience, qualifications for the position, and references should be included (Evenden, 2020; Gibson, 2018; Indeed.com, 2020; Zedlitz, 2003):

- **Standard** The standard résumé is organized by categories. By clearly stating your personal information, job objective, work experience, education, work skills, memberships, honors, and special skills, you give the employer a "snapshot" of the person requesting entrance into the workforce. This is a useful résumé for first-time employees or recent graduates.
- **Chronological** The chronological résumé lists work experiences in order of time, with the most recent experience listed first. This style is useful in showing stable employment without gaps or many job changes. The objective and qualifications are listed at the top.
- **Functional** The functional résumé also lists work experience but in order of importance to your job objective. List the most important work-related experience first. This is a useful format when you have gaps in employment or lack direct experience related to your objective.
- **Combination** The combination résumé is a popular format, listing work experience directly related to the position but in chronological order.

Most professional recruiters and placement services agree on the following tips in preparing a résumé (Korkki, 2010; Uzialko, 2018):

- **Make sure your résumé is readable** Is the type large enough for easy reading? Are paragraphs indented or bullets used to set off information, or does the entire page resemble a gray blur? Using bold headings and appropriate spacing

can offer relief from lines of gray type, but be careful not to get so carried away with graphics that your résumé becomes a new art form. Use a TrueType font when writing your résumé, such as Arial, Calibri, or Cambria (Uzialko, 2018). The paper should be an appropriate color, such as cream, white, or off-white. Use easily readable fonts and a laser printer. If a good computer and printer are not available, most printing services prepare résumés at a reasonable cost. Résumés may also be sent electronically. Some organizations require applicants to upload their résumés into their application system. Another way is to attach a résumé to an introductory e-mail. It is often recommended that you convert your résumé to a portable document format (PDF). This format is readable by most systems and also allows for greater protection, as word processing documents (Microsoft Word, WordPerfect) are easily altered.

- **Make sure the important facts are easy to spot** Education, current employment, responsibilities, and facts to support the experience you have gained from previous positions are important. Put the strongest statements at the beginning. Avoid excessive use of the word "I." If you are a new nursing graduate and have little or no job experience, list your educational background first. Remember that positions you held before you entered nursing might support experience that will be relevant in your nursing career. Be sure to let your prospective employer know how to contact you.
- **Do a spelling and grammar check** Use simple terms, action verbs, and descriptive words. Check your finished résumé for spelling, style, and grammar errors. If you are not sure if the grammar or style is correct, get another opinion.
- **Follow the do nots** Do not include pictures, fancy binders, salary information, or hobbies (unless they have contributed to your work experience). Do not include personal information such as weight, marital status, and number of children. Do not repeat information just to make the résumé longer. A good résumé is concise and focuses on your strengths and accomplishments.

No matter which format you use, it is essential to include the following:

- A clearly stated job objective
- Highlighted qualifications

▪ Directly relevant skills and experience
▪ Chronological work history
▪ Relevant education and training

Optional sections, if relevant, may include:

▪ Fluency in a foreign language
▪ Community service (if this is a focus of the organization's mission and vision)
▪ Hobbies or outside interests (only include one or two that address your personality)

How to Begin

Start by writing down every applicable point you can think of in the preceding five categories. Work history is usually the easiest place to begin. Arrange your work history in reverse chronological order, listing your current job first. Account for all your employable years. Short lapses in employment are acceptable, but give a brief explanation for longer periods (e.g., "maternity leave"). Include employer, dates worked (years only, e.g., 2001–2002), city, and state for each employer you list. Briefly describe the duties and responsibilities of each position. Emphasize your accomplishments, any special techniques you learned, or changes you implemented. Use action verbs, such as those listed in Table 14-1, to describe your accomplishments. Also cite any special awards or committee chairs you have earned. If a previous position was not in the health field, try to relate your duties and accomplishments to the position you are seeking.

Education

Next, focus on your education. Include the name and location of every educational institution you attended; the dates you attended; and the degree, diploma, or certification attained. Start with your most recent degree. It is not necessary to include your license number because you will give a copy of the license when you begin employment. If you are still waiting to take NCLEX®, you need to indicate when you are scheduled for the examination. If you are seeking additional training, such as for intravenous certification, include only what is relevant to your job objective.

Your Objective

It is now time to write your job objective. Write a clear, brief job objective. To accomplish this, ask yourself: What do I want to do? For or with whom? When? At what level of responsibility? For example (Hart, 2006; Indeed, 2020; Parker, 1989):

▪ **What** RN
▪ **For whom** Pediatric patients
▪ **Where** Large metropolitan hospital
▪ **At what level** Staff

A new graduate's objective might read: "Position as staff nurse on a pediatric unit" or "Graduate nurse position on a pediatric unit." Do not include phrases such as "advancing to neonatal intensive care unit." Employers are trying to fill current openings and are not interested in acting as a stepping stone in your career.

table 14-1			
Action Verbs			
Management Skills	**Communication Skills**	**Accomplishments**	**Helping Skills**
Attained	Collaborated	Achieved	Assessed
Developed	Convinced	Adapted	Assisted
Improved	Developed	Coordinated	Clarified
Increased	Enlisted	Developed	Demonstrated
Organized	Formulated	Expanded	Diagnosed
Planned	Negotiated	Facilitated	Expedited
Recommended	Promoted	Implemented	Facilitated
Strengthened	Reconciled	Improved	Motivated
Supervised	Recruited	Instructed	Represented
		Reduced (losses)	
		Resolved (problems)	
		Restored	

Source: Adapted from Parker, Y. (1989). The damn good résumé guide. Ten Speed Press.

Skills and Experience

Relevant skills and experience are included in your résumé not to describe your past but to present a "word picture of you in your proposed new job, created out of the best of your past experience" (Impollonia, 2004; Papandrea, 2018; Parker, 1989, p. 13). Begin by jotting down the major skills required for the position you are seeking. Include five or six major skills such as:

- Administration or management
- Teamwork or problem-solving
- Patient relations
- Specialty proficiency
- Technical skills

Other

Academic honors, publications, research, and membership in professional organizations may be included. Were you active in your school's student nurses association, or in a church or community organization? Were you on the dean's list? What if you were "just a housewife" for many years? First, do an attitude adjustment: You were not "just a housewife" but rather a family manager. Explore your role in work-related terms such as *community volunteer, personal relations, fund-raising, counseling,* or *teaching.* A college career office, women's center, or professional résumé service can offer you assistance with analyzing the skills and talents you shared with your family and community. A student who lacks work experience has options as well. Examples of nonwork experiences that show marketable skills include (Eubanks, 1991; Parker, 1989):

- Working on the school paper or yearbook
- Serving in the student government
- Holding leadership positions in clubs, bands, or church activities
- Being a community volunteer
- Coaching sports or tutoring children in academic areas

After you have jotted down everything relevant about yourself, develop the highlights of your qualifications. This area could also be called the *Summary of Qualifications,* or just *Summary.* The highlights should be immodest one-liners designed to let your prospective employer know that you are qualified and talented and the best choice for the position. A typical group of highlights might include (Parker, 1989):

- Relevant experience
- Formal training and credentials, if relevant
- Significant accomplishments, very briefly stated
- One or two outstanding skills or abilities
- A reference to your values, commitment, or philosophy, if appropriate

A new graduate's highlights could read:

- Five years of experience as a licensed practical nurse in a large nursing home
- Excellent patient and family relationship skills
- Experience with chronic psychiatric patients
- Strong teamwork and communication skills
- Special certification in rehabilitation and reambulation strategies

Tailor the résumé to the job you are seeking. Include only relevant information, such as internships, summer jobs, intersemester experiences, and volunteer work. Even if your previous work experience is not directly related to nursing, it can show transferable skills, motivation, and your potential to be a great employee.

Regardless of how wonderful you sound on paper, if the résumé itself is not high quality, it may end up in a trash can. Also let your prospective employer know whether you wish to have a response on an answering machine or fax.

Job Search Letters

The most common job search letters are the cover letter, thank-you letter, and acceptance letter. Job search letters should be linked to your SWOT analysis. Regardless of their specific purpose, letters should follow basic writing principles (Banis, 1994):

- State the purpose of your letter.
- State the most important items first, and support them with facts.
- Keep the letter organized.
- Group similar items together in a paragraph, and then organize the paragraphs to flow logically.

Business letters are formal, but they can also be personal and warm but professional.

- Avoid sending an identical form letter to everyone. Instead, personalize each letter to fit each individual situation.
- As you write the letter, keep it work-centered and employment-centered, not self-centered.

- Be direct and brief. Keep your letter to one page.
- Use the active voice and action verbs and have a positive, optimistic tone.
- If possible, address your letters to a specific individual, using the correct title and business address. Letters addressed to "To Whom It May Concern" do not indicate much research or interest in your prospective employer.
- A timely (rapid) response demonstrates your knowledge of how to do business.
- Be honest. Use specific examples and evidence from your experience to support your claims.

Cover Letter

You have spent time carefully preparing the résumé that best sells you to your prospective employer. The cover letter will be your introduction. If it is true that first impressions are lasting ones, the cover letter will have a significant impact on your prospective employer. The purposes of the cover letter include (Beatty, 1989):

- Acting as a transmittal letter for your résumé
- Presenting you and your credentials to the prospective employer
- Generating interest in interviewing you

Regardless of whether your cover letter will be read first by human resources personnel or by the individual nurse manager, its effectiveness cannot be overemphasized. A poor cover letter can eliminate you from the selection process before you even have an opportunity to compete. A sloppy, disorganized cover letter and résumé may suggest you are sloppy and disorganized at work. Likewise, a lengthy, wordy cover letter may suggest a verbose, unfocused individual (Beatty, 1991). Your cover letter should do the following (Anderson, 1992):

- **State your purpose in applying and your interest in a specific position** Also identify how you learned about the position.
- **Emphasize your strongest qualifications that match the requirements for the position** Provide evidence of experience and accomplishments that relate to the available position, and refer to your enclosed résumé.
- **Sell yourself** Convince this employer that you have the qualifications and motivation to perform in this position.
- **Express appreciation to the reader for consideration**

If possible, address your cover letter to a specific person. If you do not have a name, call the health-care facility and obtain the name of the human resources supervisor. If you still can't get a name, create a greeting that includes the word *manager:* for example, Dear Human Resources Manager or Dear Personnel Manager (Zedlitz, 2003, p. 19).

Thank-You Letter

Thank-you letters are important but seldom used tools in a job search. You should send a thank-you letter to everyone who has helped in any way in your job search. As stated earlier, promptness is important. Thank-you letters should be sent within 24 hours to anyone who has interviewed you. The letter (Banis, 1994, p. 4) should:

- Express appreciation.
- Reemphasize your qualifications and the match between your qualifications and the available position.
- Restate your interest in the position.
- Provide any supplemental information not previously stated.

Acceptance Letter

Write an acceptance letter to accept an offered position; confirm the terms of employment, such as salary and starting date; and reiterate the employer's decision to hire you. The acceptance letter often follows a telephone conversation in which the terms of employment are discussed.

Rejection Letter

Although not as common as the first three job search letters, you should send a rejection letter if you are declining an employment offer. When rejecting an employment offer, indicate that you have given the offer careful consideration but have decided that the position does not fit your career objectives and interests at this time. As with your other letters, thank the employer for their consideration and offer.

Using the Internet

Today, most job searches are conducted through the Internet. Performing Internet searches for positions offers greater opportunities and the ability to see what types of positions are available within various geographic locations. Numerous sites either post positions or assist potential employees

table 14-2

Do's and Don'ts of Internet Job Searching

Do	Don't
Focus on selling yourself: "My clinical practicum in the ICU at a major health center and my strong organizational skills fit with the entry-level ICU position posted in Nursing Spectrum."	Use many "I"s in the message: "I saw your job posting in Nursing Spectrum, and I have attached my résumé."
Use short paragraphs; keep the message short.	Long messages probably will not even be read.
Use highlighting and bullets.	Forget to format for e-mail.
Use an appropriate e-mail address: jdoe@. . .	Use a silly or inappropriate e-mail: smartypants@. . . or partyanimal@. . .
Use an effective subject: ICU RN position.	Use subjects used by computer viruses or junk e-mailers: Hi, Important, Information.
Send your message to the correct e-mail address.	Assume; if the address is not indicated, call to see what person or address is appropriate.
Send messages individually.	Send a blast message to many recipients; it may be discarded as junk mail.
Treat e-mail with the same care you treat a traditional business application.	Slip into informality—remember spelling and grammar checks.
Keep your résumé "cyber-safe."	Remove your standard contact information and replace it with your e-mail address.
Change the format of your résumé: save your Word document as an HTML file or an ASCII text file.	Assume that everyone is using the same word processing program.

Source: Adapted from Job Hunt. (2018). The online job search guide. Retrieved from http://www.job-hunt.org/

in matching their skills with available employment. Corporations, private companies, and recruiters use the Internet to reach wider audiences. If you use the Internet in your search, it is always wise to follow up with a hard copy of your résumé if an address is listed. Mention in your cover letter that you sent your résumé via the Internet and the date you did so. If you are using an Internet-based service, follow up with an e-mail to ensure that your résumé was received. Table 14-2 summarizes the major "do's and don'ts" when using the Internet to job search.

The Interview Process

Initial Interview

Your first interview may be with the nurse manager, someone in the human resources office, or an interviewer at a job fair or even over the telephone. Many employers use virtual interviews through Skype, ZOOM, or other electronic media. Prepare for these interviews the same way you prepare for an interview in someone's office. These are still face-to-face interviews conducted in real time (Moon, 2018). Be cognizant of this. Regardless of with whom or where you interview, preparation is the key to success.

You began the first step in the preparation process with your SWOT analysis. If you did not obtain any of the following information regarding your prospective employer at that time, it is imperative that you do it now (Impollonia, 2004):

- Key people in the organization
- Number of patients and employees
- Types of services provided
- Reputation in the community
- Recent mergers and acquisitions
- Other recent news

Much of this information will be available on the prospective employer's Web site. Other potential sources of information are local newspapers and magazines, either in print or on the publications' Web sites.

You also need to review your qualifications for the position. What does your interviewer want to know about you? Consider the following:

- Why should I hire you?
- What kind of employee will you be?
- Will you get things done?
- How much will you cost the company?
- How long will you stay?
- What have you not told us about your weaknesses?

Answering Questions

The interviewer may ask background questions, professional questions, and personal questions. Many employers use the *STAR* method, which focuses on behaviors. Be prepared to discuss a situation and describe the task, the action taken, and the result (Zhang, 2018). If you are especially nervous about interviewing, role-play your interview with a friend or family member acting as the interviewer. Have this person help you evaluate not just what you say but how you say it. Voice inflection, eye contact, and friendliness are demonstrations of your enthusiasm for the position.

Whatever the questions, know your key points and be able to explain in the interview how you will provide an added value to the agency or institution 4 years from now. Refrain from criticizing any former employers. Personal and professional integrity will follow you from position to position. Many companies count on personal references when hiring, including those of faculty and administrators from your nursing program. When leaving positions you held during school or on graduating from your program, it is wise not to take parting shots at someone. Doing a professional program evaluation is fine, but "taking cheap shots" at faculty or other employees is unacceptable (Costlow, 1999).

Background Questions

Background questions usually relate to information on your résumé. If you have no nursing experience, relate your prior school and work experience and other accomplishments in relevant ways to the position you are seeking without going through your entire autobiography with the interviewer. However, you may be asked to expand on the information in your résumé about your formal nursing education. Here is your opportunity to relate specific courses or clinical experiences you enjoyed, academic honors you received, and extracurricular activities or research projects you pursued. The background questions are an invitation for employers to get to know you. Be careful not to appear inconsistent with this information and what you say later.

Professional Questions

Many recruiters are looking for specifics, especially those related to skills and knowledge needed in the position available. They may start with questions related to your education, career goals, strengths, weaknesses, nursing philosophy, style, and abilities.

Interviewers often open their questioning with phrases such as "review," "tell me," "explain," and "describe," followed by "How did you do it?" or "Why did you do it that way?" (Mascolini & Supnick, 1993). How successful will you be with these types of questions?

When answering "How would you describe?" questions, it is especially important that you remain specific. Cite your own experiences, and relate these behaviors to a demonstrated skill or strength. Examples of questions in this area include the following (Bischof, 1993):

- **What is your philosophy of nursing?** This question is asked frequently. Your response should relate to the position you are seeking.
- **What is your greatest weakness? Your greatest strength?** Do not be afraid to present a weakness, but present it to your best advantage, making it sound as if it is a desirable characteristic. Even better, discuss a weakness that is already apparent, such as lack of nursing experience, stating that you recognize your lack of nursing experience but that your own work or management experience has taught you skills that will assist you in this position. These skills might include organization, time management, team spirit, and communication. If you are asked for both strengths and weaknesses, start with your weaknesses and end on a positive note with your strengths. Do not be too modest, but do not exaggerate. Relate your strengths to the prospective position. Skills such as interpersonal relationships, organization, and leadership are usually broad enough to fit most positions.
- **Where do you see yourself in 5 years?** Most interviewers want to gain insight into your long-term goals as well as some idea whether you are likely to use this position as a brief stop on the path to another job. It is helpful for you to know some of the history regarding the position. For example, how long have others usually remained in that job? Your career planning should be consistent with the organization's needs.
- **What are your educational goals?** Be honest and specific. Include both professional education, such as RN or bachelor of science in nursing, and continuing education courses. If you want to pursue further education in related areas, such as a foreign language or computers, include this as a goal. Indicate schools to which you have

applied or in which you are already enrolled. Discuss your plans for professional development (Narayanasamy & Penney, 2014).

- **Describe your leadership style** Be prepared to discuss your style in terms of how effectively you work with others, and give examples of how you have implemented your leadership in the past.
- **What can you contribute to this position?** *What unique skill set do you offer?* Review your SWOT analysis as well as the job description for the position before the interview. Be specific in relating your contributions to the position. Emphasize your accomplishments. Be specific and convey that, even as a new graduate, you are unique.
- **What are your salary requirements?** You may be asked about a minimum salary range. Try to find out the prospective employer's salary range before this question comes up. Be honest about your expectations, but make it clear that you are willing to negotiate.
- **What-if questions** Prospective employers are increasingly using competency-based interview questions to determine people's preparation for a job. There is often no single correct answer to these questions. The interviewer may be assessing your clinical decision-making and leadership skills. Again, be concise and specific, aligning your answer with the organizational philosophy and goals. If you do not know the answer, tell the interviewer how you would go about finding the answer. You cannot be expected to have all the answers before you begin a job, but you can be expected to know how to obtain answers once you are in the position.

Personal Questions

Personal questions deal with your personality and motivation. Common questions include the following:

- **How would you describe yourself?** This is a standard question. Most people find it helpful to think about an answer in advance. You can repeat some of what you said in your résumé and cover letter, but do not provide an in-depth analysis of your personality.
- **How would your peers describe you?** Ask them. Again, be brief, describing several strengths. Do not discuss your weaknesses unless you are asked about them.

- **What would make you happy with this position?** Be prepared to discuss your needs related to your work environment. Do you enjoy self-direction, flexible hours, and strong leadership support? Now is the time to cite specifics related to your ideal work environment.
- **Describe your ideal work environment** Give this question some thought before the interview. Be specific but realistic. If the norm in your community is two RNs to a floor with licensed practical nurses and other ancillary support, do not say that you believe a staff consisting only of RNs is needed for good patient care (Kuokkanen et al., 2014).
- **Describe hobbies, community activities, and recreation** Again, brevity is important. Many times this question is used to further observe the interviewee's communication and interpersonal skills.

Never pretend to be someone other than who you are. If pretending is necessary to obtain the position, then the position is not right for you.

Additional Points About the Interview

Federal, state, and local laws govern employment-related questions. Questions asked on the job application and in the interview must be related to the position advertised. Questions or statements that may lead to discrimination on the basis of age, gender, race, color, religion, or ethnicity are illegal. If you are asked a question that appears to be illegal, you may wish to take one of several approaches:

- You may answer the question, realizing that it is not a job-related question. Make it clear to the interviewer that you will answer the question even though you know it is not job-related.
- You may refuse to answer. You are within your rights but may be seen as uncooperative or confrontational.
- Examine the intent of the question and relate it to the job.

Just as important as the verbal exchanges of the interview are the nonverbal aspects. These include appearance, handshake, eye contact, posture, and listening skills.

Appearance

Dress in business attire. For women, a skirted suit, pants suit, or tailored jacket dress is appropriate. Men should wear a classic suit, light-colored shirt, and conservative tie. For both men and women, gray or navy blue clothing is rarely wrong. Shoes should be polished, with appropriate heels. Nails and hair for both men and women should reflect cleanliness, good grooming, and willingness to work. The 2-inch red dagger nails worn on prom night will not support an image of the professional nurse. In many institutions, even clear, acrylic nails are not allowed. Paint stains on the hands from a weekend of house maintenance are equally unsuitable for presenting a professional image.

Handshake

Arrive at the interview 10 minutes before your scheduled time. (Allow yourself extra time to find the place if you have not previously been there.) Introduce yourself courteously to the receptionist. Stand when your name is called, smile, and shake hands firmly. If you perspire easily, wipe your palms just before handshake time.

Eye Contact

During the interview, use the interviewer's title and last name as you speak. Never use the interviewer's first name unless specifically requested to do so. Use good listening skills (all those leadership skills you have learned). Smile and nod occasionally, making frequent eye contact. Do not fold your arms across your chest, but keep your hands at your sides or in your lap. Pay attention, and sound sure of yourself.

Posture and Listening Skills

Phrase your questions appropriately and relate them to yourself as a candidate: "What would be my responsibility?" instead of "What are the responsibilities of the job?" Use appropriate grammar and diction. Words or phrases such as "yeah," "uh-huh," "uh," "you know," or "like" are too casual for an interview.

Avoid phrases such as "I guess" or "I feel" about anything. These words make you sound indecisive. Remember your action verbs—I analyzed, organized, developed. Do not evaluate your achievements as mediocre or unimpressive.

Asking Questions

At some point in the interview, you will be asked if you have any questions. Knowing what questions you want to ask is just as important as having prepared answers for the interviewer's questions.

The interview is as much a time for you to learn the details of the job as it is for your potential employer to find out about you. You will need to obtain specific information about the job, including the type of patients for whom you would care, the people with whom you would work, the salary and benefits, and your potential employer's expectations of you. Be prepared for the interviewer to say, "Is there anything else I can tell you about the job?" Jot down a few questions on an index card before going for the interview. You may want to ask a few questions based on your research, demonstrating knowledge about and interest in the company. In addition, you may want to ask questions similar to the ones listed next. Above all, be honest and sincere (Bhasin, 1998; Bischof, 1993; Johnson, 1999).

- What is this position's key responsibility?
- What kind of person are you looking for?
- What are the challenges of the position?
- Why is this position open?
- To whom would I report directly?
- Why did the previous person leave this position?
- What is the salary for this position?
- What are the opportunities for advancement?
- What kind of opportunities are there for continuing education?
- What are your expectations of me as an employee?
- How, when, and by whom are evaluations done?
- What other opportunities for professional growth are available here?
- How are promotion and advancement handled within the organization?

The following are a few additional tips about asking questions during a job interview:

- *Do not* begin with questions about vacations, benefits, or sick time. This gives the impression that these are the most important part of the job to you, rather than the work itself.
- *Do* begin with questions about the employer's expectations of you. This gives the impression that you want to know how you can contribute to the organization.
- *Do* be sure you know enough about the position to make a reasonable decision about accepting an offer if one is made.
- *Do* ask questions about the organization as a whole. The information is useful to you and

demonstrates that you are able to see the big picture.

■ *Do* bring a list of important points to discuss as an aid to you if you are nervous.

During the interview process, there are a few red flags to be alert for (Tyler, 1990):

■ Much turnover in the position
■ A newly created position without a clear purpose
■ An organization in transition
■ A position that is not feasible for a new graduate
■ A "gut feeling" that things are not what they seem

The exchange of information between you and the interviewer will go more smoothly if you review Box 14-3 before the interview.

After the Interview

If the interviewer does not offer the information, ask about the next step in the process. Thank the interviewer, shake hands, and exit. If the receptionist is still there, you may quickly smile and say thank you and good-bye. Do not linger and chat, and do not forget to send your thank-you letter.

The Second Interview

Being invited for a second interview means that the first interview went well and that you made a favorable impression. Second visits may include a tour of the facility and meetings with a higher-level executive or a supervisor in the department in which the job opening exists, as well as with several colleagues.

In preparation for the second interview, review the information about the organization and your own strengths. It does not hurt to have a few résumés and potential references available. Pointers to make your second visit successful include the following (Green, 2016):

■ Dress professionally. Do not wear "trendy" outfits, sandals, or open-toed shoes. Minimize jewelry and makeup.
■ Be professional and pleasant with everyone, including administrative assistants and housekeeping and maintenance personnel.
■ Do not smoke.
■ Remember your manners.
■ Avoid controversial topics for small talk.
■ Obtain answers to questions you might have considered since your first visit.

In most instances, the personnel director or nurse manager will let you know how long it will be before you are contacted again. It is appropriate to ask for this information before you leave the second interview. If you do receive an offer during this visit, graciously say "thank you" and ask for a little time to consider the offer (even if this is the offer you have anxiously been awaiting).

If the organization does not contact you by the expected date, do not panic. It is appropriate to call your contact person, state your continued interest, and tactfully express the need to know the status of your application so that you can respond to other deadlines.

---

box 14-3

Do's and Don'ts for Interviewing

Do:
Shake the interviewer's hand firmly, and introduce yourself.
Know the interviewer's name in advance, and use it in conversation.
Remain standing until invited to sit.
Use eye contact.
Let the interviewer take the lead in the conversation.
Talk in specific terms, relating everything to the position.
Support responses in terms of personal experience and specific examples.
Make connections for the interviewer. Relate your responses to the needs of the individual organization.
Show interest in the facility.
Ask questions about the position and the facility.

Come across as sincere in your goals and committed to the profession.
Indicate a willingness to start at the bottom.
Take any examinations requested.
Express your appreciation for the time.

Do Not:
Place your purse, briefcase, papers, and so on, on the interviewer's desk. Keep them in your lap or on the floor.
Slouch in the chair.
Play with your clothing, jewelry, or hair.
Chew gum or smoke, even if the interviewer does.
Be evasive, interrupt, brag, or mumble.
Gossip about or criticize former agencies, schools, or employees.

Source: Adapted from Bischof, J. (1993). Preparing for job interview questions. Critical Care Nurse, 13(4), 97–100. https://doi.org/10.4037/ccn1993.13.4.97; Krannich, C., & Krannich, R. (1993). Interview for success. Impact Publications; Mascolini, M., & Supnick, R. (1993). Preparing students for the behavioral job interview. Journal of Business and Technical Communication, 7(4), 482–488; and Zedlitz, R. (2003). How to get a job in health care. Delmar Learning.

Making the Right Choice

You have interviewed well, and now you have to decide among several job offers. Your choice will not only affect your immediate work but also influence your future career opportunities. The nursing shortage has led to greatly enhanced workplace enrichment programs and nurse residencies as a recruitment and retention strategy. Career ladders, shared governance, participatory management, staff nurse presence on major hospital committees, decentralization of operations, and a focus on quality interpersonal relationships are among some of these features. Be sure to inquire about the components of the professional practice environment (Kuokkanen et al., 2014). There are several additional factors to consider.

Job Content

The immediate work you will be doing should be a good match with your skills and interests. Although your work may be personally challenging and satisfying this year, what are the opportunities for growth? How will your desire for continued growth and challenge be satisfied?

Development

You should have learned from your interviews whether your initial training and orientation seem sufficient. Inquire about continuing education to keep you current in your field. Is tuition reimbursement available for further education? Is management training provided, or are supervisory skills learned on the job?

Direction

Good supervision and mentors are especially important in your first position. You may be able to judge prospective supervisors throughout the interview process, but you should also try to get a broader view of the overall philosophy of supervision. You may not be working for the same supervisor in a year, but the overall management philosophy is likely to remain consistent.

Work Climate

As a nurse, you need to feel comfortable in the daily work climate. Your preference may be formal or casual, structured or unstructured, complex or simple. It is easy to observe the way people dress, the layout of the unit, and lines of communication. It is more difficult to observe company values, as well as other factors that will affect your work comfort and satisfaction through the long term. Try to look beyond the work environment to get an idea of values. What is the unwritten message? Is there an open-door policy sending a message that "everyone is equal and important," or does the nurse manager appear too busy to be concerned with the needs of the employees? Is your supervisor the kind of person for whom you could work easily?

Compensation

In evaluating the compensation package, starting salary should be less important than the organization's philosophy on future compensation. What is the potential for salary growth? How are individual increases determined? Can you live on the wages being offered? Also review the organization's package regarding retirement and health insurance.

I Cannot Find a Job (Or I Moved)

Many say that finding the first job is the hardest part of the job search. Many employers prefer to hire seasoned nurses who do not require a long orientation and mentoring, particularly in specialty areas. Some require new graduates to do postgraduate internships or even provide these to help ensure longevity in their employees (Walsh, 2018). Changes in skill mix with the implementation of various types of care delivery influence the market for the professional nurse. The new graduate may need to be armed with a variety of skills, such as intravenous certification, home assessment, advanced rehabilitation skills, and various respiratory modalities, to even warrant an initial interview. Keep informed about the demands of the market in your area, and be prepared to be flexible in seeking your first position. Even with the continuing nursing shortage, hiring you as a new graduate will depend on you selling yourself.

After all this searching and hard work, you still may not have found the position you want. You may be focusing on work arrangements or benefits rather than on the job description. Your lack of direction may come through in your résumé, cover letter, and personal presentation. As a new graduate, you may also have unrealistic expectations or be trying to cut corners, ignoring the basic rules of marketing yourself discussed in this chapter. Go back to your SWOT analysis. Take another look at your résumé and cover letter. Become more assertive as you start again.

The Critical First Year

Why does this chapter include a section on the "first year"? Working hard is important; however, some of the behaviors deemed important and rewarded in school are not necessarily rewarded on the job. Employers do not supply syllabi, study questions, or extra-credit points. Only an "A" is acceptable, and often there is not a correct answer. Quality is the expectation with little room for error. Discovering this has been called "reality shock" (Sparacino, 2016). Voluminous concept maps and meticulous medication cards are out; multiple responsibilities and thinking on your feet are in. What is the new graduate to do?

Your first year will be a transition year. You are no longer a college student. You are a novice nurse. You are "the new kid on the block," and people will respond to you differently and judge you differently than when you were a student. To be successful, you have to respond differently. You may be thinking, "Oh, they always need nurses—it doesn't matter." Yes, it does matter. Many of your career opportunities will be influenced by the early impressions you make. The following section addresses what you can do to help ensure first-year success.

Attitude and Expectations

Adopt the right attitudes, and adjust your expectations. Now is the time to learn the art of being new. You felt as if you were the most important, special person during the recruitment process. Now, in the real world, neither you nor the position may be as glamorous as you once thought. In addition, although you thought you learned much in school, your decisions and daily performance do not always warrant an A. Above all, people shed the company manners they displayed when you were interviewing, and organizational politics eventually surface. Your leadership skills and commitment to teamwork will get you through this transition period.

Impressions and Relationships

Manage a good impression, and build effective relationships. Remember, you are being watched: by peers, subordinates, and superiors. Because you as yet have no track record, first impressions are magnified. Although every organization is different, most are looking for someone with good judgment, a willingness to learn, a readiness to adapt, and a respect for the expertise of more experienced employees.

Most people expect you to "pay your dues" to earn respect from them.

Organizational Savvy

Develop organizational savvy. An important person in this first year is your immediate supervisor. Support this person. Find out what is important to your supervisor and what this individual needs and expects from the team. Become a team player. When confronted with an issue, present solutions, not problems, as often as you can. You want to be a good leader someday; learn first to be a good follower. Finding a mentor is another important goal of your first year. Mentors are role models and guides who encourage, counsel, teach, and advocate for their mentee. In these relationships, both the mentor and mentee receive support and encouragement (Beal, 2016; Shellenbarger & Robb, 2016).

"The spark that ignites a mentoring relationship may come from either the protégé or the mentor. Protégés often view mentors as founts of success, a bastion of life skills they wish to learn and emulate." Likewise, mentors often see the future that is hidden in another's personality and abilities (Klein & Dickenson-Hazard, 2000, pp. 20–21; Shellenbarger & Robb, 2016).

Skills and Knowledge

Master the skills and knowledge of the position. Technology is constantly changing, and, contrary to popular belief, you did not learn everything in school. Be prepared to seek out new knowledge and skills on your own. This may entail extra hours of preparation and study, but remember that no one ever said learning stops after graduation. Lifelong learning is the key to being a successful nurse.

Advancing Your Career

Many of the ideas presented in this chapter will continue to be helpful as you advance in your nursing career. Continuing to develop your leadership and patient care skills through practice and further education will be the keys to your professional growth. The RN is expected to develop and provide leadership to other members of the health-care team while providing safe, effective, and quality care to patients. According to the Health Resources and Services Administration (HRSA, 2017, 2021), the number of licensed RNs in the United States has increased to a record high level. This increase reflects a larger number of younger nurses entering the workforce along with older experienced nurses. Because of the increased demand for nurses, getting your first job within this environment may not be so difficult, but you hold the responsibility for advancing your career.

Conclusion

Finding your first position is more than being in the right place at the right time. It is a complex combination of learning about yourself and the organizations you are interested in and presenting your strengths and weaknesses in the most positive manner possible. Keeping the first position and using the position to grow and learn are also part of a planning process. Recognize that the independence you enjoyed through college may not be the skill you need to keep your first position. There is an important lesson to be learned: becoming a team player and being savvy about organizational politics are as important as becoming proficient in nursing skills. Take the first step toward finding a mentor—before you know it, you will become one yourself.

Study Questions

1. Using the SWOT analysis worksheet developed for this chapter, how will you articulate your strengths and weaknesses during an interview?

2. Design a one- to two-page résumé to use in seeking your first position. Are you able to "sell yourself" in one or two pages? If not, what adjustments are you going to make?

3. Develop a cover letter, thank-you letter, acceptance letter, and rejection letter that you can use during the interview process.

4. Using the interview preparation worksheet developed for this chapter, formulate responses to the questions. How comfortable do you feel answering these questions? Share your responses with other classmates to get additional ideas.

5. Using the STAR technique, consider the following question: "Tell me about the time you took the lead on a group project."

6. Evaluate the job prospects in the community where you now live. What areas could you explore in seeking your first position?

7. What plans do you have for advancing your career? What plans do you have for finding a mentor?

Case Study to Promote Clinical Judgment

Peter James is interviewing for his first nursing position after obtaining his RN license. He interviewed with the nurse recruiter and was asked back for a second interview with the nurse manager on the pediatric floor. After a few minutes of social conversation, the nurse manager begins to ask some specific nursing-oriented questions: How would you respond if a mother of a seriously ill child asks you if her child will die? What attempts do you make to understand different cultural beliefs and their importance in health care when planning nursing care? How does your philosophy of nursing affect your ability to deliver care to children whose mothers are HIV-positive?

Peter becomes very flustered by these questions and responds with "it depends on the situation," "it depends on the culture," and "I don't ever discriminate."

1. What responses would have been more appropriate in this interview?

2. How could Peter have used these questions to demonstrate his strengths, experiences, and skills?

3. Using the SWOT format, how would you prepare for this interview?

NCLEX®-Style Review Questions

1. A nursing student is graduating in 3 months. The student is looking for a position. Where should the student begin the search? **Select all that apply**.
   1. Health-care organizations
   2. Online job boards
   3. National Council of State Boards of Nursing
   4. American Association of Colleges of Nursing
   5. Recommendations from peers and professionals

2. A nursing student is preparing for a first job interview. What should the nursing student research about the organization before going to the interview?
   1. Review the salary scale.
   2. Research the benefits package offered to employees.
   3. Become familiar with the organization's mission and core values.
   4. Ask nurses who work at the agency how many patients they are assigned.

3. A nursing student is preparing a résumé to send to prospective employers. What qualities should the nursing student emphasize? **Select all that apply**.
   1. Responsibility and accountability
   2. Integrity
   3. Interpersonal skills
   4. Social skills
   5. Family values

4. What type of résumé is useful in showing stable employment without gaps or many job changes?
   1. Standard
   2. Chronological
   3. Functional
   4. Combination

5. A nursing student who is graduating in a few weeks is preparing a résumé. What should the nursing student highlight first? **Select all that apply**.
   1. Family status
   2. Educational degrees
   3. Community service
   4. Employment experience
   5. Leadership experiences in school

6. What is the purpose of a cover letter when applying for a position?
   1. Introduces the applicant.
   2. States the employment goal.
   3. Outlines the applicant's position in the community.
   4. Describes the reason for entering nursing.

7. What is the STAR method of interviewing?
   1. Focuses on communication.
   2. Emphasizes behaviors.
   3. Allows the employer to ask personal questions.
   4. Creates a relaxed interviewing environment.

8. When conducting a SWOT analysis, the "T" represents
   1. Time spent in education
   2. Threats to obtaining a position
   3. Terminal degree expectations
   4. Talking points for the interview

9. Which of the following represents the "S" in a SWOT analysis?
   1. Flexibility
   2. Difficulty adapting to change
   3. Nursing shortage
   4. Competition among health-care facilities

10. A new graduate plans on moving into nursing administration. What steps should the graduate take to ensure this goal is reached? **Select all that apply**.
    1. Further professional education.
    2. Meet the specific requirements for the entry-level job position.
    3. Seek new experiences.
    4. Volunteer to work on committees.
    5. Find a mentor.

chapter 15

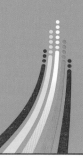

Advancing Your Career

Graduation is not the end of learning but rather the beginning of a journey toward becoming an expert nurse (Benner, 2001). As a career, nursing is full of challenges, opportunities, and possibilities. You can care for newborns in the nursery, adolescents with drug problems, adults with cancer, and older adults with Alzheimer's disease. You can become an operating room nurse, a diabetes educator, health coach, nurse–midwife, nurse executive, or researcher. All these begin with basic preparation in professional nursing.

Levels of Educational Preparation Within Professional Nursing

There are several paths you can take to become a professional registered nurse (RN). These are the bachelor of science degree in nursing (BSN), associate degree in nursing (AD), and a diploma from an approved program (U.S. Bureau of Labor Statistics [BLS], 2022). The diploma is usually offered by a hospital-based school of nursing and was the most common path in years past. Many of them now have affiliations with a college so students can earn college credits or even an AD along with their hospital diploma (nursingexplorer.com, 2022). There are far fewer diploma programs in the United States today. The AD is typically a 2-year degree offered in community colleges and at some hospital-based schools of nursing. It is meant to prepare graduates for RN licensure and for employment within the technical scope of practice. The BS or BSN is a 4-year degree obtained through colleges and universities that prepare graduates for licensure and professional nursing practice. Bachelor's degree programs typically are a combination of liberal arts, science, and nursing-specific courses. There are also RN to BSN programs for those who are already RNs but want to earn their 4-year degree. If done full-time, they can usually be completed in 2 years.

Future job prospects for RNs are promising. The median salary for RNs in the United States in 2021 was $75,330 a year ($36.22 an hour). In addition, positions for RNs are expected to increase faster than the average for all occupations. This is because of several trends including the increasing numbers of older adults whose large numbers alone will increase demand for health care, an emphasis on preventive care, and an increasing number of individuals with multiple chronic conditions such as diabetes, hypertension, and dementia (BLS, 2022).

Advanced degrees in nursing are also available at both the master's and doctoral level. Most master's degrees prepare the student for specialized roles in nursing. These may include certified midwife, clinical nurse specialist, certified nurse anesthetist, clinical nurse educator, and several nurse practitioner roles (Nurse Journal, 2018).

Many nurses work for several years or more before pursuing these advanced degrees. The reasons for this delay are many, including the cost of advanced education, the time demand, developing practice skills, and allowing time to choose a specialty. Most of these programs are an additional 2 years in length.

The highest degree in nursing is the doctoral degree. In nursing, there are two primary choices at this level: the doctor of nursing practice (DNP) or the doctor of philosophy (PhD) in nursing. DNP programs focus on highly specialized advanced practice; PhD programs focus on the preparation of nurse researchers, especially for clinical nursing research. There are even opportunities in nursing to pursue postdoctoral studies by honing research skills and seeking grant funds to support one's research.

Non-nursing degrees may be an attractive alternative to the high standards and time demands (especially for clinical courses) of nursing degrees. Given the highly complex nature of health care and expectations of practicing nurses today, however, the advanced preparation in nursing provided by nursing degree programs is becoming an essential part of higher education for nurses.

Transition From Student to Nurse

Transitions are challenging. They can shock and stress you if you are not prepared for them. But they also provide opportunity. Your first RN position provides you with an opportunity to test yourself, to put what you learned into practice, and to earn a salary for the work you are doing.

It has been known for some time that the transition from student to nurse is difficult. In fact, Marlene Kramer brought this to our attention almost 50 years ago, calling the experience of new nurses "reality shock" (Kramer, 1974; Rush et al., 2014; Strauss et al., 2016). It is generally agreed that the difficulties encountered during this important transition are because of a gap between nursing education and nursing practice as the new graduate is expected to have sufficient "know-how" to provide nursing care on entry into a nursing position and the fact that it is difficult to develop a "professional self" at the same time (Murphy & Janisse, 2017).

Employers expect new graduates to come to the work setting able to provide safe care, organize their work, set priorities, and provide leadership to ancillary personnel. Even though nursing programs are designed to help students prepare for the multiple demands of the work setting, new nurses still need to continue to learn and practice their skills on the job. Experienced nurses say that what they learned in school is only the foundation for practice and that school provided them with the fundamental knowledge and skills they needed to continue to grow and develop as they practice nursing in various capacities and work settings.

Here is an example: In most AD programs, students are assigned to care for one to three patients a day, working up to six or seven patients under a preceptor's supervision by the end of their program. Compare this with your first real job as a nurse: You might work 7 days in a row, sometimes on 8- or 12-hour shifts, caring for 10 or more patients. You may also have to supervise several licensed practical nurses (LPNs), technicians, and nursing assistants. This is a big change from the patient care assignments you had in school.

Another source of some shock to new nurses is that many of the behaviors that brought rewards in school, such as crafting detailed care plans, taking extra time to prepare a patient for discharge, or delaying another task to look up the side effects of a new medication, are not necessarily valued by the organization. Some of these behaviors may even be criticized.

When efficiency is the goal, the speed and amount of work done may be rewarded rather than the quality of the work. This creates a conflict for the new graduate who, while in school, was allowed to take as much time as needed to provide good care. The following is an example:

Brenda, a new graduate, was assigned to give medications to all of her team's patients. Because this was a fairly light assignment, she spent some time looking up the medications and explaining their actions to the patients receiving them. Brenda also straightened up the medicine cart and restocked the supplies, which she thought

would please her task-oriented team leader. At the end of the day, Brenda reported these activities with some satisfaction to the team leader. She expected the team leader to be pleased with the way she used the time. Instead, the team leader looked annoyed and told her that whoever passes out medications always does the blood pressures as well and that the other nurse on the team, who had a heavier assignment, had to do them. Also, because supplies were always ordered on Fridays for the weekend, it would have to be done again tomorrow, so Brenda had in fact wasted her time. Brenda had just encountered these differences in expectations and discovered how much more she needed to learn about the routines in her workplace.

Solutions

One of the goals of leadership courses, immersion experiences, and clinical intensives in school is to prepare you to meet the expectations of your first employer. You can also use independent study opportunities to further immerse yourself in the clinical world of patient care. If possible, these clinical placements should match your preferences for future employment.

Part-time or full-time employment in a health-care setting is another way to prepare yourself for the realities of clinical practice. However, you need to be sure that this work does not interfere with your schoolwork and that you distinguish the work you might do as an LPN or nursing assistant from the work you will do as an RN. If your instructors discourage you from doing this, it is probably because of these concerns.

Transition to Practice Programs (TPPs)

It's not just your instructors in school who are concerned that your transition to practicing nurse goes well. Your potential employer also wants it to go well. Unless you are aware of this, you might be surprised at the great effort many employers have invested in designing postgraduation transition programs. We will consider a few examples to give you an idea what is available in some health-care organizations.

Formal Mentoring Programs

Mentors can provide the support needed to increase new nurses' clinical success, job satisfaction, and retention (Burr et al., 2011; Cottingham et al., 2011; Weng et al., 2010). New graduates need help with organizing their work; time management; communicating with other members of the health-care team, especially with physicians; and recognition of critical changes in their patients. Even experienced nurses, when newly hired or transferred to different positions, need to learn the culture of the new organization, their role on the new team, and new skills (Ellisen, 2011). For example:

> The Veterans Administration (VA) requires that each VA medical center have an RN Transition-to-Practice (RNTTP) residency program if they hire RNs with less than 1 year of experience. This is a 12-month program that includes veteran-centric content. Each new trainee is assigned a trained preceptor as part of the program (va.gov, n.d.).
>
> Children's National Hospital in Washington, D.C. has a TPP that has been accredited by the American Nurses Credentialing Center (ANCC). This 12-month program includes didactic, simulation, and hands-on training. The program is offered twice a year (childrensnational.org, 2022).

At Sharp Mary Birch Hospital for Women and Newborns in San Diego, new graduates, nurses returning to work after some time away, and nurses entering a new specialty area are matched with an experienced mentor for their first year. The program includes a 3-hour orientation for mentors and mentees, quarterly support workshops, and ongoing support. This program not only reduced their new graduate turnover rate but also helped to recruit new nurses (Burr et al., 2011).

A mentor–mentee relationship may be formal, as in the previous example, or it may develop informally through time. Formal relationships usually include some training for the mentor and mentee, have specific objectives, and often have mentors assigned to mentees, whereas those in informal mentoring relationships usually choose each other

(Harrington, 2011). Either approach can be a valuable and rewarding experience for both mentor and mentee.

Internships and Residency Programs

Internships and residency programs for new graduates average 6 months to 1 year in length. Some require licensure before acceptance. Others may offer lower salaries to offset the cost to the employer of offering both learning sessions and work experience to the new nurse (Cappel et al., 2013). The content of the programs varies but may include (a) patient-centered care skills (i.e., the technical skills to provide safe, high-quality care, emergency care, and end-of-life care); (b) organizational skills, including organizing work, delegating, prioritizing, and time management; (c) clinical leadership skills; and (d) communicating with members of the interprofessional team, patients, and families (Cappel et al., 2013; Goode et al., 2009).

Development of a support network for the new graduate is considered an essential part of these programs. This network may include peers (other new graduates), a preceptor or mentor, and a nurse manager. New graduates typically begin these programs feeling very positive and confident but hit a low point halfway through them when they realize how much they still have to learn and how demanding nursing can be. However, they gradually regain their confidence and show a satisfactory level of competence, caring for even very ill patients by the end of their 12-month residencies, having achieved technical skills, decisional competence, and self-confidence (Goode et al., 2009; Jones-Bell et al., 2018).

Orientation Programs

Orientation programs for new graduates typically offer classroom, online, and on-unit training. Programs that are tailored to the individual's learning needs and provide consistent preceptors or mentors are usually the most effective. Traditional orientation programs are shorter in length than are internships or residency programs.

Ohio Health, a not-for-profit health-care system, developed a simulation-enhanced orientation program divided into three distinct stages: JumpStart week, Assessments, and Unit-based orientation. JumpStart week includes a series of skill stations (such as blood administration) and simulation scenarios. The new graduates work in groups of five to seven nurses. Two participate in each scenario while the others watch via live video, followed by debriefing. During the Assessment phase, orientees were identified as "green" if they were ready to function as staff, "yellow" if they needed more time to learn, and "red" if they were assessed as unsafe or below standard. Assessments included the evaluation of procedural skills, critical thinking, medication administration, documentation, prioritization of care, telemetry, time management, and safety (Zigmont et al., 2015).

A systematic review of these TPP programs by Edwards and colleagues (2015) indicated that they had beneficial effects for both the new nurse and the employer, including higher confidence and competence, lower stress and anxiety, and increased job satisfaction. They suggest that it is the focus on the new graduate rather than the specific approach that is the source of the program's success. If they are correct, then it is more important to seek a first position that offers a well-developed TPP than it is to find a particular type of program.

In some cases, the orientation program may be cut short and the new nurses may be required to function on their own very quickly. One way to minimize initial work stress is to ask questions about the orientation program before accepting a position: How long will it be? With whom will I be working? When will I be on my own? What happens if at the end of the orientation I still need more assistance?

Additional Suggestions to Facilitate the Transition

Instead of focusing on the stress, new nurses can also manage their transition from student to practicing nurse by taking responsibility for their own successful transition.

- **Develop a professional identity** Opportunities to challenge one's competence and develop an identity as a professional can begin in school. Success in meeting these challenges can immunize the new graduate against the loss of confidence that accompanies the shocks of the transition to practice.

- **Learn about the organization** The new graduate who understands how organizations operate will not be as shocked as the naïve individual. When you begin a new job, it is important to learn as much as you can about your new organization and how it really operates.

- **Use your energy wisely** Much energy goes into learning a new job. You may see many things that you think need to be changed, but you need to recognize that to implement change requires your time and energy, so choose your targets wisely.

- **Communicate effectively** Confront problems that might arise with coworkers. Use the problem-solving and negotiating skills you've learned in this course to do this constructively.

- **Seek feedback often and persistently** Seeking feedback pushes the people you work with to be more specific about their expectations of you and any concerns they might have. It also engages your coworkers in helping you make the transition successfully.

- **Develop a support network** A support network is a source of strength when resisting pressure to give up professional ideals and a source of power when attempting to bring about change. Identify colleagues who have held onto their professional ideals with whom you can share your problems and the work of improving the organization. Their recognition of your work can keep you going when rewards from the organization are meager.

- **Give yourself some time** Above all, give yourself time to make this transition. Do engage actively in this process of professional development, but don't expect it to happen overnight.

Ineffective Coping Strategies

Some less successful ways of coping with the transition from student to practicing nurse are provided in the list that follows.

- **Abandon professional ideals** When faced with reality shock, some new graduates abandon their professional ideals. This may eliminate the conflict but puts the needs of the organization before their own needs or the needs of the patient, which is not a satisfactory resolution.

- **Leave the profession** A significant proportion of those who do not want to give up their professional ideals escape these conflicts by leaving their jobs and abandoning their profession. There would probably be fewer recurring shortages of nurses if more health-care organizations met these professional ideals (Kramer & Schmalenberg, 1993).

When you have made it through the first 6 months of employment and are finally starting to feel as if you are a "real" nurse, you are probably beginning to realize that a completely stress-free work environment is unrealistic. Shift work, overtime, staff shortages, and pressure to do more with less continue to place demands on nurses. Another way to respond constructively to these challenges is to join a professional organization.

Professional Organizations

American Nurses Association (ANA)

In 1896, delegates from 10 nursing schools' alumni associations met to organize a national professional association for nurses. The first issue of the *American Journal of Nursing* was distributed in 1900. The constitution and bylaws were completed in 1907, and the Nurses Associated Alumnae of the United States and Canada was created. The name was changed in 1911 to the ANA, which in 1982 became a federation of constituent state nurses associations. Similarly, the Canadian Association of Nursing Education created the Canadian National Association of Trained Nurses in 1908, which became the Canadian Nurses Association (CNA) in 1924 (Mansell & Dodd, 2005).

The ANA's purpose is to "lead the profession to shape the future of nursing and healthcare" (ANA, 2022). The ANA advances the profession by "fostering high standards of nursing practice, promoting a safe and ethical work environment, bolstering the health and wellness of nurses, and advocating on health-care issues that affect nurses and the public" (ANA, 2022). The ANA's Strategic Goals for 2020 to 2023 are:

■ Elevate the profession of nursing globally.
■ Engage all nurses to ensure operational success.
■ Evolve the practice of nursing to transform health.
■ Enable transformational capability and health care through operational excellence.

The ANA uses Professional Issues Panels (ANA, 2022) to engage members in active dialogue on

---

box 15-1
American Nurses Association (ANA) Position Statements

Drug and Alcohol Abuse	Patient Safety
Electronic Health Records	Privacy and Confidentiality
Ethics and Human Rights	Role of the Registered
HIV and Viral Hepatitis	Nurse
Nursing Practice	Work Place Advocacy

Source: American Nurses Association. (2022). Official ANA position statements. Retrieved from http://www.nursingworld.org/practice-policy /nursing-excellence/official-position-statements/

---

specific practice and policy questions as approved by the ANA Board of Directors. You need to be an RN and a member of the ANA to serve on one of these panels. The topics addressed by these Professional Issues Panels in 2022 give you an idea of the scope of issues facing our profession and our health-care system:

■ End Nurse Abuse
■ Professional Issues
■ Revisions of the Code of Ethics for Nurses With Interpretive Statements
■ Barriers to RN Scope of Practice
■ Care Coordination Quality Measures
■ Connected Health/Telehealth
■ Moral Resilience
■ Palliative and Hospice Issues
■ Workplace Violence and Incivility

A list of the ANA Position Statements, which can be found on the ANA Web site, is in Box 15-1.

Canadian Nurses Association (CNA)

As of June 2018, the CNA became the national organization for RNs, nurse practitioners, practical nurses, and registered psychiatric nurses in Canada. The purpose of the CNA is "Registered nurses contributing to the health of Canadians and the advancement of nursing" (CNA, 2022). The CNA's mission includes:

■ Unifying the voices of RNs
■ Strengthening nursing leadership
■ Promoting nursing excellence and a vibrant profession
■ Advocating for healthy public policy and a quality health system
■ Serving the public interest

A list of the CNA Position Statements, which can be found on their Web site, is in Box 15-2.

box 15-2

Canadian Nurses Association (CNA) Position Statements

Joint Statement on Breastfeeding
Climate Change and Health
Environmentally Responsible Activity in the Health-Care
  Sector
Global Health and Equity
Harm Reduction and Substance Use
Influenza Immunization of Nurses
International Trade and Labor Mortality
Interprofessional Collaboration
Intraprofessional Collaboration
Mental Health Services
Nurses and Environmental Health
Nurses and Midwives Collaborate on Client-Centered Care
Nurses Health and Human Rights
Nursing Information
Nursing Leadership
The Palliative Approach to Care and the Role of the Nurse
  Pan-Canadian Health
Human Resources Planning
Patient Safety
Practice Environments

Maximizing Outcomes for Clients, Nurses,
  and Organizations
Primary Health Care
Promoting Continuing Competence for Registered Nurses
Promoting Cultural Competence in Nursing
The Role of Health Professionals in Tobacco Cessation
Scopes of Practice
Social Determinants of Health
Spirituality, Health, and the Nursing Practice
Staff Decision-Making Framework for Quality Care
Taking Action on Nurse Fatigue
Toward an Environmentally Responsible Canadian Health
  Sector
The Value of Nursing History Today
Workplace Violence and Bullying
Global Health Issues
Global Health Partnerships
Global Health and Equity
International Trade and Labor Mobility
Peace and Health
Registered Nurses, Health and Human Rights

Source: Canadian Nurses Association. (2022). CNA position statements. https://www.cna-aiic.ca/en
/policy-advocacy/policy-support-tools/position-statements

Why Join Your National Organization?

Although there are about 4.2 million nurses in the United States, only 10% are members of their professional organization. The many different nursing subgroups and numerous specialty nursing organizations contribute to this fragmentation, making it difficult to present a united front from which to advocate for nursing and for the public's health. As the ANA works on the goal of preparing nurses for the demands of the 21st century, nurses need to work together in their efforts to identify and promote their unique, autonomous role within the health-care system.

Membership in the ANA offers benefits such as informative publications, group life and health insurance, access to malpractice insurance, and continuing education courses. As the primary voice of nursing in the United States, the ANA lobbies legislators to influence the passage of laws that affect the practice of nursing and the safety of consumers. The power of the ANA was apparent when nurses lobbied against the American Medical Association's (AMA) proposal to create a new category of health-care worker, the registered care technician, as an answer to the nursing shortage of the 1980s. The registered care technician category was never established despite the AMA's vigorous support.

The ANA frequently publishes position statements outlining the organization's position on particular topics important to the health and welfare of the public or the nurse, which can be accessed on the ANA Web site (www.nursingworld.org/positionstatements). Likewise, the CNA publishes position statements on such issues as education, ethics, public health policy, leadership, practice, primary health care, protection of the public, and research (CNA, 2022).

The ANA also offers certification in various specialty areas through its subsidiary, the ANCC. Certification is a formal but voluntary process by which the professional nurse demonstrates knowledge of and expertise in a specific area of practice. It is a way to establish the nurse's expertise beyond the basic requirements for licensure and is an important part of peer recognition for nurses. In many facilities, certification entitles the nurse to salary increases and position advancement. Some specialty nursing organizations also have certification programs.

National League for Nursing (NLN)

Another large nursing organization in the United States is the NLN, the "Voice of Nursing Education." Unlike ANA membership, NLN membership is open to other health professionals and interested consumers, who number 45,000 altogether. More than 1,100 nursing schools and health-care agencies are members of the NLN (NLN, 2022). The NLN was formed to promote excellence in nursing education in order to build a strong and diverse nursing workforce, thereby improving health care.

The NLN participates in test services, research, and publication. It also lobbies actively for nursing issues and works cooperatively with the ANA and other nursing organizations on health-care issues. To do such things more effectively, the ANA, NLN, American Association of Colleges of Nursing (AACN), and American Organization of Nurse Executives (AONE) have formed a coalition called the TriCouncil for the purpose of dealing with issues that are important to all nurses.

The NLN formed a separate accrediting agency, the National League for Nursing Accrediting Agency (NLNAC), which is now called the Accreditation Commission for Education in Nursing (ACEN) (acenursing.org, n.d.). The ACEN provides for the specialized accreditation of nursing education schools and programs, both postsecondary and higher degree (master's degree, baccalaureate degree, AD, diploma, and practical nursing programs). The ACEN has entered into a partnership with the Organization for Associate Degree Nursing (OADN) to increase support for AD programs and their students (acenursing.org, 2022).

Organization for Associate Degree Nursing (OADN)

AD programs prepare the largest number of new graduates for RN licensure. Many of these individuals would never have had the opportunity to become RNs without the access afforded by the community college system. The move to begin a national organization to address AD issues began in 1986. The organization identified two major goals: to maintain eligibility for licensure for AD graduates and to interact with other nursing organizations. The current mission continues to reflect the OADN's purpose: "to ensure that the voices of associate degree nurses are heard . . ." (OADN, 2022). Today, the goals of the OADN are to:

▪ Ensure that policy makers understand the important role of AD nursing programs in providing access to safe, quality nursing care across the country.
▪ Collaborate with other organizations and influential leaders to create opportunities

and advancement for nursing educators and AD graduates.
▪ Promote diversity and inclusion in the nursing workforce to improve health equity for patients and communities.

The OADN notes U.S. Department of Health and Human Services (HHS) data that 57% of U.S. nurses begin their career with an AD. Many then continue their education to earn the BSN degree. The OADN supports the development of RN to BS degree programs at community colleges, which are available in some parts of the United States.

National Student Nurses Association (NSNA)

The NSNA is an organization you can join and become a leader in right now. The NSNA has 60,000 members across the United States. Students enrolled in AD, baccalaureate, and diploma programs are eligible for membership. The NSNA offers opportunities to meet students from other programs, prepare for initial licensing, develop leadership skills and career planning, and advocate for high-quality, affordable, accessible health care (NSNA, 2022).

American Academy of Nursing (AAN)

The AAN consists of more than 2,800 nursing leaders called fellows in practice, education, management, and research. Its mission is to advance health policy through organizational excellence and nursing leadership. Fellows are expected to contribute to the work of the AAN (for example, through membership on expert panels) and to "engage with other health leaders outside the Academy to transform existing healthcare systems" (aannet, n.d.). The mission of the AAN is to "serve the public and the nursing profession by advancing health policy, practice, and science." *Nursing Outlook* is the AAN's official journal. Membership is through nomination and election by current fellows of the Academy (aannet, n.d.).

National Institute for Nursing Research (NINR)

The NINR, unlike the other associations described here, is an arm of the federal government, one of the 27 institutes and centers of the National Institutes of Health (NIH). NINR supports and conducts basic and clinical research through the lenses of health equity, social determinants of health, population and community health, prevention and health promotion, and systems and models of care, as well as promoting innovation and developing nurse scientists for the 21st century (ninr.nih.gov, n.d.).

Specialty Organizations

In addition to the national nursing organizations, nurses may join specialty practice organizations focused on practice areas (e.g., critical care, nephrology, obstetrics) or special interest groups (e.g., male nurses, Hispanic nurses, Philippine nurses, Aboriginal nurses). These organizations provide nurses with information regarding evidence-based practice, trends in the field, and standards of specialty practice. Links to nursing organizations in the United States may be found at www.nursingworld .org/ana/org-affiliates/.

Your Future Career in Nursing

You have begun your nursing journey by applying for admission to a formal educational program and taking the courses required to qualify you to sit for the RN licensure examination. What comes next?

Stages of a Nursing Career

Upon graduation, perhaps even sooner, you will begin your search for your first nursing position. Your transition to practice begins when you assume that first position, which will require most of your attention during your first year as a practicing nurse. However, hopefully you will have some time to join your state nurses association and to think about your future career, that is, the specialty you would prefer to pursue and what you want to do within that specialty, whether it involves focusing on advancing in practice, becoming a manager and eventually an administrator, becoming an educator or a researcher in your specialty, or even a combination of these. This is your long-term career trajectory.

Shirey (2009) notes that common elements for a successful career are the ability to recognize one's strengths, align them with one's passions, and build upon them. This takes some thought and insight. She has applied a framework from Citron and Smith (2003) to nursing careers that divides a career into three phases: promise, momentum, and harvest:

Promise phase This is the time when you identify your strengths and build your knowledge and skill base.

Momentum phase This is the time when you achieve mastery in your specialty and become recognized for your expertise.

Harvest phase This is when you reach your prime in your profession but need to continue to grow and develop to retain your position and status. There is a possibility of establishing a legacy for nurses following you.

Paths to Advancement

Most health-care organizations offer advancement opportunities, a career ladder you can climb from staff level to management and administration along an administrative track or to preceptor, clinical specialist, and educator along a clinical track. There are usually specific criteria for moving up these levels within the organization and several optional activities and responsibilities you can offer to take on to add to your accomplishments and to your value to the organization. This includes serving as a mentor to new graduates, chairing committees, obtaining extra training, working on quality improvement or research projects, and so forth.

Jakubik (2008) suggests thinking of all these activities as *tools* to promote career advancement that should be collected in a tool box for building your career. There are four core compartments in your career "tool box":

1. **Continuing education** Your state may require that you complete a minimum number of hours of continuing education to renew your license. This requirement is just a minimum accomplishment. In addition, you can attend local and national conferences in your specialty area, attend training sessions offered by your employer, and take online courses offered by your nursing association. You can also pursue formal education, progressing through the levels of education described earlier from earning your BSN degree to master's level programs and a doctorate in nursing.

2. **Certification** Certification is a formal acknowledgement by a recognized nursing association that you have achieved either a basic

or advanced level in your specialty area. There is also required certification for advanced practice (nurse practitioner).

3. **Mentoring** Experienced nurses often find it very satisfying to be able to share their experience with new nurses. Most health-care organizations not only offer training for the mentoring role but also reward employees for taking on this additional responsibility. From the perspective of the mentor, this activity provides satisfaction, recognition, and reward.

4. **Professional activities** This last compartment in your career-building tool box can be filled with a great variety of activities. The following are just a few examples:

▪ Join one of the committees of your local or state nursing association or specialty association. Even better, become a chair of one of these committees.

▪ Offer to serve on the innumerable committees that form in almost every work environment. For career advancement purposes, seek opportunities to serve on committees concerned with practice issues such as patient safety, design of a new unit, or quality improvement.

▪ Lead or participate in a research study or quality improvement project.

▪ Volunteer to speak at local schools of nursing, at organizational meetings, and at research conferences.

▪ Join interprofessional initiatives where you can showcase nursing's contributions to health care.

Finally, be sure to keep detailed records of all these activities so that you can include them in your annual evaluations and list them on your employment applications.

Conclusion

In this chapter, we reviewed the multiple paths to entry into the nursing profession and the additional levels of education and degrees that nurses can achieve from master's to doctoral level. The transition from student to practicing nurse and the TPPs (transition to practice programs) designed to facilitate this transition were discussed, including mentoring, internships and residency programs, and other orientation programs. Once the transition has been successfully accomplished, the practicing nurse can look forward to the many career opportunities available in nursing. Phases of a successful career and the development of a tool box for career advancement were discussed. Finally, the many important nursing organizations that support the profession, members of the profession, and students preparing to enter the profession were reviewed.

Study Questions

1. Describe the three educational paths to entry into professional nursing.

2. What advanced levels of education are available to nurses? What type of preparation does each one provide?

3. Describe the challenges of making the transition from student to practicing nurse.

4. What types of TPP programs are available to new graduates? How do they differ?

5. What can you, as a new graduate, do to help yourself make the transition to practicing nurse?

6. Why have nurses created professional nursing organizations?

7. Review the mission, purpose, and member benefits of the ANA, CNA, or another national nursing organization on its Web site. Do you believe that nurses should belong to these organizations? Why or why not? Explain your answer.

8. Visit the Web site of the ANA or CNA. What do these organizations offer to practicing nurses?

9. What is the purpose of the NLN? Why should nurses support it?

10. What is the purpose of the OADN? Why is this organization important to you?

11. Search for a specialty nursing organization that you might join in the future. Describe the functions of the organization and why you might join.

12. List 12 different advanced nursing positions and specialties that might interest you. Name the three that interest you the most and explain why.

13. Explain what a career tool box is. What are the compartments of this tool box? What would you put in each compartment?

Case Study to Promote Clinical Judgment

Charles Christoph is currently in the last semester of a 2-year AD program. He is actively preparing for the licensure examination that he will take after graduation but not certain what else he should be doing to prepare for his first nursing position. He is very excited about graduation but also concerned because he has student loans he must begin to pay back as soon as possible and a family to support. Charles and a classmate are doing their last-semester immersion experience at a large teaching hospital near their college. On their lunch break, Charles asked his classmate Stephanie if she had begun her job search and how it was going. "Of course," she said, "haven't you?"

"I need to get started," he answered, "but I have a lot of questions."

"What questions?" she asked.

"What should I look for other than salary levels?" asked Charles.

1. Charles wants to know how important a TPP program is and what he should look for. Prepare an answer Stephanie could give him.

2. Charles also wants to know how much he should be thinking about his future career in nursing: Should he plan to continue his education? Join a nursing organization? Look for a promotion? What would help him make a long-term plan?

3. Some educators argue that all nursing students should be in a BS or BSN program. Prepare a debate, pro and con, in response to this argument.

NCLEX®-Style Review Questions

1. Which of the following organizations supports nursing education?
   1. NINR
   2. NLN
   3. AMA
   4. ANA

2. What is an important contribution of the nursing specialty organizations?
   1. Setting standards for specialty practice
   2. Improving nursing's image on television
   3. Supporting the AD education
   4. Providing collective bargaining agreements

3. Benefits of membership in the ANA include all but which one of the following?
   1. Advocacy for nurses' rights
   2. Provision of lower-cost health insurance
   3. Work toward a safer workplace
   4. Improvement of patient safety

4. What does the NSNA provide to its members?
   1. Help in improving course grades
   2. Guidance in choosing a good nursing school
   3. Career development information
   4. Opportunities for graduate school

5. Who may become a member of the NSNA? **Select all that apply**.
   1. AD program students
   2. Graduates of AD programs
   3. Diploma school students
   4. Baccalaureate degree students

6. Jean Paul has practiced nursing for 5 years and wants to continue his education. He has an AD and is trying to decide whether to pursue a nursing degree or a non-nursing degree. Which of the following is an advantage of choosing a nursing degree?
   1. Higher time demand of the non-nursing degree
   2. Opportunity to learn about other professions outside nursing
   3. Broader focus of the non-nursing degree
   4. Opportunity to advance knowledge and skills in his profession

7. Which of the following characterize the transition from nursing student to practicing nurse? **Select all that apply**.
   1. Increased number of assigned patients
   2. Higher productivity expectations for the student compared with the practicing nurse
   3. Greater emphasis on efficiency in practice
   4. Shorter hours and fewer workdays back-to-back in practice

8. As a new graduate, what features should you look for in a TPP program?
   1. Match with an experienced nurse mentor
   2. Shortest transition time possible
   3. Rapid movement to full assignment
   4. Opportunities to network with peers

9. What can the new graduate do to make a successful transition from student to practicing nurse?
   1. Try to maintain one's student identity.
   2. Move into nursing management as soon as possible.
   3. Learn about the organization as a whole as well as about your assigned unit.
   4. Focus on the stress of making this difficult transition.

10. Professional careers typically go through several phases. Which of the following would be the final phase of a successful career?
    1. Promise phase
    2. Harvest phase
    3. Transition phase
    4. Momentum phase

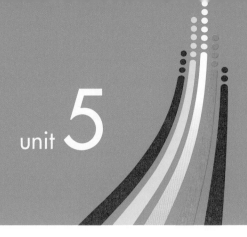

Looking to the Future

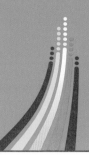

What the Future Holds

As a new graduate nurse, you are about to enter a proud profession that ranks high in the public's trust and fills an essential societal need. Although most of your attention will be focused on learning your new role and caring for your patients in the first year or two of practice, we encourage you to join your professional organization and at least become aware of the many political and economic issues that affect nurses, the nursing profession, and, ultimately, the health of our patients. You will be introduced to them in this chapter.

Most nurses, most of the time, see their patients and the health-care system up close. In fact, most nurses work within the health-care system, experiencing its effects both personally and through their patients. Sometimes this leads to acceptance of current practices even when they could hurt patients. Other times, however, alert nurses draw attention to solvable problems. Here is an example of an alert nurse's action during the flu epidemic of 2017 to 2018:

> Katherine Lockler, a Florida nurse, posted a 6-minute video after a 12-hour shift during which she saw multiple instances of failure to take action to protect people from the spread of the flu virus during a flu season when the flu shot was only about 35% effective. In the video, she demonstrates how to sneeze into your arm, calling it a "magic trick" to keep others well. She also scolded a softball coach for bringing the whole team to visit a teammate in the emergency department (ED). At the time the article about her video was printed in a Florida paper, it had already been viewed 4.8 million times (Bever, 2018). Since then, we have encountered many instances of heroic nurses, particularly during the COVID-19 pandemic, where nurses worked to the point of mental and physical exhaustion to provide care to many very sick patients.

What has the COVID-19 pandemic shown us? For all its devastating effects, the COVID-19 pandemic also stimulated nimbleness and agility uncharacteristic of the health-care industry. Suddenly health-care facilities were locked down and totally reliant on themselves to address the challenges of this novel and life-threatening virus. The triaging and prioritizing of our work pushed all non-essential activity out. For example, we were challenged to keep as much of the testing and diagnosing of COVID-19 away from our facilities as possible. Once welcoming of visitors and family, hospitals and nursing homes found themselves cutting their patients off from their loved ones. Patients died with no family present, saying goodbye on cell phones or tablets. Among the saving graces during this time were our nation's nurses. They kept coming to work, consoling their colleagues and patients, and letting their own safety take a backseat to the needs of the patients and communities who needed them.

Nurses have demonstrated their ingenuity and agility by being proactive across a variety of settings. Some of the inventions in acute care hospitals were really revisited "old school" nursing interventions that date back to years gone by . . . back to a time when we didn't have technology or automated equipment to treat our patients. An example of this is the practice of proning (turning patients onto their stomachs) patients with COVID to ease their breathing and keep their airways open. This method of positioning improved patient comfort and, in many cases, reduced the morbidity and mortality of COVID-19 for these patients. Nurses also quickly repurposed technology to provide better care. An example is the use of tablet technology for both families and nurses to stay in constant communication with COVID-19 patients, which was a comfort to patients and enhanced nursing surveillance of these patients while reducing the use of personal protective equipment (PPE). In addition, many nurses shared their ideas to improve protection of staff and partnered in biodesign initiatives to confront the challenges of dwindling PPE supplies. Academic medical centers with access to engineers, scientists, and nurses combined their talents to build what they were having trouble purchasing. Items such as face shields were designed and produced using 3D printers. Workflows were redesigned to accommodate better care and management of PPE. Moving patient equipment such as IV pumps outside the isolation rooms allowed nurses to easily adjust medication doses and troubleshoot equipment without unnecessary exposure. This list of simple fixes and inventions could be endless, but one thing that is constant has been the contribution and creativity of practicing nurses.

Each of us can act individually when we see situations that concern us. We can also work collectively through our nursing organizations on behalf of the nursing profession and the people we care for.

Innovation

Defined as "the design, invention, development, and/or implementation of new or altered products, services, systems, organizational structures, or system models" (Cianelli et al., 2016, p. 4), innovation is a natural part of providing the highest quality nursing care, yet it receives far too little attention in most leadership and management textbooks. As you just read, the examples of Katherine Lockler and many nurses during the pandemic showed some of the best innovative ideas that arose from challenges encountered in clinical practice. Generally speaking, health-care organizations are risk-averse in order to protect their patients and the people caring for them. Within this cautionary environment, however, nurse leaders and managers are still able to introduce what Cianelli and colleagues (Cianelli et al., 2016, p. 5) call the "spirit and practice of innovation." To do this, leaders need to promote thinking "outside the box" (i.e., considering new ways to solve problems and to improve care). They also need to be able to tolerate taking some risk as many new ideas or solutions may not succeed the first time they are tried. Along with these important characteristics, they also need to exercise flexibility, as opposed to rigidity, and autonomy, thinking for oneself instead of thinking the same way as everyone around you.

Health Care Today

Health Concerns

This section on the many health problems today in the United States begins with a remarkably long list of current concerns. Despite its length, it only highlights some of our current concerns and is not by any means exhaustive. It will, however, give you an idea of the number and scope of these issues.

- The opioid crisis has been responsible for many potentially preventable deaths across the country. Life expectancy in the United States declined for the second year in a row in 2016 because of the increase in fatal opioid overdoses, whereas the decline in deaths because of heart disease seemed to have leveled off (Stein, 2017). Drug overdose deaths exceeded 100,000 annually as of April 2021 (CDC, 2021).
- Health-care–associated (i.e., nosocomial) infections have "escaped" from hospitals and now can be found occurring in nursing homes and in the community.
- Adverse drug events, including prescribing errors, medication administration errors, and serious side effects, have harmed many patients.
- Health-care providers have been forced to cancel surgeries, diagnostic scans, and other procedures because of cyberattacks, making it clear that increased security measures and regulation are called for (hhs.gov, 2022).
- More Americans died from gun-related violence in 2020 than in any preceding year according to Pew Research (2022).
- LGBTQ (lesbian, gay, bisexual, transgender, and queer) individuals face a number of mental health issues and distress related to the effects of discrimination (healthypeople.gov, 2022).

Demographics and Diversity

Increased numbers of older adults, longer life expectancy, a more ethnically and racially diverse population, and recognition of serious inequities in the U.S. health system present challenges that need to be met to improve access to care for all members of society. Older adults and ethnic minorities include many at-risk, vulnerable individuals who suffer disadvantages in access to care, payment for care, and quality of care (Affordable Care Act [ACA], 2010; Anderson et al., 2003).

Social Determinants of Health (SDOH)

Much has been written about health disparities and inequities, with some groups receiving less or poorer quality care and subsequent poorer outcomes, including being ill more often, having more chronic illnesses, and experiencing shorter life expectancies.

SDOH are those conditions or situations in a person's environment that affect health, function, and quality of life (see Figure 16-1). The many social determinants are grouped into the following categories:

Education (access and quality)
Health care (access and quality)
Neighborhood and home environment
Social and community climate

The current *Healthy People 2030* goals include many SDOH-related goals.

Many conditions included in the SDOH, such as high levels of pollution, living in a food desert where fruits and vegetables are expensive or hard to find, and encountering discrimination based on age,

Social Determinants of Health

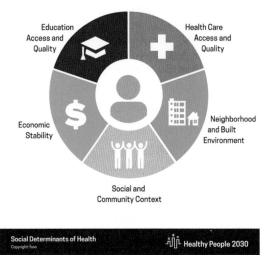

Figure 16.1 Social Determinants of Health.
*Retrieved from https://health.gov/healthypeople
/objectives-and-data/social-determinants-health*

race, religion, sexual preference, or other factors, are called "upstream" factors that affect a person's health and well-being (Health.gov, 2022).

Addressing SDOH

Most of the programs and policies designed to address SDOH are community-based, addressing a wide range of these upstream factors. Here are a few examples:

> The Centers for Disease Control and Prevention (CDC) has several programs addressing SDOH. These include prevention of lead poisoning in children, culturally tailored interventions, and the prevention of youth violence.
> Green Cart in New York City brings fresh fruits and vegetables to underserved communities using mobile carts.
> Boston Center for Independent Living negotiated greater access to medical equipment for people with disabilities.

Current Trends in Care

The following are trends in the provision of health care that present some challenges but have the potential to improve care:

- Increased use of electronic health-care records, which eliminates paper and allows remote access to patient information but requires increased

attention to cybersecurity. Health-care providers have been forced to cancel surgeries, radiology examinations, and other services because of cyberattacks, making it clear that increased regulations are called for (hhs.gov, 2022).
- Reduction of unnecessary hospital admissions
- Increase in surgical procedures done on an outpatient basis
- Attention to providing patient-centered care, reducing the ineffectiveness of fragmented, uncoordinated, unresponsive, and inaccessible care (Alkema, 2016)
- Using "big data" from many sources, including patient data from large health-care systems, to identify trends that otherwise would not have been noted
- Integrated health-care systems that provide community-based primary care and home health care as well as acute care and long-term care within a single coordinated system
- Keeping the caring in nursing in a highly technological setting
- Continuing the efforts to reduce health disparities in people who are poor or members of minority groups
- Continuing increase in the use of alternative and complementary modalities such as meditation, massage, and nutraceuticals

U.S. Health-Care System Challenges

Victor Fuchs (2018) remarked that the United States "already spends so much so badly" that we could use these misspent funds to catch up with or even outdo everyone else in creating a system of universal health care (p. 15). The United States has technologically advanced, highly sophisticated health care but has been spending more per capita (per person) on health care than most countries without achieving the highest quality outcomes. Among the industrialized countries of the world, the United States is the only one that does not provide basic health insurance coverage to every citizen. Before the ACA, 81 million Americans ages 19 to 64 were underinsured or uninsured (Schoen et al., 2011). Many reported going without care, skipping doses of medication, or not filling a prescription because they could not afford it. One-third reported using credit card debt or a loan to pay health-care bills. Sixty-two percent of personal bankruptcies in the United States (2007 figures) were because of individuals' health problems, even though 78% of these individuals had health insurance (ANA, 2009). To address this, the ACA provides subsidies to lower the costs of health insurance for people whose incomes are 400% or less than the federal poverty level (healthcare.gov, 2022).

Concerns About the U.S. Health-Care System

The diverse interests of consumers, providers, insurance companies, government, and regulators also present challenges to those trying to redesign the current system to make it more cost-effective as well as more responsive to health-care consumers' needs.

The three primary problems with the U.S. health-care system are the number of uninsured, high costs, and less-than-ideal outcomes (Fuchs, 2018). If the United States has the most advanced knowledge and equipment and spends a great deal of money on health care, then why the cause for concern? What is wrong? The answer is not simple.

For most people, health insurance comes through their place of employment. A serious problem with this is that if one loses their job, health insurance is also lost. If not eligible for Medicaid or Medicare, purchasing health insurance on one's own can be very expensive. Another is that many employers are motivated to keep the cost as low as possible or transfer much of the cost to the employee. But most consumers are relatively satisfied with their job-related insurance and, so long as they have it, are reluctant to trade it for an untested plan (Capretta, 2017).

The term *universal health care* means that every individual has access to affordable, high-quality health care. One model used in Canada employs a single payer, usually a government agency. A second model uses a two-payer system, which also allows people to have private insurance as well as government-supported health care if they can afford it (Redwanski, 2007). Redwanski describes the effect that a universal health-care system would have on prescription drugs:

> All pharmacies would be reimbursed the same amount and expected to have the same drugs in their formulary. To adjust to the lower prices, however, pharmaceutical manufacturers may reduce their budgets for developing new drugs.

Managed care was originally designed to reduce the amount spent on health care by emphasizing prevention. However, some believe that it has become a way to limit care choices and ration care (Mechanic, 2002) rather than prevent illness. As managed care plans grew and spread across the country, these companies became powerful enough to negotiate reduced rates (discounts) from local hospitals (Trinh & O'Connor, 2002). They could, in effect, say, "We can get an appendectomy for $2,300 at hospital A; why should we pay you $2,700?" If hospital B does not agree, the hospital may lose all the patients enrolled in that managed care plan. This pressures hospital B to reduce costs and spread staff thinner than before.

With the upsurge in for-profit health plans and the purchase of not-for-profit hospitals by for-profit companies, U.S. health care has become increasingly "corporatized." It was thought that this would yield a highly efficient, responsive system ("the customer is always right"). That has not happened, however, because the "customer" who pays for insurance coverage is usually the employer or the government, not the individual.

Furthermore, the United States is facing what Buchan called a "demographic double whammy" of an aging population that will need more health care and, at the same time, an aging workforce (Hewison & Wildman, 2008, pp. 1-3).

In Canada, a debate regarding privatization versus public funding of health care continues (Villeneuve & MacDonald, 2006). Health care is still illness- and disease-focused there as in the United States. Although there is interest in complementary and alternative treatments, they have not been integrated into general care. Disparities in the care of members of minority groups threaten to increase if not addressed more effectively.

Global interconnectedness has brought new concerns about how quickly and easily infectious diseases can cross national borders. Human immunodeficiency virus (HIV), severe acute respiratory syndrome, Ebola, Chikungunya, and the annual waves of influenza that cross the globe are just a few reminders of how vulnerable populations remain. These risks create an increased need for health-care provider surveillance across continents. A broader view of global health encompasses concern for the health of all people (Wilson et al., 2016).

Health-Care Reform and the Affordable Care Act

After lengthy arguments and despite some strenuous opposition, the Patient Protection and Affordable Care Act, known familiarly as Obamacare after

table 16-1	

Major Provisions of the Affordable Care Act 2010 to 2015

2010	Young adults can be covered by parents' health insurance to age 26 instead of 19. Insurers will eventually be prohibited from denying coverage for preexisting conditions. In the meantime, the government will provide coverage.
2011	Insurers are required to spend 80% of their premiums on patient care or reimburse policyholders for the excess. Reimbursement for Medicare Advantage plans (HMOs) is frozen at 2010 rates.
2012	Hospitals with high readmission rates will be penalized by Medicare. States are expected to submit plans for insurance exchanges.
2013	Tax increases on medical devices and for Medicare are applied on high-income wage earners. States will begin enrolling people through their insurance exchanges.
2014	State health exchanges will be up and running. Preexisting condition rule is now effective. Medicaid is expanded to those earning 133% of poverty-level wage. Businesses with more than 50 employees must provide health insurance. Uninsured individuals will pay increased taxes.
2015	Added tax on so-called "Cadillac" insurance plans offered by employers.

Source: Adapted from Leonard, D. (2012, October 11). Obamacare is not an epithet. Bloomberg/BusinessWeek.
Additional references from www.nursingworld.org/practice-policy/health-policy/health-system-reform

the president who promoted it, was enacted in 2010 (Rosenbaum, 2011). This complex legislation contained provisions for sweeping changes in health care (see Table 16-1). The following are some of the changes of most interest to nurses:

- Insurance reforms that prohibit cancellation if the person is ill, eliminate preexisting condition clauses, and prohibit lifetime limits
- Creation of state health insurance exchanges to offer affordable insurance coverage
- Support for nursing education and nursing students
- Nurse-managed clinics eligible for federal funding
- Expansion of school-based health centers
- Support for transitional care and chronic disease management
- Creation of accountable care organizations and medical homes that bridge the gap between hospital, nursing home, and home and medical office care (Webb & Marshall, 2010)
- Free preventive care services for women, including HIV screening, contraception, breastfeeding, and domestic violence services
- A standardized report of health insurance coverage so that consumers can compare different plans (ANA, 2013)

Provisions of the ACA were not universally welcomed. Fewer people than expected applied for coverage of preexisting conditions, and some insurers threatened to drop individual policies for children if they had to cover preexisting conditions (Adamy & Radnofsky, 2012). Several states also resisted setting up the proposed health exchanges (Anonymous, 2013).

Some call the ACA socialized medicine and are strongly opposed to it; others think it is a much-needed step in the direction of ensuring that everyone can receive the health care they need. Some even say it did not go far enough. The second opinion seems to be in line with the World Health Assembly resolution supporting universal coverage:

[E]nsuring that all people have access to needed health services—prevention, promotion, treatment and rehabilitation—without facing financial ruin because of the need to pay for them. (World Health Organization, 2012, p. 38)

If the ACA were completely withdrawn, several major benefits would be lost; these are illustrated in Figure 16-2.

Nursing Issues

Issues of high workloads, mandatory overtime, incivility, workplace violence, and lack of professional autonomy contribute to these concerns, along with an aging nurse workforce. On the bright side, there are indications of increasing interest in a nursing career as salaries improve and job opportunities expand.

Safe staffing, defined as the appropriate number and mix of nursing staff, is a critical issue for nurses and the people who need their care. A series of research studies has demonstrated the importance of adequate nurse staffing. There is powerful evidence that nurses save lives: for each additional

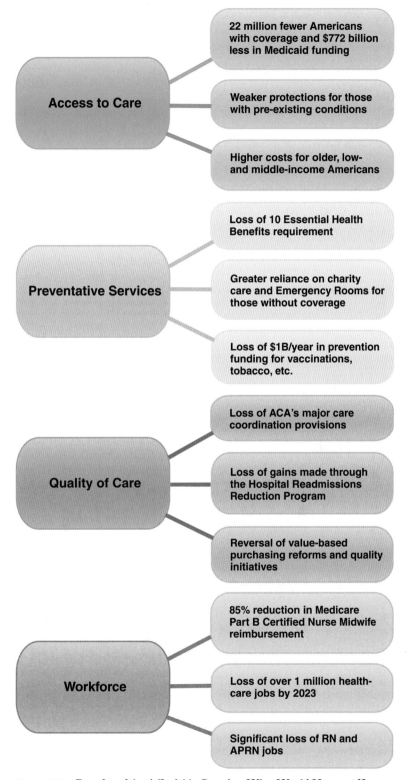

Figure 16.2 Benefits of the Affordable Care Act: What Would Happen if It Were Withdrawn? *Adapted from http://nursingworld.org/healthcarereform*

patient assigned to a nurse, there is a 7% increase in the likelihood of a patient dying within 30 days of admission (Aiken et al., 2002; Potter & Mueller, 2007). Nurses cannot gain in-depth understanding of their patients, protect their patients, or catch early warning signs if they are overloaded by the number of patients for whom they are responsible. Adequate numbers of nurses affect patient mortality, length of stay, prevalence of urinary tract infections, fall rates, incidence of hospital-acquired pneumonia, and more.

Trends in Nursing and Health Care

Change and innovation are constants in health care. The following are trends that are expected to affect the nursing profession and the care nurses provide to their patients in the near future:

- Efforts to ensure patient safety, especially in acute care, will continue to be emphasized, including reduction of nosocomial infections, medication errors, failure to rescue, and other serious adverse events.
- The use of a variety of technological innovations (computerized order entry, telehealth, mobile devices, sensors, webcams, etc.) are becoming standard practice in health care.
- The beneficial effects of alternative and complementary approaches (such as meditation, herbs, use of nutraceuticals, yoga, visual and musical arts, etc.), already widely accepted by many members of the public, will be integrated into standard medical and nursing practice (Fleischer & Grehan, 2016).
- Increased focus on care transitions (from hospital to home, from the nursing home back to the hospital, etc.) will involve nurses in better preparing patients for these transitions.
- Whenever and wherever possible, care will move out of the hospital and into the community.
- Continued use of "physician extenders" (nurse practitioners and physician assistants, etc.), although this may also put additional strain on current nursing staff.

What does all this mean for the new nurse? Many opportunities for nurses will open up in community-based care, transitional care, quality improvement efforts, telehealth, and nontraditional roles. However, there will also be challenges ahead as cost cutting increases the demand on individual staff members and the tolerance of errors that threaten patient safety and well-being becomes very limited.

Health Care in the Future

One of the fundamental reasons why the United States has not achieved successful health-care reform is that there hasn't been agreement on whether access to health care is a privilege or a right. Citizens of the United States are guaranteed access to basic education, fire and police protection, mail, parks, and many other benefits but not health care (Bauchner, 2017). Ideally, a new model of health care is needed that offers the following:

- Holistic, person-centered care
- Seamless connections across community, acute-care, and long-term care settings (Pogue, 2007)
- Elimination of health disparities
- Guaranteed accessible, affordable care for everyone
- Safe care that heals and does not harm the patient
- Equivalent support for prevention, health promotion, and mental health care as for acute and primary care
- Creation of a healthy environment, from green buildings to the elimination of air, water, soil, and other forms of pollution
- Attention to global health concerns: climate change, hunger, poverty, and disease at home and in developing countries

Although there were provisions in the ACA that addressed some of these concerns, there is still much work to do on health-care reform.

Advocating for Nursing's Future

Within the nursing profession, there is also much work to do. One issue to address is image-related challenges (Motshedisi et al., 2015). Too often, members of the public and colleagues in other professions think of nurses in only an assistive role, as "perpetual servants of heroic physicians" based on impressions from the media (Bleich, 2012, pp. 180-184; Summers & Summers, 2014). This limited view ignores our unique perspective that encompasses the whole person within that individual's family and community. Nurses think differently from other health-care providers.

Michael Bleich (2012, p. 184) says we need to "publicly give voice to the value of this perspective," particularly during this time of debate regarding the shape of our health-care system in the future. If we do not participate in the debate, we "will be left to react to models that may stymie our capacity to influence health" and the future of the nursing profession.

Another concern is external appearance. Cohen (2007) quotes Dumont on the question of dress, particularly wearing uniforms covered with cartoon characters: "You're the only thing between the patient and death, and you're covered in cartoons. No wonder you have no authority." The following are some additional suggestions to improve nursing's image:

- Always introduce yourself as an RN.
- Define professional appearance appropriate to your workplace and enforce it.
- Define professional behavior and enforce it.
- Take every opportunity to speak to the public about nursing.
- Document what nurses do and how important they are (Cohen, 2007).

What else can nurses do? It is important that more members of minority groups be brought into nursing so that nursing better reflects the increasing diversity of the population. Collaboration with colleagues in other health professions is also vital to improving health care. Physicians, therapists, social workers, psychologists, aides, assistants, and technicians are also concerned about the quality of care provided. Patients and their families, too, are concerned and personally affected by the quality of care provided. All these groups together would have a strong voice in health-care reform.

Nurses are the largest professional group within health care in terms of numbers. They spend the most time with patients and receive top ranking for having the public's trust according to Gallup polls. These are significant accomplishments. However, a national Gallup poll of 1,500 opinion leaders revealed a serious lack of nursing representation and influence at the highest policy levels. These opinion leaders thought that government and health insurance executives have the most influence on health-care reform. Only 14% of them thought that nurses would be influential. It was also noted that nurses did not have a single, unified voice and

seemed disinterested and uninvolved for the most part (Khoury et al., 2011). There was a more positive side to these disturbing survey results. Many of the opinion leaders interviewed thought more nurses should get involved. Given their number and unique position within health care, nurses should be full partners in health-care reform (Hassmiller & Reinhard, 2015). Issues on which nurses should have a say include patient safety, quality of care, reducing medical errors, health promotion, and prevention (Hassmiller, 2011). The urgency of making our voices heard is undisputable. Hassmiller (2011) wrote that "right now is the right time to tackle the difficult and essential work of bringing nursing perspectives, knowledge, and voices into health policy decision making" (p. 308). This is still true today.

An example of political activism in support of improving health care and making it more accessible from Canada follows:

The Canadian Federation of Nurses Unions released the results of a public opinion poll on various health-care issues. One issue was access to prescription drugs: 77% of people responding to the poll supported a universal drug plan so that everyone could obtain the medications they need. It was estimated that in the previous year one in five Canadians did not fill a prescription because they could not afford it (Close-Up Media, 2016).

The following are some specific actions you can take to exert leadership in supporting your profession and improving health care:

- Be sure you are registered to vote if you are eligible. Every county has a supervisor of elections office that you can visit, call, or connect with online to register.
- Learn more about the health-care system and your role in it.
- Take advantage of legislative days when your state nurses' organization or your college organizes groups of nurses and nursing students to visit their legislators either locally or at the state capitol building to discuss nursing issues and ask for their support.
- Another excellent learning experience supported by many community colleges involves service learning programs. In these programs, students commit

up to 20 hours a week to engage in community projects of endless variety: urban gardens, autism programs, Special Olympics, health screenings, care kits for hospital patients or nursing home residents, and so forth. You can gain an appreciation of the needs of people in your community, learn how health and social welfare programs do and do not work well, and gain leadership skills. Evangeline Manjares, dean of academic and student service at Nassau Community College in New York, added another benefit of these programs, stating, "Everyone is too involved with looking at our cell phones. It's time to maybe share some of their cell phone time with the community" (Finkel, 2017, p. 29). Here are some ways to get involved:

■ Join both your professional association and specialty association and support their efforts to improve care.

■ Talk about these issues with everyone and anyone who will listen.

■ Write letters to the editor, speak on local radio and television programs, and participate in online discussions.

■ Send e-mail messages to your legislators, sign petitions if you support them, and communicate your position through social media.

■ Speak to your local, state, and national representatives about these concerns.

■ Consider supporting the ANA or your specialty organization's political action committee (PAC) even if you can only afford a small amount. These funds make it possible for the organization's staff to be visible and speak with key legislators on issues important to nursing.

In summary, "be visible, be vocal" in your support of nursing and improved health care (Davis, 2015).

The ANA Web site features some of the many ways in which the ANA advocates for nurses and patients in the political arena. Just a few examples:

Capitol Beat Blog: analysis of national issues
Advocacy Toolkit: educational materials for nurse advocates
ANA Political Action Committee: supports nursing-friendly candidates for Congress
Nurses Vote: encourages political action

Issues of practical importance include:

Retirement of nurses is occurring faster than the rate of entry into the profession.

The median age of nurses nationally is 52 years of age.

At the same time, the demand for nurses is increasing as the population ages and the number of individuals with chronic diseases increases. The BLS predicts there will be 195,000 openings annually over the next 5 years.

Insufficient support for nurses in the workforce reduces retention.

Given these very important issues facing the nursing profession, it is no surprise that the advocacy groups try to:

Increase the supply of nurses.
Create healthy work environments for nurses.
Support the quality of health care.
Support regulations and policies that allow nurses to practice "at the fullest extent of their education and licensure" (Nursingworld.org/practice-policy/workforce/2022).

Conclusion

Although our health care is technologically advanced, it is also very expensive when compared with other industrialized countries. The United States is also one of the few industrialized countries that does not provide basic health-care coverage to every citizen. However, some would argue that universal access to health care is not a right that should be guaranteed and paid for by the government. There are also questions about the quality of care provided and the outcomes of that care. Issues of particular interest to nurses include equal access to care, drug-resistant infections, fragmented care, and a continuing struggle to provide holistic, patient-centered care. The provisions of the ACA were intended to address some of these problems but continue to generate some controversy. Issues related to nurses themselves include high workloads, mandatory overtime, incivility, workplace violence, safe staffing, and periodic nurse shortages. A new patient-centered model that allows seamless transitions from one setting to another, provides safe care, and emphasizes prevention and a healthy environment for all is needed. Actions nurses can take to address these concerns were discussed in this chapter.

Study Questions

1. Identify a health-care concern that you have observed in your clinical assignments. Describe how you as an individual and as a member of a nursing organization could address this concern.

2. Describe your ideal health-care system of the future. Compare it with the current system operating today. What is different? What is similar?

3. Write an "elevator speech" (30 seconds to 2 minutes in length) that describes the value of the care nurses provide. (An elevator speech or elevator pitch is designed to be very short but persuasive so that it can be delivered during an elevator ride.)

4. Debate arguments in support for (pro) and against (con) the principle that health care is a right for all, not a privilege for some.

Case Study to Promote Clinical Judgment

Alina went to nursing school on a U.S. Air Force scholarship. She has been directed to lead the planning for establishing a comprehensive primary care and health promotion program on board the newest international space station. The crew is expected to remain on board the station for 6 months at a time. The crew will consist of military men and women from three countries.

1. What type of care will be needed by the crew of the space station? How much of this will be provided by nurses?

2. What medical and nursing technology and equipment should Alina plan to have in this center?

3. Develop a nursing research study topic for this situation that Alina could actually do when the space station becomes a reality.

NCLEX®-Style Review Questions

1. A good description of the present U.S. health-care system would be
   1. The best in the world
   2. Efficient and effective
   3. Needs improvement
   4. Meets everyone's needs

2. In the U.S. health-care system, who is the real "customer"? That is, who actually pays most of the health-care bill?
   1. The U.S. government
   2. The head of the household
   3. Government entities and employers
   4. Employees and their families

3. In the United States, health-care insurance can best be described as
   1. Universal
   2. Available to all
   3. Free
   4. Expensive

4. Which of the following best describes the nurse of today?
   1. Assistant to the physician
   2. Member of the largest health-care profession
   3. Member of the most powerful lobby group in health care
   4. Woman in white

5. What does "be visible and vocal" mean? **Select all that apply**.
   1. Take a course on health-care policy.
   2. Speak out on issues important to nursing.
   3. Write letters to the editor, and e-mail your state and federal representatives.
   4. Look for opportunities to appear on radio or television.

6. Which of the following health and safety concerns is NOT one of our greatest concerns currently?
   1. "Escape" of health-care–acquired infections into the community
   2. Spread of poliomyelitis and smallpox
   3. Increase in opioid-related deaths
   4. Health disparities (poorer health and treatment outcomes in minority, limited-income, and other groups)

7. Which of the following are the primary current problems with the U.S. health-care system? **Select all that apply**.
   1. Increased use of electronic health records (EHRs)
   2. Less-than-optimum outcomes (quality issues)
   3. Number of people who are uninsured
   4. High cost of care

8. Janice Mendoza is settled in her nursing position and wants to devote some time to one of the issues facing the nursing profession. Which of the following activities would probably have the LEAST impact on advocating for the nursing profession?
   1. Contribute to the ANA's PAC.
   2. Visit the representatives when the state legislature is in session.
   3. Talk with her friends, explaining her concerns.
   4. Speak on radio and television programs.

9. Which of the following is a current concern related to the nursing profession?
   1. Aging of the nursing workforce
   2. Oversupply of nurses versus decreasing demand for nursing care
   3. Emphasis on evidence-based practices
   4. Expansion of EHR use into the community

10. Health-care reform encompasses many issues and concerns. Which of the following is probably the most controversial goal?
    1. Requiring everyone to have some form of health insurance
    2. Developing school-based health-care centers
    3. Eliminating preexisting condition rules in insurance coverage
    4. Eliminating lifetime limits to insurance coverage

Standards Published by the American Nurses Association*

- Addictions Nursing Practice: Scope and Standards of Practice
- Cardiovascular Nursing: Scope and Standards of Practice (2nd edition)
- Clinical Research Nursing: Scope and Standards of Practice
- Correctional Nursing: Scope and Standards of Practice (2nd edition)
- Faith Community Nursing: Scope and Standards of Practice (3rd edition)
- Genetics and Genomics: Scope and Standards of Practice (2nd edition)
- Gerontological Nursing: Scope and Standards of Practice
- Holistic Nursing: Scope and Standards of Practice (2nd edition)
- Home Health Nursing: Scope and Standards of Practice
- Hospice and Palliative Nursing: Scope and Standards of Practice
- Intellectual and Developmental Disabilities Nursing: Scope and Standards of Practice (2nd edition)
- Neonatal Nursing: Scope and Standards of Practice (2nd edition)
- Neuroscience Nursing: Scope and Standards of Practice
- Nursing Administration: Scope and Standards of Practice (2nd edition)
- Nursing Informatics: Scope and Standards of Practice (2nd edition)
- Nursing Professional Development: Scope and Standards of Practice
- Pain Management Nursing: Scope and Standards of Practice (2nd edition)
- Pediatric Nursing: Scope and Standards of Practice (2nd edition)
- Pediatric Oncology Nursing: Scope and Standards of Practice
- Plastic Surgery Nursing: Scope and Standards of Practice (2nd edition)
- Psychiatric–Mental Health Nursing: Scope and Standards of Practice (2nd edition)
- Public Health Nursing: Scope and Standards of Practice (2nd edition)
- Radiologic and Imaging Nursing: Scope and Standards of Practice
- Rheumatology Nursing: Scope and Standards of Practice
- School Nursing: Scope and Standards of Practice (3rd edition)
- Transplant Nursing: Scope and Standards of Practice (2nd edition)
- Vascular Nursing: Scope and Standards of Practice (2nd edition)

---

*https://www.nursingworld.org/continuing-education/ce-subcategories/scope-and-standards-of-practice

Guidelines for the Registered Nurse in Giving, Accepting, or Rejecting a Work Assignment*

Registered nurses (RNs), as licensed professionals, share the responsibility and accountability, along with their employer, to ensure that safe, quality nursing care is provided. The scope of professional nurses' accountability involves legal, ethical, and professional guidelines for ensuring safe, quality patient care. Legal responsibility for the provision, delegation, and supervision of patient care is specified in the Nurse Practice Acts and the Administrative Rules. The American Nurses Association (ANA) *Code for Nurses With Interpretive Statements* (2015b) guides the ethical conduct and decision making of professional nurses. In contrast, the *ANA Standards and Scope of Practice* (2015a) provides a systematic application of the nursing process for patient care management across patient care settings. Lastly, the employer requirements for safe, competent staffing are outlined in facility policies and guidelines.

Within ethical and legal parameters, the nurse exercises informed judgment and uses individual competence and qualifications as criteria in seeking consultation, accepting responsibilities, and delegating nursing activities to others. The nurse's decision regarding accepting or making work assignments is based on the legal, ethical, and professional obligation to assume responsibility for nursing judgment and action.

The document offers strategies for problem-solving as the staff nurse, nurse manager, chief nurse executive, and administrator practice within the complex environment of the health-care system.

Nursing Care Delivery

Only an RN will assess, plan, and evaluate a patient's or client's nursing care needs. No nurse shall be required or directed to delegate nursing activities to other personnel in a manner inconsistent with the Nurse Practice Act, the standards of The Joint Commission (TJC) on Accreditation of Health Organizations, the ANA Standards of Practice, or hospital policy. Consistent with the preceding sentence, the individual RN has the autonomy to delegate (or not delegate) those aspects of nursing care the nurse determines appropriate based on the patient assessment.

When a nurse is floated to a unit or area and receives an assignment that is considered unsafe to perform independently, the RN has the right and obligation to request and receive a modified assignment, which reflects the RN's level of competence.

The ANA, the American Organization of Nurse Executives (AONE), and the state Labor Employee Relations Commission (LERC) recognize that changes in the health-care delivery system have occurred and will continue to occur while emphasizing the common goal to provide safe, quality patient care. The parties also recognize that RNs have a right and responsibility to participate in decisions affecting the delivery of nursing care and related terms and conditions of employment. All parties have a mutual interest in developing systems that will provide quality care on a cost-efficient basis without jeopardizing patient outcomes. Thus, commitment to measuring the impact of staffing and assignments to patient outcomes is a shared commitment of all professional nurses irrespective of organizational structure.

Assignment Despite Objection (ADO)/Documentation of Practice Situation (DOPS)

Staff nurses today often face untenable assignments that need to be documented as such. Critical, clinical judgment should be utilized when evaluating the appropriateness of an assignment. Refusal to accept an assignment without appropriate discussion within the chain of command can be defined as insubordinate behavior. Each RN should become familiar with organizational policies, procedures, and documentation regarding refusal to accept an unsafe assignment. The ANA has recently adopted a position statement and model ADO form available for use by state nurses association (SNA) members. (Please contact your state nurses association for further information.)

Staffing

In the event an RN determines in their professional opinion that they have been given an assignment that does not allow for appropriate patient care, the RN shall notify the supervisor or designee, who shall review the RN's concerns. If these concerns cannot be resolved by telephone, the supervisor or designee, except in instances of compelling business reasons that preclude them from doing so, will then come to the unit within 4 hours of being contacted by the nurse to assess the staffing. Such assessment shall be documented, with a copy given to the nurse. Nothing herein shall prohibit an RN from completing and submitting a protest of assignment form.

Scenario

- Suppose you are asked to care for an unfamiliar patient population or to go to a unit for which you feel unqualified—what do you do?
- Suppose you are approached by your supervisor and asked to work an additional shift. Your immediate response is that you don't want to work another shift—what do you do?

Such situations are familiar and emphasize the rights and responsibilities of the RN to make informed decisions. Yet all members of the health-care team, from staff nurses to the administrator, share a joint responsibility to ensure that quality patient care is provided. At times, though, a difference in the interpretation of legal or ethical principles may lead to conflict.

Guidelines for decision making are offered to help RNs problem-solve work assignment issues. Applications of these guidelines are presented in the form of scenarios, examples of unsafe assignments experienced by RNs.

Guidelines for Decision Making

The complexity of the delivery of nursing care is such that only professional nurses with appropriate education and experience can provide nursing care. Upon employment with a health-care facility, the nurse contracts or enters into an agreement with that facility to provide nursing services in a collaborative practice environment.

It Is the RN's Responsibility to:

- Provide competent nursing care to the patient.
- Exercise informed judgment and use individual competence and qualifications as criteria in seeking consultation, accepting responsibilities, and delegating nursing activities to others.
- Clarify assignments, assess personal capabilities, and jointly identify options for patient care assignments when they do not feel personally competent or adequately prepared to carry out a specific function.
- Refuse an assignment that they do not feel prepared to assume after appropriate consultation with a supervisor.

It Is Nursing Management's Responsibility to:

- Ensure competent nursing care is provided to the patient.
- Evaluate the nurse's ability to provide specialized patient care.
- Organize resources to ensure that patients receive appropriate nursing care.
- Collaborate with the staff nurse to clarify assignments, assess personal capabilities, and jointly identify options for patient care assignments when the nurse does not feel personally competent or adequately prepared to carry out a specific function.
- Take appropriate disciplinary action according to facility policies.
- Communicate in written policies to the staff the process to make assignment and reassignment decisions.
- Provide education to staff and supervisory personnel in the decision-making process regarding patient care assignments and reassignments, including patient placement and allocation of resources.
- Plan and budget for staffing patterns based on patient requirements and priorities for care.
- Provide a clearly defined written mechanism for immediate internal review of proposed

assignments, which includes the participation of the staff involved, to help avoid conflict.

Issues Central to Potential Dilemmas Are:
- The right of the patient to receive safe, professional nursing care at an acceptable level of quality
- The responsibility for an appropriate utilization and distribution of nursing care services when nursing becomes a scarce resource
- The responsibility for providing a practice environment that ensures adequate nursing resources for the facility while meeting the current socioeconomic and political realities of shrinking health-care dollars

Legal Issues

Behaviors and activities relevant to giving, accepting, or rejecting a work assignment that could lead to disciplinary action include:

- Practicing or offering to practice beyond the scope permitted by law or accepting and performing professional responsibilities that the licensee knows or has reason to believe that they are not competent to perform
- Performing, without adequate supervision, professional services that the licensee is authorized to perform only under the supervision of a licensed professional, except in an emergency situation in which a person's life or health is in danger
- Abandoning or neglecting a patient or client who is in need of nursing care without making reasonable arrangements for the continuation of such care
- Failure to exercise supervision over persons who are authorized to practice only under the supervision of the licensed professional

Of the previous list, the issue of abandonment or neglect has thus far proven the most legally devastating. Abandonment or neglect has been legally defined to include such actions as insufficient observation (frequency of contact), failure to ensure competent intervention when the patient's condition changes (qualified physician not in attendance), and withdrawal of services without provision for qualified coverage. Because nurses at all levels most frequently act as agents of the employing facility, the facility shares the risk of liability with the nurse.

Application of Guidelines for Decision Making

Two clinical scenarios are presented for the RN to demonstrate appropriate decision making when faced with an unsafe assignment. Sometimes an example or two can help the RN objectively examine legal, ethical, and professional issues before making a final decision. Additional resources are listed following the scenarios.

Scenario—A Question of Competence

An example of a potential dilemma is when an evening supervisor pulls a psychiatric nurse to the coronary care unit (CCU) because of a lack of nursing staff. The CCU census has risen, and there is not additional qualified staff available.

Suppose you are asked to care for an unfamiliar patient population or to go to a unit for which you feel unqualified—what do you do?

1. CLARIFY what it is you are being asked to do.
   - How many patients will you be expected to care for?
   - Does the care of these patients require you to have specialty knowledge and skills in order to deliver safe nursing care?
   - Will there be qualified and experienced RNs on the unit?
   - What procedures or medications will you be expected to administer?
   - What kind of orientation do you need to function safely in the unfamiliar setting?
2. ASSESS yourself. Do you have the knowledge and skill to meet the expectations that have been outlined for you? Have you had experience with similar patient populations? Have you been oriented to this unit or a similar unit? Would the perceived discrepancies between your abilities and the expectations lead to an unsafe patient care situation?
3. IDENTIFY OPTIONS and implications of your decision.
   a. If you perceive that you can provide safe patient care, you should accept the assignment. You would now be ethically and legally responsible for the nursing care of these patients.
   b. If you perceive there is a discrepancy between your abilities and the expectations of the assignment, further dialogue with the nurse

supervisor is needed before you reach a decision. At this point it may be appropriate to consult the next level of management, such as the house supervisor or the chief nurse executive.

In further dialogue, continue to assess whether you are qualified to accept either a portion or the whole of the requested assignment. Also point out options that might be mutually beneficial. For example, obviously it would be unsafe for you to administer chemotherapy without prior training. However, if someone else administered the chemotherapy, perhaps you could provide the remainder of the required nursing care for that patient. If you feel unqualified for the assignment in its entirety, the dilemma becomes more complex.

At this point, the RN must be aware of the legal rights of the facility. Even though the RN may have legitimate concerns for patient safety and one's own legal accountability in providing safe care, the facility has legal precedent to initiate disciplinary action, including termination, if you refuse to accept an assignment. Therefore, it is important to continue to explore options in a positive manner, recognizing that both the RN and the facility have a responsibility for safe patient care.

4. POINT OF DECISION AND IMPLICATIONS: If none of the options is acceptable, you are at your final decision point.
   a. Accept the assignment, documenting carefully your concern for patient safety and the process you used to inform the facility (manager) of your concerns. Keep a personal copy of this documentation, and send a copy to the manager(s) involved. Once you have reached this decision, it is unwise to discuss the situation or your feelings with other staff or patients. Now you are legally accountable for these patients. From this point, withdrawal from the agreed-upon assignment may constitute abandonment.
   b. Refuse the assignment, being prepared for disciplinary action. Document your concern for patient safety and the process you used to inform the facility (manager) of your concerns. Keep a personal copy of this documentation, and send a copy to the nurse executive. Courtesy suggests that you also send a copy to the manager(s) involved.

c. Document the steps taken in making your decision. It may be necessary for you to use the facility's grievance procedure.

Scenario—A Question of an Additional Shift

An example of another potential dilemma is when a nurse experiencing personal fatigue and its potential for patient harm is required to work an additional shift.

Suppose you are approached by your supervisor and asked to work an additional shift. Your immediate response is that you don't want to work another shift—what do you do?

1. CLARIFY what it is you are expected to do.
   ▪ For example, would the additional shift be with the same patients you are currently caring for, or would it involve a new patient assignment?
   ▪ Is your reluctance to work another shift because of a new patient assignment you do not feel competent to accept? (If the answer is yes, then refer to the previous example, "A Question of Competence.")
   ▪ Is your reluctance because of work fatigue, or do you have other plans?
   ▪ Is this a chronic request caused by poor scheduling, inadequate staffing, or chronic absenteeism?
   ▪ Are you being asked to work because there is no relief nurse coming for your present patient assignment? Because your unit will be short of professional staff on the next shift? Because another unit will be short of professional staff on the next shift?
   ▪ How long are you being asked to work—the entire shift or a portion of the shift?
2. ASSESS yourself.
   ▪ Are you really tired, or do you just not want to work? Is your fatigue level such that your care may be unsafe? Remember, you are legally responsible for the care of your current patient assignment if relief is not available.
3. IDENTIFY OPTIONS and implications of your decision.
   a. If you perceive that you can provide safe patient care and are willing to work the additional shift, accept the assignment.
   b. If you perceive that you can provide safe patient care but are unwilling to stay because of other plans or the chronic nature of the

request, inform the manager of your reasons for not wishing to accept the assignment.

c. If you perceive that your fatigue will interfere with your ability to safely care for patients, indicate this fact to the manager.

If you do not accept the assignment and the manager continues to attempt to persuade you, it may be appropriate to consult the next level of management, such as the house supervisor or the nurse executive.

In further dialogue, continue to weigh your reasons for refusal versus the facility's need for an RN. If you have a strong alternate commitment, such as no child care, or if you seriously feel your fatigue will interfere with safe patient care, restate your reasons for refusal.

At this point, it is important for you to be aware of the legal rights of the facility. Even though you may have legitimate concerns for patient safety and your own legal accountability in providing safe care, or a legitimate concern for the safety of your children or other commitments, the facility has a legal precedent to initiate disciplinary action, including termination, if you refuse to accept an assignment. Therefore, it is important to continue to explore options in a positive manner, recognizing that both you and the facility have a responsibility for safe patient care.

4. POINT OF DECISION AND IMPLICATIONS

  a. Accept the assignment, documenting your professional concern for patient safety and the process you used to inform the facility (manager) of your concerns. Keep a personal copy of this documentation, and send a copy to the nurse executive. Courtesy suggests that you also send a copy to the manager(s) involved. Once you have reached this decision, it is unwise to discuss the situation or your feelings with other staff or patients.

  b. Accept the assignment, documenting your professional concerns for the chronic nature of the request and possible long-term consequences in reducing the quality of care. Documentation should follow the procedures outlined in the first item of this list.

  c. Accept the assignment, documenting your personal concerns regarding working conditions in which management decides the legitimacy of employee personal commitments. This documentation should go to your manager. You may wish to request a meeting with your manager to discuss the incident and your concerns regarding future requests.

  d. Refuse the assignment, being prepared for disciplinary action. If your reasons for refusal were patient safety or an imperative personal commitment, document this carefully, including the process you used to inform the facility (nurse manager) of your concerns. Keep a personal copy of this documentation, and send a copy to the chief nurse executive. Courtesy suggests that you also send a copy to the manager(s) involved.

  e. Document the rationale for your decision. It may be necessary to use the facility's grievance procedure.

Summary

Two scenarios of how an RN may apply the guidelines for decision making in the actual work situation have been presented. Staffing dilemmas will always be present and mandate that active communication between staff nurses and all levels of nursing management be maintained to ensure patient safety. The likelihood of a satisfactory solution will increase if there is prior consideration of the choices available. This consideration of available alternatives should include recognition that professional nurses are intelligent adults who should be involved in the decision-making process. Professional nurses are accountable for nursing judgments and actions regardless of the personal consequences. Providing safe nursing care to the patient is the ultimate objective of the professional nurse and the health-care facility.

Resources

To maintain current and accurate information on accountability of RNs for giving, accepting, or rejecting a work assignment, the following resources are suggested:

- **Health-Care Facility:** Nurses are encouraged to seek consultation with their nurse manager or executives to discuss the facility's missions and goals as well as policies and procedures.
- The **ANA** serves as the national clearinghouse of information and offers publications on

contemporary issues, including standards of practice and nursing ethics, as well as legal and regulatory issues. Contact the ANA for a complimentary copy of the Publications Catalogue.

- *ANA Basic Guide to Safe Delegation* is available through the ANA.

- *ANA Code of Ethics for Nurses* (2015b) is available through the ANA.
- *ANA Standards and Scope of Practice* (2015a) is available through the ANA.
- Board of Nursing. A complimentary copy of the Nurse Practice Act is available to each RN upon request.

---

*Reproduced with permission of Florida Nurses Association, 1999, Orlando, Florida.
Revised 07/2018

National Council of State Boards of Nursing Guidelines for Using Social Media Appropriately*

Nursing organizations are beginning to develop social media guidelines so that social media can be used to its fullest potential in communicating with patients. National Council of State Boards of Nursing (NCSBN) guidelines can be found online and are summarized as follows:

- Nurses must recognize that they have an ethical and legal obligation to maintain patient privacy and confidentiality at all times.
- Nurses must not transmit, by way of any electronic media, any patient-related information or image that is reasonably anticipated to violate patient rights to confidentiality or privacy or to otherwise degrade or embarrass the patient.
- Nurses must not share, post, or otherwise disseminate any information, including images, about a patient or information gained in the nurse–patient relationship with anyone unless there is a patient care-related need to disclose the information or other legal obligation to do so.
- Nurses must not identify patients by name or post or publish information that may lead to the identification of a patient. Limiting access to postings through privacy settings is not sufficient to ensure privacy.
- Nurses must not refer to patients in a disparaging manner, even if they are not identified.
- Nurses must not take photos or videos of patients on personal devices, including mobile devices.
- Nurses must maintain professional boundaries in the use of electronic media.
- Nurses must consult employer policies or an appropriate leader within the organization for guidance regarding work-related postings.
- Nurses must promptly report any identified breach of confidentiality or privacy.
- Nurses must be aware of and comply with employer policies regarding the use of employer-owned computers, cameras, and other electronic devices and the use of personal devices in the workplace.
- Nurses must not make disparaging remarks about employers or coworkers (NCSBN, 2011).

---

*https://www.nursingworld.org/~4af4f2/globalassets/docs/ana/ethics/social-networking.pdf

Answers to NCLEX® Review Questions

Chapter 1 Questions

1. Answer: 3

Rationales:

1. Florence Nightingale formalized nursing practice.
2. The Knights of Columbus was an organization but not a religious order.
3. **Religious orders such as the Sisters of Mercy assumed the role of "nursing" the sick and infirm.**
4. Wars and battles required nurses.

2. Answer: 4

Rationales:

1. Henderson built on Nightingale's theory.
2. Rogers developed a theory of nursing known as the Science of Unitary Human Beings.
3. Robb was the first superintendent of nurses at Johns Hopkins School of Nursing.
4. **Florence Nightingale defined nursing function in both the sick and well state.**

3. Answer: 4

Rationales:

1. Although good communication is expected, it is not considered an "ethical code."
2. Protecting autonomy is part of the ethical code.
3. All individuals are entitled to equitable care; however, nursing care is patient-centered, so care, although equitable, may not be identical.
4. **Codes of ethics provide guidelines for appropriate professional behaviors and guide practice.**

4. Answer: 4

Rationales:

1. The examination ensures minimally safe practice.
2. Standards of care are designated by evidence-based practice.
3. Honest and ethical care is expected and guided by the Code of Ethics.
4. **The NCLEX® examination ensures that the registered nurse has achieved the minimum knowledge and skills necessary to enter practice.**

5. Answer: 1, 5

Rationales:

Although advanced practice registered nurses (APRNs) work in a variety of settings, they all:
1. **Function independently as guided by the nurse practice acts of the individual states.**
2. Are educated to provide higher level patient care.
3. May work in acute care settings.
4. May work in university settings.
5. **Are educated at the master's level or higher.**

6. Answer: 3

Rationales:

1. Continuing education furthers knowledge and skills within the professional domain.
2. Graduate education leads to a higher level degree such as a master's or doctorate.
3. **In-service education takes place within an institution or agency. It is usually directed at teaching nurses who work in the institution about a new policy, standard, or type of equipment.**
4. Professional registered nurse education is the basic nursing education to sit for licensure.

7. Answer: 1, 2

Rationales: **Professional behaviors include accountability and sound decision-making abilities.**

1. **Professionals look at risks and benefits before making a decision.**
2. **They analyze choices in order to make sound decisions.**
3. Concrete thinking is literal and focuses on the physical world.
4. Professional decision making occurs independently.

8. Answer: 1

Rationales:

1. **Health-care reform and nursing practice focus on client- or patient-centered care.**
2. The nursing process is a scientific method used by nurses to ensure the quality of patient care.
3. Cultural diversity is the understanding that various cultures exist within populations.
4. The health-care facility is the physical place where care occurs.

9. Answer: 1, 2, 3

Rationales:

1. **Accountability for one's work and responsibilities is a professional behavior.**
2. **Advocating for patients and families is a professional behavior.**
3. **Autonomy in making decisions within the scope of practice is a professional behavior.**
4. Social networking is not considered a knowledge or skill unique to professional nursing.
5. Participation in nursing blogs is not considered a knowledge or skill unique to professional nursing.

10. Answer: 1, 2, 3, 4

Rationales:

1. **To provide a basis for ethical decision making is a characteristic of professional accountability.**
2. **To respect the decision of the patient is a characteristic of professional accountability.**
3. **To maintain standards of health is a characteristic of professional accountability.**
4. **To evaluate new professional practices and reassess existing ones is a characteristic of professional accountability.**
5. Belonging to a professional organization demonstrates commitment to the profession, but not necessarily accountability.

Chapter 2 Questions

1. Answer: 5

Rationales:

People are more likely to complete advance directives about their care when they are informed and they understand the ramifications of doing so. Studies have shown that certain populations are more likely to follow through with completing advance directives when compared with others; these populations include those who have higher levels of socioeconomic status, those with higher levels of education, and people who have already suffered from a chronic disease.

2. Answer: 1

Rationales:

1. **The ANA Code of Ethics is designed to guide nurses toward quality, ethical care of patients. There may be times when it is difficult to discern the most ethical action, particularly when the lines are blurred as to the correct decision. The Code of Ethics provides some guidance that nurses can follow as part of the profession of nursing to uphold standards of ethical care.**
2. Improving care environments is important but does not address the ANA Code.
3. Maintaining professional boundaries comes under professional behaviors.
4. Caring for self is important; however, it does not address quality and ethical care.

3. Answer: 2, 3

Rationales:

1. The health information of incarcerated patients is still protected under the Health Insurance Portability and Accountability Act (HIPAA).
2. **Although HIPAA provides protections for patient privacy, there are some cases in which health-care providers can disclose patient**

information to other providers and caregivers. These exceptions typically include care related to criminal acts, such as child or elder abuse, or when a patient is injured because of a firearm or some other weapon.

3. Although HIPAA provides protections for patient privacy, there are some cases in which health-care providers can disclose patient information to other providers and caregivers. These exceptions typically include care related to criminal acts, such as child or elder abuse, or when a patient is injured because of a firearm or some other weapon.

4. Individual occupations and vocations are protected.

5. Any breach of information, intentional or unintentional, violates HIPAA.

4. Answer: 2

Rationales:

1. Beneficence is to do good.

2. **The principle of autonomy indicates that the client has independence to make decisions and take personal action. When the nurse asks the patient about his concerns, the nurse is exploring the reasons and allowing the patient to make his own decision.**

3. Veracity is to be truthful.

4. Justice is to treat all patients equally.

5. Answer: 2

Rationales:

1. Confidentiality is an expectation of anyone who is under treatment.

2. **Privacy is the condition of being free from being observed or disturbed by other people. Confidentiality has to do with the sharing of someone else's information.**

3. Technology often causes breaches in confidentiality.

4. Confidentiality goes beyond verbal exchanges; breaches can occur electronically or in writing.

6. Answer: 2

Rationales:

1. Although important to be able to support reasons, lists do not help with this.

2. **Creating a list of positives and negatives helps when difficult choices need to be made. The list outlines the positive and negative aspects of a decision. It allows the nurse to compare the benefits of making a choice versus the potential disadvantages. When compared side by side, it could help the nurse to make a difficult decision through an easier method.**

3. Communicating the choice occurs after the list is created.

4. Providing care should always be based on policies and standards.

7. Answer: 3

Rationales:

1. To affirm means to strongly state a fact, not indicating satisfaction with the choice.

2. Choosing is to decide what is important.

3. **Prizing a value means being satisfied with a choice and being willing to declare the choice to others. The patient made her choice clear to her family and provider.**

4. Reflecting a value means considering it.

8. Answer: 4

Rationales:

1. Calling the supervisor does not demonstrate speaking or advocating for the patient.

2. Values and ethics are beliefs.

3. Documenting clinical changes is important; however, this is not advocating.

4. **Nurses strengthen their ability to advocate for a client when nurses are able to identify personal values and then accurately identify the values of the client and articulate the client's point of view.**

9. Answer: 2

Rationales:

1. Being an employee does not give permission to access the chart.

2. **Unless the significant other has authorized any access to information, the only people entitled to information without written consent are the client and those providing direct care.**

3. The patient still needs to give consent.

4. The surgeon cannot discuss the patient's health without consent from the patient.

10. Answer: 1

Rationales:

1. **All patients are entitled to the best possible care regardless of their socioeconomic status, culture, or situations.**
2. Veracity refers to truthfulness.
3. Autonomy is the right to make one's own decisions.
4. Nonmaleficence means to do no harm.

Chapter 3 Questions

1. Answer: 1

Rationales:

1. **Giving out information about a patient without permission is an invasion of privacy.**
2. Providing information about the patient to those who will be caring for the patient is appropriate.
3. Sharing information with those who are responsible for the patient's care in order to ensure safe and effective care is appropriate.
4. Patients sign release of information forms to allow this; if a form has not been signed, third-party payers will not reimburse.

2. Answer: 1, 3

Rationales:

1. **Because nurses have greater ability to provide care, their obligation to provide care is higher than that of laypersons.**
2. The nurse has not made an inflammatory or false statement.
3. **According to the Code of Ethics, nurses need to care for patients without judgment.**
4. Caring for a patient is an expectation of the role. Nurses do not establish contracts with patients to deliver care.

3. Answer: 1

Rationales:

1. **Nurses must be held accountable for errors but should be treated in a professional and assistive manner.**
2. Dismissal for incompetence fails to demonstrate ethical or supportive behavior.

3. Advising a professional not to discuss the error is unethical.
4. Reassigning is punitive.

4. Answer: 3

Rationales:

1. Assault is a threat to do harm.
2. Wrongful publication refers to erroneous information in writing.
3. **Charting or saying unsupported defamatory statements can lead to tort litigation.**
4. Slander is making an untrue statement that causes harm to someone's reputation.

5. Answer: 3

Rationales:

1. The incident occurred outside of the hospital.
2. A good faith agreement implies that a contract exists.
3. **The Good Samaritan law protects persons who assist at an accident scene if they act in good faith. Professional insurance is not in effect because the actions were not performed while on duty.**
4. Professional liability insurance does not necessarily cover this type of litigation.

6. Answer: 4

Rationales:

1. Although this was performed without malice and is considered an unintentional tort, harm occurred, making the action malpractice.
2. The licensed practical nurse (LPN) did not intend to hurt the patient.
3. Negligence falls in the category of an unintentional tort.
4. **Malpractice occurs when an unintentional tort causes an injury to a client.**

7. Answer: 1, 5

Rationales:

1. **1, 5. Before surgery, the nurse needs to ensure that the patient fully understands what the physician explained about the procedure and that the consent form has been signed before any preoperative sedation is administered.**

2. The physician needs to provide the information so that the patient is fully informed; the nurse may obtain the signature but needs to ensure that the patient is aware and understands.

3. The nurse acts as the witness.

4. Although the signature should be in ink, often electronic signatures are obtained.

8. Answer: 1

Rationales:

1. **Malpractice occurs when an unintentional tort causes an injury to a client.**

2. Malpractice falls under negligence.

3. Nonmaleficence is an ethical principle.

4. The nurse failed to open the valve; there is not any evidence that the equipment malfunctioned.

9. Answer: 1, 2, 3, 5

Rationales:

The advance directive provides instructions for future health-care decisions if the patient becomes unable to make personal treatment choices.

10. Answer: 4

Rationales:

1. 1, 2, and 3 are all steps the nurse needs to take; however, verifying the order is the most important action to take first.

4. **The Joint Commission on National Safety Goals requires that all telephone orders be written down and read back. This ensures the accuracy of the order. Failure to follow this procedure leaves the nurse and the facility open to negligence because it is a standard of care.**

Chapter 4 Questions

1. Answer: 3

Rationales:

1. Inflexibility is not a leadership competency. In fact, it impedes leadership effectiveness.

2. Leaders who ignore negative feedback may lose opportunities to improve their leadership effectiveness.

3. **Ability to communicate effectively with other people is one of the three competencies identified by Hersey and Campbell.**

4. Nurse leaders need to be critical thinkers. There are times when they are obligated as caring professionals to question directions, requests, or medical orders.

2. Answer: 2

Rationales:

1. Democratic leaders are active leaders, not passive leaders.

2. **Laissez-faire leaders are passive, inactive leaders who would not provide direction.**

3. Autocratic leaders are often too directive and controlling.

4. Situational leaders are adaptive but will spell out team members' responsibilities.

3. Answer: 3

Rationales:

1. Democratic leaders do not set goals without consulting with or recognizing the group's goals.

2. Democratic leaders are active, not passive.

3. **Democratic or participative leaders are characterized by their inclusion of team members in important decisions.**

4. Autocratic leadership squelches creativity, whereas democratic leadership fosters it.

4. Answer: 1

Rationales:

1. **The situational leadership approach considers the complexity of a situation, which would include followers and the task at hand.**

2. A focus only on the task(s) to be done is too limited for the situational approach.

3. Likewise, a focus only on the follower would be too limited.

4. Behavior is an important, but not the only, focus of situational leadership.

5. Answer: 4

Rationales:

1. Emotionally intelligent leaders understand and manage their own emotions.

2. Emotionally intelligent leaders are able to juggle multiple demands.
3. Emotionally intelligent leaders actively work with members of their team rather than alone.
4. **Emotionally intelligent leaders welcome criticism that is constructive and acknowledges other team members' perspectives.**

6. Answer: 3

Rationales:

1. An effective leader would increase the positivity of the team, not its negativity.
2. Transformational leaders work with others, not alone.
3. **Transformational leaders help their teams define their mission and see how their work helps them achieve their mission.**
4. Transformational leaders do not focus their attention on team members' weaknesses.

7. Answer: 1, 2, 3, 4

Rationales:

1. **Integrity and courage are qualities of an effective leader.**
2. **Thinking critically is a behavior of effective leaders.**
3. **Setting priorities is another behavior of effective leaders.**
4. **Skillful communication includes providing constructive feedback.**

8. Answer: 1, 2

Rationales:

1. **Every leader is at times a follower.**
2. **Effective leaders work with their teams on shared goals.**
3. Although they are not always able to act on their ideas, effective leaders do so as much as they can if the ideas are constructive.
4. Earning a master's degree would be helpful but is not required for effective leadership.

9. Answer: 2

Rationales:

1. Effective followers are actively involved in the work of the team.
2. **The most effective followers are not only competent but self-directed.**

3. Effective followers are very valuable employees.
4. Although they cannot be expected to support every new idea, effective followers support constructive new ideas.

10. Answer: 3

Rationales:

1. Postponing decision making is a characteristic of laissez-faire leaders; autocratic leaders are more active.
2. Autocratic leaders make decisions independently; they generally do not share decision making with their teams.
3. **Autocratic leaders frequently give orders and make decisions without consulting with team members.**
4. Encouraging creativity when problem-solving is more characteristic of democratic (participative) leaders.

Chapter 5 Questions

1. Answer: 2

Rationales:

1. Budgets are a concern of nurse managers but not their major focus.
2. **Everyone can exert leadership at various times, but *manager* is a designated position, assigned by upper-level administration.**
3. Nurse leaders are definitely concerned that the work of the team gets done.
4. Both management and leadership focus on people.

2. Answer: 1

Rationales:

1. **A Theory Y manager employs staff guidance, staff development, and rework as opposed to Theory X's emphasis on control, close monitoring, and punishment, if needed.**
2. Theory Y is a management theory, not a leadership theory.
3. These are the focus of Theory X, not Theory Y.
4. Time studies are used primarily by those managing in the scientific management mode.

3. Answer: 3

Rationales:

1. Helping patients care for themselves is a nursing care approach, not a management approach.
2. Removal or demotion is sometimes necessary but not the focus of servant leadership.
3. **Servant leadership employs a "people first" approach to improving how employees are treated.**
4. Resolving conflicts as quickly as possible would not be the goal of a servant leader or manager, who would try to come to a resolution that is best for all, even if it takes some time.

4. Answer: 1, 2, 3, 4

Rationales:

1, 2, 3, and 4. To be maximally effective, nurse managers need a constellation of skills: people skills (leadership), expertise (clinical experience), and financial skills (business sense and budget savvy).

5. Answer: 4

Rationales:

1. Evaluation is one of the decisional activities of a nurse manager.
2. Resource allocation is also a decisional activity.
3. Being a coach is one of the interpersonal activities of a nurse manager.
4. **Being a spokesperson for staff, patients, and administration is an informational activity.**

6. Answer: 2

Rationales:

1. Very few new graduates have either the preparation or experience to assume management responsibilities soon after graduation.
2. **Development of clinical expertise is an essential part of preparing to be a nurse manager.**
3. It is the amount of preparation and experience gained, not the number of years, that is critical in making this decision.
4. Nurse managers need to have leadership expertise.

7. Answer: 2

Rationales:

1. Pretending to have experience is likely to cause him to lose credibility and the trust of his staff.
2. **This is an accurate description of his situation and is likely to engage staff in supporting his growth and development as a nurse manager.**
3. Staff need to contribute to the leadership of the team but are not expected to "manage themselves."
4. It is preferable to take a positive approach, emphasizing a willingness to learn.

8. Answer: 1

Rationales:

1. **Managing people is probably the most challenging task for nurse managers. It is fundamental to good management.**
2. The unit budget is important but not as complex as managing people.
3. Planning for the future is also important but not as fundamental as managing people.
4. Redesigning the unit's workflow is usually a task that should be done only after gaining familiarity with all aspects of the unit's operation.

9. Answer: 4

Rationales:

1. Interpersonal relations are not the focus of scientific management.
2. Servant leadership is also more focused on interpersonal relations than is scientific management.
3. Likewise, staff development is not emphasized in scientific management.
4. **The focus on increasing efficiency is the hallmark of scientific management.**

10. Answer: 3

Rationales:

1. Newly licensed nurses face many challenges, but poor pay is usually not the reason for resignation.
2. Needlestick injuries are a concern, of course, but most facilities have developed adequate prevention programs.

3. **Newly licensed nurses, in particular, need supportive management and may resign if it is not present.**
4. A lack of advancement opportunities becomes more important after the initial adjustment to this new role.

Chapter 6 Questions

1. Answer: 1

Rationales:

1. **The gloves are contaminated and should be removed before answering the phone.**
2. Log rolling is an appropriate action.
3. Using an incontinence diaper is an appropriate action.
4. Keeping the head elevated is an appropriate action.

2. Answer: 1, 2, 3, 5

Rationales:

1. **1, 2, 3, and 5. These are appropriate to the care of a patient receiving anticoagulants.**
4. This is inappropriate. Although a patient is receiving anticoagulation therapy, it is important to avoid trauma to the rectal tissue, which could cause bleeding (e.g., avoid rectal thermometers and enemas).

3. Answer: 1

Rationales:

1. **Assisting patients with positioning and activities of daily living is within the educational preparation and scope of practice of a nursing assistant.**
2. Instructing requires additional education and skills and is more appropriate for a licensed nurse.
3. Teaching patients requires additional education and skills and is more appropriate for a licensed nurse.
4. Assessing patients requires additional education and skills and is more appropriate for a licensed nurse.

4. Answer: 3

Rationales:

1. Discussing weight-loss strategies requires additional education and training.

2. Teaching requires additional education and training. These actions are within the scope of practice of the registered nurse (RN).
3. **The nursing assistant can remind patients about actions that have already been taught by the nurse and are part of the patient's plan of care.**
4. The RN can delegate the administration of medication to a licensed practical nurse (LPN) or licensed vocational nurse (LVN).

5. Answer: 4

Rationales:

1. This patient's needs are not urgent or emergent.
2. In chronic obstructive pulmonary disease (COPD), patients' pulse oximetry oxygen saturations of more than 90% are acceptable.
3. The IV needs to be started; however, there is not an indication that the patient is in an urgent or emergent situation.
4. **The patient with asthma did not achieve relief from shortness of breath after using the bronchodilator and is at risk for respiratory complications. This patient's needs are urgent.**

6. Answer: 4

Rationales:

1. Suctioning will increase the heart rate. This needs reporting and reassessment and may be related to the increased temperature.
2. Respiratory rate is often increased with a fever.
3. Pulse oximetry of 95% is acceptable.
4. **The patient has a tracheostomy and is at risk for infection. A tympanic temperature of 101.4°F (38.6°C) indicates an infection and needs to be reported immediately.**

7. Answer: 1, 2

Rationales:

1. **1, 2. The experienced licensed practical nurse (LPN) is capable of gathering data and making observations, including noting breath sounds and performing pulse oximetry. Administering medications, such as those delivered via metered dose inhalers (MDIs), is within the scope of practice of the LPN.**

3. Independently completing the admission assessment is within the scope of practice of the professional registered nurse (RN).

4. Initiating the nursing care plan is within the scope of practice of the professional RN.

5. Evaluating a patient's abilities requires additional education and skills. These actions are within the scope of practice of the professional RN.

8. Answer: 4

Rationales:

1. To care for the patient with tuberculosis (TB) in isolation, the nurse must be fitted for a high-efficiency particulate air (HEPA) respirator mask.

2. The bronchoscopy patient needs specialized procedure care and a more experienced nurse.

3. The ventilator-dependent patient needs a nurse who is familiar with ventilator care.

4. **Many surgical patients are taught about coughing, deep breathing, and the use of incentive spirometry preoperatively.**

9. Answer: 1

Rationales:

1. **When the oxygen flow rate is higher than 4 L/min, the mucous membranes can be dried out. The best treatment is to add humidification to the oxygen delivery system. Application of a water-soluble jelly to the nares can also help decrease mucosal irritation.**

2. This does not treat the problem.

3. This does not treat the problem.

4. This does not treat the problem.

10. Answer: 1

Rationales:

1. **Experienced licensed practical nurses (LPNs) and licensed vocational nurses (LVNs) can use observation of patients to gather data regarding how well patients perform interventions that have already been taught.**

2. Planning requires additional education and skills, appropriate to a registered nurse (RN).

3. Assisting patients with activities of daily living (ADLs) is more appropriately delegated to a nursing assistant.

4. Consulting requires additional education and skills, appropriate to an RN.

Chapter 7 Questions

1. Answer: 3

Rationales:

1. Although answer 1—talking to the staff—is important, the best answer is 3.

2. This is incorrect. Laughing with staff can confuse the audience and cause them to misconstrue the seriousness of the message from Manager Jane.

3. **Listening to staff is the most critical communication skill because it helps the manager understand the situation and the staff's rationale for their actions. It also demonstrates empathy and openness, which can lead to agreement on better adherence to the policies.**

4. This is incorrect. Demonstrating emotions such as crying can confuse the audience and cause them to misconstrue the seriousness of the message from Manager Jane.

2. Answer: 4

Rationales:

1. **Physical barriers—such as the absence of the charge nurse to answer questions—could prevent the staff from following policies.**

2. **Emotional barriers—such as a nurse's fear of retribution from a colleague—can cause nurses to seek out answers, which can delay care or compromise safety.**

3. **Semantic barriers—such as acronyms or nicknames—can confuse or mislead staff unfamiliar with their meaning.**

4. **All of the above**

3. Answer: 2

Rationales:

1. 1, 4. Although answers 1 and 4 should be included in the bedside shift report, they are not the best answer.

2. **Introducing the client and his diagnosis ensures that the sender and receiver of the communication are familiar with the client and share pertinent care needs, nursing interventions, and client progress with goals of care.**

3. This is incorrect. Personal opinions may prejudice the oncoming nurse's view of the patient, which could compromise care.

4. Answer: 2

Rationales:

2. Ineffective hand-off communication or miscommunication between caregivers during the transfer of care is estimated to contribute to 80% of serious medical errors. Poor hand-offs can lead to delays in treatment, inappropriate treatment, and prolonged hospital stays.
Answers 1, 3, and 4 contribute to medical error but not to the same degree as ineffective hand-off communication.

5. Answer: 4

Rationales:

1. Implicit bias is formed during a lifetime because it is formed based on an individual's culture, which shapes attitudes, beliefs, and actions.
2. Implicit bias is automatic and subconscious during our interactions with others and can influence our clinical decision making and even treatment.
3. Implicit bias contributes to social behavior because it is derived from an individual's cultural norms.
4. All of the above

6. Answer: 2

Rationales:

1. The emergency medical responder (EMR) is readily available at the hospital where the patient was treated. Only electronic health records (EHRs) contain a comprehensive accounting of health encounters regardless of the location.
2. EMRs are usually hospital or practice specific, so Jane would not have access to the patient's hospital EMR. Recent changes in technology and the creation of health information exchanges are making EMR information available to hospital and practice affiliates.
3. EHRs can capture patient information from anywhere within a health information exchange.

4. General consents for treatment and release of information are part of primary care practice and hospital paperwork.

7. Answer: 1

Rationales:

1. Protected health information (PHI) must be protected and never shared without expressed written permission. A patient's privacy and confidentiality are paramount.
2. Nurses and other health professionals should never post stories about patients or work on social media sites. People familiar with you may easily put 2 and 2 together and surmise the situation and patient involved, which could be a breach in patient privacy. This could be grounds for disciplinary action.
3. Photos of patients or work areas should not be shared on social media. Although innocent, a photo may include an assignment board or other information that could inadvertently display PHI.
4. The time of social media posting is irrelevant; the issue is the confidentiality and privacy of the patients and the staff caring for them.

8. Answer: 4

Rationales:

1. Paging the MD to the bedside without any information may cause the MD to just add visiting the patient to his list rather than conveying the urgency of the patient's change in condition.
2. Placing a STAT page to the MD may get the MD there quickly; however, without the necessary information about the patient, the MD may think that you overreacted and dismiss the severity of the clinical change.
3. Rather than bother the MD, you medicate the patient for pain and continue to observe the patient.
4. Describing the situation, background, assessment, and recommendations (SBAR) is best. Reporting on situational change is designed to provide concise, pertinent, and factual information to members of the health-care team. This approach to a sudden change in patient condition allows you to communicate information, your concerns, and the need for action.

9. Answer: 3

Rationales:

The ISBARR is an acronym for a concise review of the client with other team members to ensure timely intervention and feedback. It includes introducing the patient, the current situation, any pertinent background that could be contributing to the situation, a clinical assessment with recommendations, and, finally, a readback of the instructions or orders to ensure accuracy.

10. Answer: 3

Rationales:

1. Unit secretaries may enter orders into a patient record; however, it is the responsibility of the professional nurse to accept or sign off on the order before it is implemented.
2. Medical students may write orders; however, they must first be signed off by the faculty physician before being accepted by the professional nurse, who can then ensure they are implemented.
3. **The professional nurse is responsible for accepting, transcribing, and implementing health-care provider orders.**
4. Medical assistants may not accept or implement physician or health-care provider orders without being accepted by a professional nurse.

Chapter 8 Questions

1. Answer: 2

Rationales:

1. Conflict does have a positive side; when managed constructively, people can develop more open, cooperative ways of working together.
2. **The use of negotiating skills can resolve conflicts more effectively by helping differing parties see each other as people with similar needs, concerns, and dreams instead of as competitors or blocks in the way of progress. Being involved in successful conflict resolution can be an empowering experience.**
3. Winning more negotiations is counterintuitive. The purpose of negotiation

is to build consensus and agreement between parties, not win more for your side.
4. Negotiations by themselves can be stressful; however, the outcome of a good negotiation would be reduced stress caused by the conflict.

2. Answer: 1

Rationales:

1. **Disrespect and incivility are the leading cause of conflict within health-care teams.**
Answers 2, 3, and 4 are less likely to cause conflict when compared with disrespect and incivility.

3. Answer: 4

Rationales:

1. **Observing daily unit activity will allow the nurse manager to see that no patient care is missed because of extraneous duties that her staff may be asked to perform because of the reorganization.**
2. **The reorganization may create a scarcity of supplies or change delivery times, which could cause hoarding or competition for limited resources.**
3. **Keeping the patient care assignments equitable will allow for prompt intervention should workloads become unmanageable or breaks are missed.**
4. **All of the above**

4. Answer: 4

Rationales:

1. There is no union or management involvement in the scenario presented.
2. Although this change in workload may eventually cause some interpersonal problems, the job cuts were an organizational decision, not a personal one.
3. This was an organizational decision, not one made because of a cultural difference.
4. **Work intensification causes everyone involved to increase their workloads to accommodate the job cuts. Nurses and respiratory therapists adjusting to this change may be unable to request service or respond to a request for service in a timely manner.**

5. Answer: 3

Rationales:

1. Win–lose infers competition; the aim of conflict resolution is to work together more effectively, not win.
2. Lose–lose makes everyone a loser and can make people angry or heighten their need to win next time. Both of these situations take attention away from the work and place it on the need to win.
3. **Win–win allows both sides to come together to identify the issue, and each side gains some benefit from the solution. Both sides walk away winners.**
4. None of the above

6. Answer: 1

Rationales:

1. **Brainwriting is a creative approach to problem-solving. Similar to brainstorming, it offers everyone a chance to share ideas; however, by writing their ideas before the discussion, there is less likelihood of being influenced by early ideas.**
2. Brainwriting is a tool that may be used for different types of negotiation; however, it is not a result of negotiation.
3. Brainwriting is not an approach to formal negotiation, but it may inform the negotiation.
4. Brainwriting is not a reaction to negotiation.

7. Answer: 2

Rationales:

1. Employee counseling may further exacerbate the conflict because employee counseling will deal with each staff member individually rather than bringing them all together to resolve the issue.
2. **Problem resolution is the best answer. Florence has addressed both of her staff members about their behavior, and there has been no improvement. Problem resolution will help the two parties identify the issue and agree on a solution to the problem.**
3. This is not a union issue. A union representative is usually only engaged when there is a dispute between employees and management, not between employees.

4. Formal negotiation would be too complex for this situation. The two team members are openly critical of one another, but the overall climate of the unit is supportive and collegial.

8. Answer: 4

Rationales:

1. **When a union has been designated as the official bargaining unit for your staff, shift differentials and salary increases are addressed as part of the collective bargaining.**
2. **Issues concerning safe working environments are usually included. They may include things such as the provision or availability of lift equipment, personal protective equipment, or protocols on the reduction of workplace violence.**
3. **Grievance procedures are part of collective bargaining agreements. These procedures ensure that staff issues are heard and reduce the possibility of unfair labor practice.**
4. **All of the above**

9. Answer: 2

Rationales:

1. Staff rights to fair treatment are protected by personnel policies, state and federal law, and the current union contract. This item is a regular part of collective bargaining.
2. **Discussion between management and union representatives about the issues may create conflict, which can be constructive or become emotional and competitive. If emotions are not managed, the interaction can become adversarial and delay resolution.**
3. Individual members of the bargaining team may display unprofessional behavior during bargaining sessions; however, this usually occurs between management and the union at the bargaining table.
4. Organization and nursing policies and procedures and nursing professional practice standards ensure that standards of care are met. Collective bargaining centers on employee rights rather than those of the patient or management.

10. Answer: 3

Rationales:

1. The free flow of feelings can cause participants to begin to feed off of each other's emotions, which can get out of control and even lead to emotional outbursts, personal attacks, and physical violence.
2. The manager should not cancel the negotiation. Canceling the negotiation will delay resolution of the problem, and underlying anger or frustration could result in outward hostility on the unit. Instead, the manager may choose to take a short recess so that people can get their feelings under control and then resume the session.
3. **The first step in any negotiation is to manage emotions. Emotions should be acknowledged and never responded to with added emotion. Once acknowledged, the team can move forward.**
4. Ignoring feelings can cause an individual to focus on personal anger rather than identifying the issues causing the conflict. When left unchecked, these emotions may follow the person into the work environment and manifest themselves in emotional outbursts and personal attacks.

Chapter 9 Questions

1. Answer: 3

Rationales:

1. Public hospitals are funded by federal, state, or local funds and are considered not-for-profit.
2. Voluntary not-for-profit hospitals are usually private or community hospitals and are privately funded.
3. **For-profit hospitals are corporately owned and listed on the stock market. Decisions are driven by the shareholders.**
4. All of the above

2. Answer: 3

Rationales:

1. Providing adequate resources such as support services makes care delivery easier, which can reduce safety risks.

2. The use of interprofessional teams improves root cause analysis, which improves problem-solving and contributes to sustained improvement.
3. **Although staffing ratios may improve patient safety, they are not required to ensure a culture.**
4. Work environments free of reprimand and punishment create an atmosphere of trust and result in open sharing to solve problems in care and practice.

3. Answer: 4

Rationales:

1. An organization's philosophy, mission, and vision are based on its values.
2. Policies and procedures are written to translate mission, vision, and values into action.
3. An organization's décor may be selected based on its mission, vision, and values.
4. **Shared values and beliefs are the foundation of organizational culture.**

4. Answer: 4

Rationales:

1. **Adequate staffing ensures that staff members have time to provide care to clients. The number of patients assigned to a nurse can affect patient clinical outcomes.**
2. **Collegial relationships contribute to staff engagement, teamwork, and morale, which are linked to better outcomes.**
3. **Staff development ensures clinical competence and promotes learning, which enhances the capabilities of nursing staff.**
4. **All of the above**

5. Answer: 3

Rationales:

1. *Organic* structure is more dynamic, more flexible, and less centralized than the static traditional hierarchical structure. In organically structured organizations, many decisions are made by the people who will implement them, not by their bosses.
2. Flexible teams are organic in nature. These teams are responsible for their own self-correction and self-control; although

they may also have a designated leader, the teams supervise and manage themselves.

3. **Rigid unit structures are characteristic of a bureaucratic organization. They are very organized and formal. Organizational charts depict each department, and decision making is a very formal, organized process.**

4. Self-correction and self-control are characteristics of an organic structure.

6. Answer: 1

Rationales:

1. **Authority is position dependent. It is assigned based on the organization's hierarchy. For example, a nurse manager has authority over the staff nurses on that unit. Unless a job description or the person hiring requires expertise, leadership, or collaboration with this manager's staff, authority is entirely dependent on where the position falls on the organizational chart. The higher the position, the more authority.**

2. This manager's authority is not derived from one's ability to lead people.

3. This manager may not be required to have expertise even though the manager may be expected to manage a group of experts.

4. Staff members reporting to this position have no formal authority over this manager based on the fact that the manager is in a position above them on the organizational chart.

7. Answer: 1

Rationales:

1. **Nurses do have the authority to control clinical resources and make patient care decisions by virtue of their position and licensure.**

2. Bedside nurses are limited in their ability to tangibly reward staff in any organization.

3. Nurses control information about their clients and daily clinical care that, if shared or withheld, can directly impact care delivery and outcomes.

4. Unfortunately, coercion—whether real or implied—exists. Threatening to report a colleague or giving someone a perception that a call light may not be answered are two examples.

8. Answer: 2

Rationales:

1. Belonging to a professional organization can offer nurses a sense of support from a larger group. It can offer ways to grow professionally through continuing education and allow the nurse to have a stronger voice on community and legislative issues.

2. **Direct control over work and the ability to influence clinical and organizational decisions are essential to feeling empowered. Participating on a unit practice council is an opportunity to contribute to the nursing unit and even the organization, make a difference in clinical practice, and know that her opinion and ideas are valued and important.**

3. Reasonable work assignments can help nurses by giving them time to accomplish tasks and may contribute to a nurse feeling empowered; however, work assignments are not essential to a nurse's ability to feel empowered.

4. Rewards and recognition programs are not necessary for nurse empowerment but can contribute by creating an environment where staff accomplishments and actions are publicly recognized, which can make a nurse feel valued.

9. Answer: 3

Rationales:

1. Professional governance rarely requires working longer hours; rather, it enhances communication and can streamline or simplify nursing practice.

2. Although meetings are necessary for professional governance, they are kept to a minimum.

3. **Nurses set nursing standards of practice for their organization. Because you are closest to the bedside, you see and experience the realities of clinical practice. Your input ensures that clinical practice standards are relevant and that nursing care is delivered in a safe, high-quality manner.**

4. Professional governance sets nursing standards that may or may not influence the culture of an organization.

10. Answer: 1

Rationales:

1. **Professional organizations create a collective voice for nurses that can be stronger and more likely to be heard, especially at the national, state, and local levels. Your membership and participation let your voice be heard.**
2. Professional organizations have no involvement in the management of hospital and health-care organizations, but they do provide opportunities for nurses to work with the professional organization membership on nursing issues.
3. Opportunities for promotion come from the health-care organization, not memberships in professional organizations. However, professional organizations may enhance nurse competence through publications, continuing education, and certifications, which can prepare a nurse for promotion.
4. Health-care and other benefits are provided by a nurse's employer. Some professional organizations may offer liability insurance for their membership but seldom, if ever, health-care benefits.

Chapter 10 Questions

1. Answer: 1

Rationales:

1. **Macro-level changes happen on a large scale. Changes to national Medicare payment policies are large and far reaching because Medicare encompasses the U.S. health-care system.**
2. Changing shift differentials is a small-scale or micro-level change. It is made at a local level such as a hospital or a nursing unit.
3. Opening a new unit is a small-scale or micro-level change.
4. Changing visiting hours is a local or micro-level change.

2. Answer: 2

Rationales:

1. A new assignment moves the nurse to the unknown even though it may occur on the same unit. She must familiarize herself with her assignment and new expectations that would put her out of her comfort zone.

2. **The nurse is accustomed to the daily routine, knows what to expect, and understands what is expected. This puts the nurse in a personal comfort zone.**
3. Moving to a shift where a nurse is unfamiliar with the surroundings, the people, or the workflow puts the nurse out of a personal comfort zone.
4. Adding new tasks or duties can put the nurse out of a personal comfort zone because the nurse may not know what to expect or how to deal with complications that arise when carrying out these duties.

3. Answer: 4

Rationales:

1. Staff receptivity is critical to the successful introduction of an important practice change. The nurse manager should involve both experienced and new staff in the process. This gives the staff an opportunity to ask questions and express their feelings about the anticipated change. It also gives them some ownership in the process, which can lower resistance to the change.
2. There is no need to apologize. Change does not automatically translate to complicating work for staff. The purpose of the change and anticipated benefits should be shared with the staff with the understanding that their work may be affected but not necessarily complicated.
3. Providing additional information about change does not address the proposed change and how it may impact the staff's daily routine. It may leave the staff with more questions and concerns.
4. **Allowing time to learn or practice the new procedure lets staff gain confidence and reduces the threat of failure. This can make the staff more receptive to the proposed change.**

4. Answer: 2

Rationales:

1. This approach discounts the staff's currently held beliefs about the schedule and may create more resistance to change. The nurse manager should have introduced information that would allow the staff to consider the benefits of this change.

2. **Sharing information about the new scheduling process and how it can benefit the staff offers them time to learn about the new process and possibly have input into the proposed change.**

3. Dictating change by posting the schedule as is can result in heightened resistance to change.

4. Providing the staff with the opportunity to come up with an alternative could be seen as passive resistance to change if the staff members are allowed to drag the process out. Disregarding the staff's efforts could threaten their psychological safety.

5. Answer: 3

Rationales:

1. Change ordered by the administration could be perceived as a threat by the staff, which could create more resistance to the new protocol.

2. Statistics will show the staff the number of infections but may not compel them to make changes to their practice.

3. **Telling a story about a patient gives the nurse manager an opportunity to appeal to the staff members' emotions, which compels staff to act, can increase receptivity to change, and may even create a sense of urgency for change.**

4. Explaining the importance of change in simple terms helps staff understand that change is necessary; however, it does not appeal to their emotions, which may affect the implementation of the protocol.

6. Answer: 4

Rationales:

1. Resistance caused by inertia or the status quo is both passive and active. Both can be acknowledged; by providing more information and involving the staff in the proposed change, resistance to the change is lowered.

2. Active resistance is direct and easy to recognize. Things such as flat-out refusal to change or a memo are examples of tangible indicators of resistance. The nurse manager can acknowledge the resistors and address their concerns as needed.

3. Passive resistance is more difficult to identify because it manifests itself in things such as staff agreeing to make the change but not adhering to their commitment or avoiding meetings on the subject. Once acknowledged, this resistance to change can be addressed.

4. **Resistance based on the fear of losing one's job is the most difficult type of resistance to overcome because the person perceives that there is a threat to that person's way of life, which the person will guard at all costs. Sometimes individuals do not feel able to speak freely without jeopardizing their job; therefore, although the individual disagrees with the change, the person keeps silent to stay employed.**

7. Answer: 2

Rationales:

1. When change is complicated, involving staff in the change can help to lower resistance and improve the adoption of the proposed change.

2. **In an emergency, there is little time for discussion or debate around taking action. In this situation, it is appropriate for someone in authority to take charge and dictate how the department will proceed. This is most common during life-threatening events such as a Code Blue, a fire, or a natural disaster.**

3. When resistance is high, it is important to share information with the staff to increase understanding, which lowers resistance to change.

4. Change is seldom unimportant. Even the smallest change can impact a person or a department in a significant way. The impact of change should be considered before implementation.

8. Answer: 2

Rationales:

1. When there is an immediate need, making a personal change is easy because the benefits are realized as soon as the change is made.

2. **If the benefits will not be realized for several years (e.g., going back to school so that you can advance your career), it makes it**

harder to make the change because there may be more at risk (e.g., your dream job may not be available).

3. Being immediately rewarded for making a change can be an easy decision, for example, receiving a sign-on bonus for taking a new job.

4. Making a change that keeps you in your comfort zone is one with little risk. You know what to expect and know the daily routine.

9. Answer: 4

Rationales:

1. **It is important to know whether the process really warrants change. If the process under review is working well as part of current practice, there may be no benefit to making a change. Rather, this would exhaust resources and create unnecessary stress.**

2. **It is important to examine whether the change is needed. Is the change part of a bigger change that will better prepare the organization for the future? Research could support the need for change and allow the department to make a more informed decision.**

3. **The proposed change should address the problem to be solved. Confirming the merit of the initiative and understanding the easiest way to make the technical change are important.**

4. **All of the above**

10. Answer: 1

Rationales:

1. **When a change has truly been incorporated into the daily routine, it has been integrated. Usually staff will no longer refer to the practice as new or a change because they have integrated it into their work. Results of the change will be present, too.**

2. A quick adoption of change can be a good sign as long as the department sustains the change over time. If the staff members still continue to discuss the change in practice, they have not truly adopted it as part of their daily routine.

3. When resistance turns from active to passive, this is indicative that the change has not been integrated. Passive resistance is more difficult

to identify, making the chance of acknowledging the staff's resistance to change more difficult.

4. Time may have little to do with the integration of change into the department's daily routine, especially if the staff members continually discuss the change and demonstrate active or passive resistance every time there is talk of the initiative in the department.

Chapter 11 Questions

1. Answer: 1

Rationales:

1. **The good catch program is a strategy designed to identify system improvement opportunities aimed at reducing risk or harm to patients by staff reporting errors or near misses without fear of punishment or reprisal.**

2. Subscribing to The Joint Commission (TJC) safety publications is a good way to stay current on trends and best practices; however, unless the hospital uses this information in practice, it would not contribute to improving patient safety.

3. Measuring quality performance may not include safety indicators.

4. All of the above

2. Answer: 4

Rationales:

1. **There are six characteristics of quality health care. The use of evidence-based research (EBR) ensures that care delivery is effective and efficient, which avoids overuse and waste.**

2. **Acting respectful and responsive to client preferences is patient-centered.**

3. **Independent double checks avoid possible injury to the patient, making the call safe.**

4. **All of the above**

3. Answer: 1

Rationales:

1. **Review of the medication administration record (MAR) with the off-going nurse allows you to review the list of medications and learn of any issues, possible reactions to medication, or missed doses.**

2. It is always safer to obtain your patient's medication yourself to ensure it is the right medication for the right patient.

3. Unless there is an issue or question about a particular medication, this may not be indicated.

4. Reviewing the medication policy is helpful; however, it will not offer specific information about your patient's possible condition or situation.

4. Answer: 3

Rationales:

1. Sentinel events are unexpected events that result in death or serious physical or psychological injury. These events are rare, and investigation and learning happen after harm to the patient.

2. Adverse events are injuries caused by the care providers and are studied after the fact.

3. **Near misses are potential errors interrupted before they occur. They are useful in identifying and remedying vulnerabilities in the system before harm can occur.**

4. Wrong-procedure events are considered sentinel events because they should never occur.

5. Answer: 4

Rationales:

1. **Events that are not the expected response or activity may constitute a near miss or adverse event and should be reported. It is better to overreport events.**

2. **Documenting in real time reduces the incidence of forgetting important patient information, which reduces risk to the patient.**

3. **Failure to communicate significant information in real time may result in harm to a patient.**

4. **All of the above**

6. Answer: 1

Rationales:

1. **A culture of safety requires a blame-free environment where error reporting is rewarded; this promotes trust, honesty, and transparency, which have been shown to reduce cases of adverse events.**

2. Honesty is important in a culture of safety, but all event reports should be studied—not just the unexpected, serious ones.

3. Event reports are protected confidential documents, but they can be shared with the organization for warning purposes.

4. A blameless environment lacks personal accountability, which is an important requirement in a culture of safety.

7. Answer: 2

Rationales:

1. The quality improvement (QI) process is dependent on teamwork.

2. **Data are used to identify opportunities for improvement and to monitor performance.**

3. Common safety indicators such as falls and infections are regularly used to evaluate the quality of care.

4. Identifying opportunities for QI is everyone's responsibility.

8. Answer: 2

Rationales:

1. Structured care methodologies (SCMs) involve interprofessional tools such as clinical pathways, guidelines, or protocols designed to facilitate care standards.

2. **SCMs facilitate the standardization of patient care and provide a mechanism for quality enhancement, outcomes measurement, and research that informs nursing practice.**

3. SCMs are tools used in the delivery of patient care.

4. Staffing assignments are based on patient acuity, staff competence, and resource availability.

9. Answer: 2

Rationales:

1. Budgets are considered to be a structural aspect of care quality because they support the organization's ability to support patient care.

2. **Preparing a patient for discharge is a care delivery process that consists of care interventions and decision making between the care team and the patient.**

3. This can be considered a quality outcome of safe care delivery.

4. Measuring the time between clinic visits can be a measure of the efficiency of care delivery.

10. Answer: 1

Rationales:

1. **Post-acute care reform is a U.S. Department of Health and Human Services (HHS) initiative aimed at reducing care fragmentation and unsafe transitions of care such as from acute care hospitals to skilled nursing facilities.**
2. Agency for Healthcare Research and Quality (AHRQ) quality indicators are designed to be used by organizations to identify and study quality concerns and track changes through time. Current quality initiatives include assessing access to health care.
3. The National Database of Nursing Quality Indicators (NDNQI) was initiated by the American Nurses Association and measures nurse-sensitive quality indicators that reflect the structure, process, and outcomes of nursing care, which lead to improved quality and safety at the bedside.
4. Health information technology (IT) is an AHRQ initiative that promotes the development and testing of IT solutions and applications designed to improve the quality of care.

Chapter 12 Questions

1. Answer: 4

Rationales:

1. The Occupational Safety and Health Administration (OSHA) focuses on safety, not on the provision of health care.
2. Many agencies provide training, not just OSHA.
3. OSHA does not focus on practice standards or nursing care.
4. **This is the best, most specific description of the purpose and focus of OSHA.**

2. Answer: 3

Rationales:

1. Coal mines are known to be dangerous work sites.
2. Cleaning the windows of high-rise buildings is known to present some risks to the workers.

3. **Few people realize the many risks encountered by individuals employed in health-care facilities.**
4. Likewise, police work is well known for the risks encountered.

3. Answer: 4

Rationales:

1. The Food and Drug Administration's policies are specific to food and drug safety.
2. The Institute of Medicine makes policy recommendations. It is not a federal agency.
3. The American Nurses Association is also not a federal agency and focuses on nursing-related issues.
4. **The Centers for Disease Control and Prevention is a federal agency that does investigate a wide range of health concerns.**

4. Answer: 1, 3

Rationales:

1. **One of the first steps in violence prevention is to identify what contributes to violence and devise ways to control these things.**
2. Allowing violence to escalate makes the situation worse.
3. **Learning how much staff members know about handling episodes of violence is essential to preparing staff education programs.**
4. Those who have a high potential for violence should not be given greater access to weapons.

5. Answer: 2

Rationales:

1. Increased appetite is not a frequent reaction to exposure to latex.
2. **Allergic contact dermatitis is a frequent reaction to latex for those who are allergic to it.**
3. Increased falls are not common allergic responses to latex.
4. An increase in violent outbursts is not associated with latex allergy.

6. Answer: 4

Rationales:

1. The term *ergonomic* refers to the design of equipment and the use of equipment and

other procedures in a safe and healthy manner. Indoor air pollution is concerned with exposure to toxic substances in the air.
2. Active shooters are human rather than equipment or procedural risks.
3. Nosocomial infections are not ergonomic risks.
4. **Back injuries are a very common ergonomic risk in health care.**

7. Answer: 1, 3

Rationales:

1. **Self-scheduling allows staff to consider both their personal needs and the unit's needs in assigning work shifts.**
2. A large meal at the end of a night shift may make it more difficult to sleep after work.
3. **Consistent days off reduce the circadian rhythm disturbance.**
4. Adjusting visiting hours to end with the end of the day shift may prevent employed visitors from seeing their loved ones and places responsibility for consulting with them entirely on the day shift.

8. Answer: 1, 4

Rationales:

1. **Modification of a work schedule is a reasonable accommodation.**
2. Salary reduction would be discriminatory.
3. Additional days off or extended vacations would be costly and unfair to nondisabled employees.
4. **Adjustment of work procedures to accommodate a person's disability is also a reasonable response.**

9. Answer: 2

Rationales:

1. Windows that can be opened by patients or visitors may present a fall risk; outdoor air may not be less polluted.
2. **Improved ventilation and filtration may reduce indoor air pollution.**
3. Polyvinyl chloride (PVC) is a source of indoor air pollution.
4. Medical waste incinerators are also potential sources of air pollution.

10. Answer: 4

Rationales:

1. Disinfection of the site is insufficient.
2. These actions are also inadequate given the risks associated with a sharps injury.
3. Hepatitis B immunization is appropriate but not sufficient.
4. **PEP (post-exposure prophylaxis) includes the necessary actions to be taken.**

Chapter 13 Questions

1. Answer: 1, 4

Rationales:

1. **Many people would find this behavior offensive in a workplace environment.**
2. Separate restrooms are the norm in our society.
3. Providing coffee and doughnuts to everyone on the staff would not constitute harassment.
4. **Demanding a daily kiss for writing a favorable evaluation could be interpreted as a quid pro quo.**

2. Answer: 1, 4

Rationales:

1. **One of nurses' greatest sources of satisfaction derived from their work is providing high-quality care.**
2. High workloads, especially insufficient numbers of RNs, have been shown to reduce the quality of care and even increase patient mortality.
3. Working in an environment where conflict is virtually continuous is a source of stress for most staff.
4. **On the other hand, showing civility and respect to one another creates an environment in which most nurses can thrive.**

3. Answer: 1

Rationales:

1. **Opportunities to express ideas and make suggestions are empowering.**
2. Discouraging the development of working relationships creates isolation and a sense of powerlessness.
3. Negativity, especially if it is frequent, can create an atmosphere of powerlessness, inadequacy, and hopelessness.

4. Endangering a client's health or safety is not an acceptable strategy.

4. Answer: 3

Rationales:

1. The IHI is concerned with quality of care provided; staff issues are not an issue they are prepared to address.
2. ANA can provide nurses with useful information about the issue of sexual harassment (some state associations can provide some support and guidance as well).
3. **The EEOC is the government agency charged with investigating employment issues such as sexual harassment.**
4. The CDC is concerned with the health of the population but would not be in a position to investigate a specific incident.

5. Answer: 1

Rationales:

1. **Expressions of frustration or powerlessness are clear warnings of burnout.**
2. These may be related to burnout but to other factors as well.
3. This is clearly not a symptom of burnout.
4. Efficiency is not a symptom of burnout, although inefficiency might be.

6. Answer: 4

Rationales:

1. Colleagues rarely criticize a brand new nurse in the first few weeks or "honeymoon" period.
2. New graduates are not usually assigned long hours. Their pay may reflect the amount of training time they require, however.
3. Most new graduates find themselves welcomed by their colleagues.
4. **Excitement about the new (usually first) registered nurse (RN) position is common in the honeymoon phase.**

7. Answer: 1

Rationales:

1. **Providing equal opportunities for raises and promotions is an excellent approach to managing a diverse team.**
2. Ignoring cultural differences does not help staff work with them.

3. Promoting uniformity may appear to be an attempt to diminish diversity.
4. An English-only policy may be troublesome for non-English-speaking patients.

8. Answer: 1, 2, 3

Rationales:

1. **Unprepared equipment should not be used, as it may cause injury or death.**
2. **This represents a Health Insurance Portability and Accountability Act (HIPAA) violation of patient privacy.**
3. **This is an example of an impaired employee.**
4. Although an accident occurred, no one was hurt, and the risk to others (wet floor) was addressed immediately.

9. Answer: 4

Rationales:

1. Verbal abuse may also become very harmful and should not be ignored.
2. A nurse manager's bullying behavior may confuse staff. It may appear that the manager is encouraging it.
3. Presenting these concerns at the annual evaluation delays dealing with it for too long.
4. **Direct but carefully worded confrontations will make it clear that bullying is not tolerated.**

10. Answer: 3

Rationales:

1. Although time away from work may help address fatigue, it is more likely to be an escape from the causes of burnout instead of a solution to it.
2. It is likely that your colleague will encounter the same concerns at the next hospital and will not have learned anything about managing stress or preventing burnout.
3. **These are good opening questions to lead into learning how to manage stress and burnout.**
4. Although it may help to know others have the same problem, it does not solve the problem.

Chapter 14 Questions

1. Answer: 1, 2, 5

Rationales:

   1. **1, 2, 5. Today, job seekers look to online job boards. Contacting specific health-care institutions and organizations and filling out a job application lets employers know that you are interested in working with them.**
   3. The National Council of State Boards of Nursing (NCSBN) is responsible for the National Council Licensure Examination (NCLEX®) and regulatory efforts.
   4. The American Association of Colleges of Nursing provides information for collegiate nursing education and accreditation of schools.

2. Answer: 3

Rationales:

   1. Reviewing the salary scale does not show an interest in the organization.
   2. Researching the benefits package is important when comparing organizations but does not show a prospective employer your interest.
   3. **Before attending an interview, review the organization's philosophy, mission, and values. This demonstrates to the prospective employer that you have an interest in the position and the organization.**
   4. Asking other nurses about the number of patients is not relevant.

3. Answer: 1, 2, 3

Rationales:

   1. **1, 2, 3. In addition to passing the National Council Licensure Examination (NCLEX®), employers cite responsibility, integrity, and interpersonal skills, along with oral and written communication skills, as qualities to emphasize.**
   4. Social skills are not qualities of interest for an employer.
   5. Family values are not of interest to an employer.

4. Answer: 2

Rationales:

   1. A standard résumé in a professional, modern format gives specific details about your skills and experience.

2. **The chronological résumé lists work experiences in order of time, with the most recent experience listed first. This style is useful in showing stable employment without gaps or many job changes. The objective and qualifications are listed at the top.**
   3. Functional résumés focus on your skills and experience, rather than on chronological work history.
   4. A combination résumé is organized into two parts or pages.

5. Answer: 2, 4

Rationales:

   1. Family status is not necessary for a résumé.
   2. **2, 4. If you are a new nursing graduate and have little or no job experience, list your educational background first. Remember that positions you held before you entered nursing might support experience that will be relevant in your nursing career.**
   3. Community service is of interest; however, your education is of primary importance.
   5. Employers are interested in your leadership abilities; however, your education is of primary importance.

6. Answer: 1

Rationales:

   1. **The cover letter will be your introduction. If it is true that first impressions are lasting ones, the cover letter will have a significant impact on your prospective employer.**
   2. Your employment goal should be on your résumé.
   3. The position in the community may be included but is not the purpose of the letter.
   4. The reason for entering nursing is more appropriate for a school application.

7. Answer: 2

Rationales:

   1. Communication is part of any interview; STAR (situation, task, action, result) is specific.
   2. **Many employers use the STAR method, which focuses on behaviors. Be prepared to discuss a situation and describe the task, the action taken, and the result.**

3. Personal questions should not be part of an interview.
4. Many interviewers attempt to create a relaxed environment, but STAR is a technique.

8. Answer: 2

Rationales:

SWOT
S = Strengths
W = Weaknesses
O = Opportunities
T = Threats
Increased competition among health-care facilities or changes in government regulation represent threats.

9. Answer: 1

Rationales:

1. Strengths include the following:
Relevant work experience
Advanced education
Product knowledge
Good communication and people skills
Computer skills
Self-managed learning skills
Flexibility
2. Difficulty adapting to change would be a weakness.
3. The nursing shortage is an opportunity.
4. Competition among health-care facilities is a threat or opportunity.

10. Answer: 1, 3, 4, 5

Rationales:

1. **Furthering professional education and obtaining advanced degrees and certifications indicates to an organization that you want to move forward with your professional career.**
2. Meeting the specific requirements for an entry-level job position does not indicate a commitment to the organization or desire to advance a career.
3. **Seeking new experiences demonstrates a commitment to the organization.**
4. **Volunteering to work on committees demonstrates a commitment to the organization.**
5. **Finding a mentor demonstrates a commitment to the organization.**

Chapter 15 Questions

1. Answer: 2

Rationales:

1. The National Institute of Nursing Research (NINR) primarily supports nursing research.
2. **The National League for Nursing (NLN) supports nursing education.**
3. The American Medical Association (AMA) supports the medical profession.
4. The American Nurses Association (ANA) supports advancement of the nursing profession.

2. Answer: 1

Rationales:

1. **Nursing specialty organizations support the interests of a defined practice area or special interest group.**
2. They may be concerned about nursing's image but are more focused on the specialty or special interest group that defines their purpose.
3. Specialty organizations do not focus on basic preparation.
4. Collective bargaining agreements are generally provided by a union or state nurses association.

3. Answer: 2

Rationales:

1. The American Nurses Association (ANA) does advocate for nurses.
2. **The ANA does not provide health insurance.**
3. The ANA has put considerable effort into making the workplace safer.
4. Improvement of patient safety is an additional concern of the ANA.

4. Answer: 3

Rationales:

1. The National Student Nurses' Association (NSNA) does not provide tutoring or similar assistance.
2. The NSNA does not provide advice in selecting a nursing school.
3. **The NSNA does provide career development information.**
4. The NSNA itself does not provide graduate education.

5. Answer: 1, 3, 4

Rationales:

1. **Associate degree students are eligible for National Student Nurses' Association (NSNA) membership.**
2. Graduates of nursing degree programs are not eligible.
3. **Diploma school students are eligible for NSNA membership.**
4. **Baccalaureate degree students are also eligible for NSNA membership.**

6. Answer: 4

Rationales:

1. Nursing degrees typically have a higher time demand than do non-nursing degrees.
2. Learning about other professions is useful but not as important as advancing knowledge and skills in one's own profession.
3. Likewise, the broader focus of non-nursing degrees fails to provide advanced preparation in nursing.
4. **Advancing one's knowledge and skills in one's own profession is the primary goal of obtaining a higher degree.**

7. Answer: 1, 3

Rationales:

1. **Students generally are assigned fewer patients.**
2. Productivity expectations for the practicing nurse are higher.
3. **Efficiency is emphasized more in practice than in school.**
4. Shorter hours and fewer back-to-back workdays characterize student assignments.

8. Answer: 1, 4

Rationales:

1. **Being matched with an experienced nurse mentor is very valuable for the new graduate.**
2. Transitions take time; there is no advantage to rushing through them.
3. Again, rushing through the transition has little advantage and may leave the new graduate unprepared for the full responsibility of a practicing nurse.
4. **Opportunities to network with peers provide support and a chance to hear others' ideas for making a successful transition.**

9. Answer: 3

Rationales:

1. Transition includes changing one's identity from student to nurse.
2. New graduates are not ready for management and may fail to mature as a practicing nurse if they move into management too quickly.
3. **The organization is the context in which a nurse practices and has an important influence on the practice environment.**
4. Focusing on one's stress may increase negativity and may impede programs through the transition. Stress needs to be managed and eventually reduced, but it is not the primary focus of your transition.

10. Answer: 2

Rationales:

1. The Promise phase is an early phase that follows transitions to practicing nurse.
2. **The Harvest phase is the time when you reach your prime, usually the final phase of your career.**
3. Transition (from student to practicing nurse) is the first phase.
4. The Momentum phase is usually the middle phase of your career.

Chapter 16 Questions

1. Answer: 3

Rationales:

1. There are health-care systems in other countries that are less expensive but have better outcomes in terms of population health indicators.
2. U.S. health care is expensive, not efficient.
3. **There are many ways in which the U.S. health-care system could be improved.**
4. Given the number of health disparities, the current conclusion is that the U.S. health-care system does not meet everyone's needs.

2. Answer: 3

Rationales:

1. The U.S. government pays a large portion of the health-care bill but not all of it.
2. The head of household may contribute to the cost of health care, but most do not pay the majority of the bill.
3. **Government entities (state and federal) and employers together pay for most of the cost of health care in the United States.**
4. Employees and their families contribute but do not pay for most of the cost of health care.

3. Answer: 4

Rationales:

1. Health-care insurance is not universally available in the United States.
2. Likewise, it is not available to everyone.
3. Neither health care nor health-care insurance is free in the United States.
4. **Health-care insurance in the United States is relatively expensive.**

4. Answer: 2

Rationales:

1. Nurses today have many independent functions.
2. **Nurses constitute the largest health-care profession by numbers.**
3. Nurses are not the most powerful lobbying group in health care but have considerable potential to influence legislation.
4. Not all nurses are women; not all wear white.

5. Answer: 2, 3, 4

Rationales:

1. Taking a course will help you be a better-informed advocate but not be "visible and vocal."
2. **Speaking out is being "vocal."**
3. **Writing letters and e-mails are also ways to be visible and vocal.**
4. **Likewise, appearing on radio or television is both visible and vocal.**

6. Answer: 2

Rationales:

1. Antibiotic-resistant infections continue to be a great concern.

2. **Both polio and smallpox are relatively well controlled.**
3. Opioid-related deaths are increasing.
4. Health disparities are a continuing concern.

7. Answer: 2, 3, 4

Rationales:

1. Increased use of electronic health records (EHRs) is occurring but is not a major problem.
2. **Outcomes that are less than optimal continue to be a concern.**
3. **The number of uninsured also continues to be a concern.**
4. **Likewise, high costs continue to be a concern.**

8. Answer: 3

Rationales:

1. The American Nurses Association's (ANA's) political action committee (PAC) actively advocates for nursing and for patients.
2. Visiting one's representatives continues to be an effective strategy.
3. **Talking only with one's friends is less likely to be effective.**
4. Speaking on public media is another effective strategy.

9. Answer: 1

Rationales:

1. **Aging of the current nurse population continues to be a concern.**
2. Demand for nursing care is not decreasing; oversupply occurs only sporadically.
3. Evidence-based practice is a positive trend.
4. The use of electronic health records (EHRs) is also a positive trend.

10. Answer: 1

Rationales:

1. **Many believe that people have a right to forego insurance if they wish.**
2. School-based centers themselves are not highly controversial, but some of the services they might offer could be.
3. There is considerable support for eliminating the preexisting condition clause.
4. There is also support for eliminating lifetime limits on insurance.

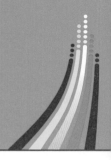

Bibliography

Chapter 1 References

Al-Rubaish, A. M. (2010). Professionalism today. *Journal of Family and Community Medicine, 17*(1), 1–2. https://doi.org/10.4103/1319-1683.68781

American Nurses Association. (2006). https://www.nursingworld.org/

Ang, S., Rockstuhl, T., & Tan, M. L. (2015). Cultural intelligence and competencies. In *International encyclopedi of the social and behavioral sciences* (2nd ed., pp. 433–439). Science Direct. https://www.sciencedirect.com/science/article/pii/B9780080970868250502?via%3Dihub

Beletz, E. (1974). Is nursing's public image up-to-date? *Nursing Outlook, 22,* 432–435. https://doi.org/10.1177/019394598801000410

Black, B. P. (2014). *Professional nursing: Concepts and challenges* (7th ed.). Saunders-Elsevier, Inc.

Bragg, J. (2014). Lead to succeed through generational differences. *American Nurse Today, 9*(10). https://www.americannursetoday.com/lead-succeed-generational-differences

Breckinridge, M. (1952). *Wide neighborhoods: A story of the Frontier Nursing Service.* University Press of Kentucky.

Bureau of Labor Statistics. (2017). *Employment projections 2016–2026.* https://www.bls.gov/news.release/pdf/ecopro.pdf

Cardillo, D. (2013). Is nursing a profession or a job? *American Nurse Today.* https://www.americannursetoday.com/blog/is-nursing-a-profession-or-a-job/

Centers for Medicare and Medicaid Services. (2017). *History of Medicare and Medicaid.* http://www.cms.gov/About-CMS/Agency-Information/History/index.html?redirect=/history/

Clarke, C. (2015). Conversations to inspire and promote a more civil workplace. *American Nurse Today, 10*(11). https://www.americannursetoday.com/cne-civility/

Dik, B. J., & Duffy, R. D. (2009). Calling and vocation at work: Definitions and prospects for research and practice. *The Counseling Psychologist, 37*(3), 424–450. https://doi.org/10.1177/0011000008316430

Feissner, T. (2015). *Grace under pressure: Professionalism and problem solving.* https://planetdepos.com/grace-under-pressure-professionalism-and-problem-solving/

Henderson, V. (1966). *The nature of nursing: A definition and its implications for practice, education and research.* MacMillan & Co.

Institute of Medicine. (2010). *The future of nursing: Leading change, advancing health.* http://books.nap.edu/openbook.php?record_id=12956&page=R1

Jeong, S., & Kim, J. (2022). Factors influencing nurses' intention to care for patients with COVID-19: Focusing on positive psychological capital and nursing professionalism. *PLoS One, 17*(1), E0262786. https://doi.org/10.1371/journal.pone.0262786

Kalisch, P. A., & Kalisch, B. J. (2004). *American nursing: A history.* Lippincott Williams & Wilkins.

Kub, J. E., Kulbok, P. A., Miner, S., & Merrill, J. A. (2017). Increasing the capacity of public health nursing to strengthen the public health infrastructure and to promote and protect the health of communities and populations. *Nursing Outlook, 65*(5), 661–664. https://doi.org/10.1016/j.outlook.2017.08.009

Luis, C., & Vance, C. (2020). A pandemic crisis: Mentoring, leadership and the millennial nurse. *Nursing Economics, 38*(3), 152–154, 163.

McKay, D. R. (2017). *Professionalism in the workplace: How to conduct yourself on the job.* https://www.thebalancecareers.com/professionalism-526248

Moore, J. M., Everly, M., & Bauer, R. (2016). Multigenerational challenges: Teambuilding for positive clinical workforce outcomes. *Online Journal of Issues in Nursing, 21*(2). http://ojin.nursingworld.org/MainMenuCategories/ANAMarketplace/ANAPeriodicals/OJIN/TableofContents/Vol-21-2016/No2-May-2016/Multigenerational-Challenges.html

National Council of State Boards of Nursing. (2012). *What you need to know about licensing and state boards of nursing.* https://www.ncsbn.org

National Council of State Boards of Nursing. (2016). *NCLEX-RN® test plan.* https://www.ncsbn.org/exams/testplans.page

National Council of State Boards of Nursing. (2018). *Licensure compacts.* https://www.ncsbn.org/compacts.htm

National Hospice and Palliative Care Organization. (2012). *Hospice: A historical perspective.* http://www.nhpco.org/history-hospice-care

Nightingale, F. (1992). *Notes on nursing: What it is and what it is not.* J. B. Lippincott. (Original work published in 1859.)

Porter-O'Grady, T. (2003). A different age for leadership, Part 1: New context, new content. *Journal of Nursing Administration, 33*(2), 105–110.

Post, P. (2014). Traits that convey character also define a professional. *Boston Globe Business.* https://www.bostonglobe.com/business/2014/08/16/just-what-does-mean-professional/MTIZfzUhw4cDphH6E99LIO/story.html

Roberts, M. (1937). Florence Nightingale as a nurse educator. *American Journal of Nursing, 37,* 775.

Rogers, M. E. (1988). Nursing science and art: A perspective. *Nursing Science Quarterly, 1,* 99–102.

Roux, G., & Halstead, J. A. (2018). *Issues and trends in nursing* (2nd ed.). Jones & Bartlett Learning.

Saks, M. (2012). Defining a profession: The role of knowledge and expertise. *Professions and Professionalism, 2*(1), 1–10.

Shohani, M., & Zamanzadeh, V. (2017). Nurses' attitude towards professionalization and factors influencing it. *Journal of Caring Sciences, 6*(4), 345–357. https://doi.org/10.15171/jcs.2017.033

Smiley, R. A., Ruttinger, C., Oliveira, C. M., Hudson, L. R., Allgeyer, R., Kyrani, A. R., Silvestre, J. H., Alexander, M., & Reneau, K. A. (2020). The 2020 National Nursing Workforce Survey. *Journal of Nursing Regulation, 12*(1), S1–S96. https://doi.org/10.1016/S2155-8256(21)00027-2

Spurlock, D. (2020). The nursing shortage and the future of nursing is in our hands. *Journal of Nursing Education, 59*(6), 303–304. https://doi.org/10.3928/01484834-20200520-0

Texas Tech University Vietnam Center and Archive. (2017). *Celebrating the nurses of the Vietnam War.* https://www.vietnam.ttu.edu/exhibits/nurses/

Warrington, J. (1839). *The nurse's guide: A series of instructions to females who wish to engage in the important business of nursing mother and child in the lying-in chamber.* Thomas Cowperthwait and Co. http://www.nursing.upenn.edu

Wheatley, C. (2017). Nursing overtime: Should it be regulated? *Nursing Economics, 35*(4), 213–217.

Chapter 2 References

Al-Jabir, A., Kerwan, A., Nicola, M., Alsafi, Z., Khan, M., Sohrabi, C., O'Neill, N., Iosifidis, C., Griffin, M., Mathew, G., & Agha, R. (2020). Impact of the coronavirus (COVID-19) pandemic on surgical practice—Part 2 (surgical prioritization). *International Journal of Surgery (London, England), 79*, 233–248. https://doi.org/10.1016/j.ijsu.2020.05.002

American Association of Critical Care Nurses. (2018). *Improving work environment could reduce moral distress.* https://www.aacn.org/newsroom/improving-work-environment-could-reduce-moral-distress

American Nurses Association. (2020). *Nurses, ethics and the response to COVID-19.* https://www.nursingworld.org/~495c6c/globalassets/practiceandpolicy/work-environment/health–safety/coronavirus/nurses-ethics-and-the-response-to-the-covid-19-pandemic.pdf

Ayanian, J. Z. (2020). Mental health needs of health care workers providing frontline COVID-19 care. *JAMA Health Forum, I*(4), e200397. https://doi.org/10.1001/jamahealthforum

Ball, P. (2015). Complex societies evolved without belief in all-powerful deity. *Nature.* https://www.nature.com/news/complex-societies-evolved-without-belief-in-all-powerful-deity-1.17040#/ref-link-2

Barker, C. F., & Markmann, J. F. (2013). Historical overview of transplantation. *Cold Spring Harbor Perspectives in Medicine, 3*(4), a014977. https://doi.org/10.1101/cshperspect.a014977

Barlow, N. A., Hargreaves, J., & Gillibrand, W. P. (2018). Nurses' contributions to the resolution of ethical dilemmas in practice. *Nursing Ethics, 25*(2), 230–242. https://doi.org/10.1177/0969733017703700

Baumane-Vitolina, I., Cals, I., & Sumilo, E. (2016). Is ethics rational? Teleological, deontological and virtue ethics theories reconciled in the context of traditional economic decision making. *Procedia Economics and Finance, 39*(2), 108–114. https://doi.org/10.1016/S2212-5671(16)30249-0

Beltran-Aroca, C. M., Girela-Lopez, E., Collazo-Chao, E., Montero-Pérez-Barquero, M., & Muñoz-Villanueva, M. C. (2016). Confidentiality breaches in clinical practice: What happens in hospitals? *BMC Medical Ethics, 17*(1), 52. https://doi.org/10.1186/s12910-016-0136-y

Benner, P., & Wrubel, J. (1989). *The primacy of caring: Stress and coping in health and illness.* Addison Wesley Publishing.

Bian, J., Li, L., Sun, J., Deng, J., Li, Q., Zhang, X., & Yan, L. (2019). The influence of self-relevance and cultural values on moral orientation. *Frontiers in Psychology, 10*, 292. https://doi.org/10.3389/fpsyg.2019.00292

Butler, J. M. (2015). The future of forensic DNA analysis. *Philosophical Transactions of the Royal Society of London. Series B, Biological Sciences, 370*(1674), 20140252. https://doi.org/10.1098/rstb.2010.0410

Capp, S., Savage, S., & Clarke, V. (2001). Exploring distributive justice in healthcare. *Australian Health Review, 24*(2), 40–44. https://doi.org/10.1071/ah010040

Carruci, R. (2016, December 16). Why ethical people make unethical choices. *Harvard Business Review.* https://hbr.org/2016/12/why-ethical-people-make-unethical-choices

Cavallari, L. H. (2021). Moving pharmacogenetics into practice: It's all about the evidence! *Clinical Pharmacology and Therapeutics, 110*(3), 649–661. https://doi.org/10.1002/cpt.2327

Centers for Disease Control and Prevention. (2015). *Health care cost measures.* https://www.cdc.gov/workplacehealthpromotion/model/evaluation

Choi, S., Jang, I., Park, S., & Lee, H. (2014). Effects of organizational culture, self-leadership and empowerment on job satisfaction and turnover intention in general hospital nurses. *Journal of Korean Academy of Nursing Administration, 20*(2), 206–214. https://doi.org/10.11111/jkana.2014.20.2.206

Ekmekci, P. E., & Arda, B. (2015). Enhancing John Rawls's theory of justice to cover health and social determinants of health. *Acta Bioethica, 21*(2), 227–236. https://doi.org/10.4067/S1726-569X2015000200009

Epstein, E. G., & Hamric, A. B. (2009). Moral distress, moral residue, and the crescendo effect. *The Journal of Clinical Ethics, 20*(4), 330–342.

Feeney, O., Cockbain, J., & Sterckx, S. (2021). Ethics, patents and genome editing: A critical assessment of three options of technology governance. *Frontiers in Political Science, 3*(9). https://doi.org/10.3389/fpos.2021.731505

Fisher, O. M., Brown, K., Coker, D. J., McBride, K. E., Steffens, D., Koh, C. E., & Sandroussi, C. (2020). Distributive justice during the coronavirus disease 2019 pandemic in Australia. *ANZ Journal of Surgery, 90*(6), 961–962. https://doi.org/10.1111/ans.16069

Fourie, C. (2015). Moral distress and moral conflict in clinical ethics. *Bioethics, 29*(2), 91–97. https://doi.org/10.1111/bioe.12064

Gong, Y., Song, H. Y., Wu, X., & Hua, L. (2015). Identifying barriers and benefits in patient safety event reporting toward user centered design. *Safety in Health, 1*(7), 1–9. https://safetyinhealth.biomedcentral.com/articles/10.1186/2056-5917-1-7

Greene, D., Hoffman, A. L., & Stark, L. (2019). Better, nicer, cleaner, fairer: A critical assessment of the movement for ethical artificial intelligence and machine learning. In *Hawaii International Conference on*

System Sciences pp. 1–10). Proceedings of the 52nd Hawaii International Conference on System Sciences.

Hagendorff, T. (2020). The ethics of AI ethics: An evaluation of guidelines. *Minds and Machines, 30*(1), 99–120.

Hamric, A. B. (2014). Case study of moral distress. *Journal of Hospice and Palliative Nursing, 16*(8), 457–463. https://doi.org/10.1097/NJH .0000000000000104

Hanel, P., Maio, G. R., Soares, A., Vione, K. C., de Holanda Coelho, G. L., Gouveia, V. V., Patil, A. C., Kamble, S. V., & Manstead, A. (2018). Cross-cultural differences and similarities in human value instantiation. *Frontiers in Psychology, 9,* 849. https://doi.org /10.3389/fpsyg.2018.00849

Henderson, L. W. (2009). A tribute to Willem Johan Kolff, M.D., 1912–2009. *Journal of the American Society of Nephrology, 20*(5), 923–924. https://doi. org/10.1053/j .jvca.2012.11.011

Hine, K. (2011). What is the outcome of applying principlism? *Theoretical Medicine and Bioethics, 32*(6), 375–388. https://doi.org/10.1007/ s11017-011-9185-x

Hume, D. (1978). A treatise of human nature. In O. A. Johnson, *Ethics* (4th ed.). Holt, Reinhart & Winston.

Huxley, A. (1932). *Brave new world.* Harper Row Publishers. Institute for Healthcare. (2018). *Patient safety.* http://www.ihi.org/Topics/PatientSafety/Pages /default.aspx

Jie, L. (2015). The patient suicide attempt: An ethical dilemma case study. *International Journal of Nursing Sciences, 2*(4), 408–413. https://doi.org/10.1016/j .ijnss.2015.01.013

Johnstone, M. J. (2011). Nursing and justice as a basic human need. *Nursing Philosophy, 12*(1), 34–44. https://doi. org/10.1111/j.1466-769X.2010.00459.x

Kant, I. (1949). *Fundamental principles of the metaphysics of morals.* Liberal Arts.

Keshta, I., & Odeh, A. (2020). Security and privacy of electronic health records: Concerns and challenges. *Egyptian Informatics Journal, 22*(2), 177–183. https://doi.org/10.1016/j.eij.2020.07.003

Kirschenbaum, H. (2011). From values clarification to character education: A personal journey. *Journal of Humanistic Counseling, 39*(1), 4–20. https://doi .org/10.1002/j.2164-490X.2000.tb00088.x

Kooli, C. (2021). COVID-19: Public health issues and ethical dilemmas. *Ethics, Medicine, and Public Health, 17,* 100635. https://doi.org/10.1016/j.jemep.2021 .100635

Leonard, K. (2018, March 15). The importance of ethics in organizations. *Small Business—Chron.com.* http:// smallbusiness.chron.com/importance-ethics -organizations-20925.html

Luzum, J. A., Petry, N., Taylor, A. K., Van Driest, S. L., Dunnenberger, H. M., &

Ma, H. K. (2013). The moral development of the child: An integrated model. *Frontiers in Public Health, 1*(57), 16–21. https://doi.org/10.3389/fpubh.2013.00057

Malone, S. (2017). Conjoined twins posed ethical dilemma for Massachusetts hospital. *Health News.* https://www.reuters.com/article/us-usa-health-ethics /conjoined-twins-posed-ethical-dilemma-for- massachusetts-hospital-idUSKBN1CU31Z

Maxwell, B., & Narvaez, D. (2013). Moral foundations theory and moral development and education. *Journal*

of Moral Education, 42(3), 271–280. https://www .tandfonline.com/toc/cjme20/42/3

McHugh, C., & Way, J. (2018). What is good reasoning? *Philosophy and Phenomenological Research, 96*(1), 153–174. https://doi.org/10.1111/phpr.12299

McLeod-Sordjan, R. (2014). Evaluating moral reasoning in nursing education. *Nursing Ethics, 21*(4), 473–483. https://doi.org/10.1177/0969733013505309

Merriam-Webster. (2017). *Value.* Retrieved November 9, 2022 from https://www.merriam-webster.com /dictionary/value

Morley, G. (2016). Perspective: The moral distress debate. *Journal of Research in Nursing, 27*(7), 570–575. https://doi.org/10.1177/1744987116666701

Morley, G., Grady, C., McCarthy, J., & Ulrich, C. M. (2020). COVID-19: Ethical challenges for nurses. *The Hastings Center Report, 50*(3), 35–39. https://doi .org/10.1002/hast.1110

National Institutes of Health. (2021). *The human genome project.* https://www.genome.gov/human-genome -project

Numminen, O., Repo, H., & Leino-Kilpi, H. (2017). Moral courage in nursing: A concept analysis. *Nursing Ethics, 24*(8), 878–891. https://doi.org/10.1177 /0969733016634155

Oh, Y., & Gastmans, C. (2015). Moral distress experienced by nurses: A quantitative literature review. *Nursing Ethics, 22*(1), 15–31. https://doi. org/10.1177/0969733013502803

Olsen, L. L., & Stokes, F. (2016). *The ANA Code of Ethics with Interpretive Statements:* Resource for nursing regulation. *Journal of Nursing Regulation, 7*(2), 9–20. https://doi.org/10.1016/S2155-8256(16)31073-0

Ostlund, U., Backstrom, B., Lindh, V., Sundin, K., & Saveman, B. I. (2015). Nurses' fidelity to theory-based core components when implementing family health conversations: A qualitative inquiry. *Scandinavian Journal of Caring Sciences, 29*(3), 582–590. https://doi .org/10.1111/scs.12178

Picker Institute. (2020). *Impact report 2019–2020.* Picker Institute.

Piergentili, R., Del Rio, A., Signore, F., Umani Ronchi, F., Marinelli, E., & Zaami, S. (2021). CRISPR-Cas and its wide-ranging applications: From human genome editing to environmental implications, technical limitations, hazards and bioethical issues. *Cells, 10*(5), 969. https://doi.org/10.3390/cells10050969

ProCon.org. (2018). *State-by-state guide to physician assisted suicide.* https://euthanasia.procon.org/view. resource.php?resourceID=000132

ProCon.org. (2021). *States with legal physician-assisted suicide.* https://euthanasia.procon.org/ states-with-legal-physician-assisted-suicide/

Quill, T. E. (2005). Terri Schiavo: A tragedy compounded. *New England Journal of Medicine, 352*(16), 1630–1633.https://doi.org/10.1056 /NEJMp058062

Rahmani, A., Ghahramanian, A., & Alahbakhshian, A. (2010). Respecting to patients' autonomy in viewpoint of nurses and patients in medical–surgical wards. *Iranian Journal of Nursing and Midwifery Research, 15*(1), 14–19.

Rainey, J. (2018). Familial DNA puts elusive killers behind bars. *NBC News.* April 28, 2018. https://www .nbcnews.com/news/us-news/familial-dna-puts-elusive -killers-behind-bars-only-12-states-n869711

Raths, L. E., Harmon, M., & Simmons, S. B. (1979). *Values and teaching.* Charles E. Merrill.

Sahebi, A., Moayedi, S., & Golitaleb, M. (2020). COVID-19 pandemic and the ethical challenges in patient care. *Journal of Medical Ethics and History of Medicine, 13*, 24. https://doi.org/10.18502/jmehm.v13i24.4955

Sakellariouv, A. M. (2015). Virtue ethics and its potential as the leading moral theory. *Discussions, 12*(1). http://www.inquiriesjournal.com/a?id=1385

Severini, E. (2021). Moral progress and evolution: Knowledge versus understanding. *Ethical Theory Moral Practice, 24*, 87–105. https://doi.org/10.1007/s10677-021-10158-8

Shahriari, M., Mohammadi, E., Abbaszadeh, A., & Bahrami, M. (2013). Nursing ethical values and definitions: A literature review. *Iranian Journal of Nursing and Midwifery Research, 18*(1), 1–8.

Silverman, H. J., Kheirbek, R. E., Moscou-Jackson, G., & Day, J. (2021). Moral distress in nurses caring for patients with COVID-19. *Nursing Ethics, 28*(7–8), 1137–1164. https://doi.org/10.1177/09697330211003217

Sivandzade, F., & Cucullo, L. (2021). Regenerative stem cell therapy for neurodegenerative diseases: An overview. *International Journal of Molecular Sciences, 22*(4), 2153. https://doi.org/10.3390/ijms22042153

Skedgel, C., Wailoo, A., & Akehurst, R. (2015). Societal preferences for distributive justice in the allocation of healthcare resources: A latent class discrete choice experiment. *Medical Decision Making, 35*(1), 94–105. https://doi.org/10.1177/0272989X14547915

Sokol, D. K. (2007). Can deceiving patients be morally acceptable? *BMJ: British Medical Journal, 334*(7601), 984–986. https://doi.org/10.1136/bmj.39184.419826.80

Taylor, J. (2012, May 12). Personal growth: Your values, your life. *Psychology Today.* https://www.psychologytoday.com/us/blog/the-power-prime/201205/personal-growth-your-values-your-life

Thompson, J., & Thompson, H. (1992). *Bioethical decision-making for nurses.* Appleton-Century-Crofts.

Toren, O., & Wagner, N. (2010). Applying an ethical decision-making tool to a nurse management dilemma. *Nursing Ethics, 17*(3), 393–402. https://doi.org/10.1177/0969733009355106

Tuckett, A. (2015). Speaking with one voice. *Nurse Education in Practice, 15*(4), 258–264. https://doi.org/10.1016/j.nepr.2015.02.004

Varelius, J. (2013). Ending life, morality, and meaning. *Ethical Theory and Moral Practice, 16*(3), 559–574. http://www.jstor.org/stable/24478619

Varkey, B. (2021). Principles of clinical ethics and their application to practice. *Medical Principles and Practice: International Journal of the Kuwait University, Health Science Centre, 30*(1), 17–28. https://doi.org/10.1159/000509119

Vincent, J. L. (2013). Critical care: Where have we been and where are we going? *Critical Care 2013, 17*(Suppl. 1), S:2. https://doi.org/10.1186/cc11500

Zahedi, F., Sanjari, M., Aala, M., Peymani, M., Aramesh, K., Parsapour, A., Madah, S. B., Cheraghi, M., Mirzabeigi, G., Larijani, B., & Dastgerdi, M. V. (2013). The code of ethics for nurses. *Iranian Journal of Public Health, 42*(Suppl. 1), 1–8.

Zimmerman, M. J., & Zalta, E. N. (2014). Intrinsic vs. extrinsic values. *Stanford Encyclopedia of Philosophy.* https://plato.stanford.edu/entries/value-intrinsic-extrinsic/

Chapter 3 References

Altman, S. H., Butler, A. S., & Shern, L. (2016). *Assessing progress on the Institute of Medicine Report: The future of nursing.* National Academies Press. https://doi.org/10.17226/21838

American Nurses Association. (1992).

American Nurses Association. (2005). *American Nurses Association statement on the Terri Schiavo case.* https://www.legis.iowa.gov/docs/publications/SD/19318.pdf

American Nurses Association. (2012). *Nursing care and Do Not Resuscitate (DNR) and Allow Natural Death (AND) decisions.* https://www.nursingworld.org/practice-policy/nursing-excellence/official-position-statements/id/nursing-care-and-do-not-resuscitate-dnr-and-allow-natural-death-and-decisions/

American Nurses Association. (2015). *Nursing scope and standards of practice.* The American Nurses Association.

American Nurses Association. (2021). *Nursing: Scope and standards of practice* (4th ed.). American Nurses Association.

American Nurses Association. (2022). ANA statement in response to the conviction of nurse RaDonda Vaught. *Nursing World.* https://www.nursingworld.org/news/news-releases/2022-news-releases/statement-in-response-to-the-conviction-of-nurse-radonda-vaught/

Bal, B. S., & Choma, T. J. (2012). What to disclose? Revisiting informed consent. *Clinical Orthopaedics and Related Research, 470*(5), 1346–1356. https://doi.org/10.1007/s11999-011-2232-0

Balestra, M. (2018). Telehealth and legal implications. *The Journal for Nurse Practitioners, 14*(1), 33-39.

Bernhardt, M., Alber, J., & Gold, R. S. (2014). A social media primer for professionals: Digital do's and don'ts. *Health Promotion Practice, 15*(2), 168–172. https://doi.org/10.1177/1524839913517235

Best, M., & Neuhauser, D. (2004). Avedis Donabedian: Father of quality assurance and poet. *Quality & Safety in Health Care, 13*(6), 472–473. https://doi.org/10.1136/qshc.2004.012591

Cantor, M., Braddock, C., Derse, A., Edwards, D., Louge, G., Nelson, W., Prudhomme, J., & Fox, E. (2003). Do not resuscitate orders and medical futility. *Archives of Internal Medicine, 163*, 2689–2694.

Catalano, L. A. (2014). What you need to know about electronic documentation. *American Nurse Today, 9*(11). https://www.americannursetoday.com/need-know-electronic-documentation/

Centers for Medicare and Medicaid Services. (2010). *The Patient's Bill of Rights.* https://www.cms.gov/CCIIO/Programs-and-Initiatives/Health-Insurance-Market-Reforms/Patients-Bill-of-Rights.html

Charters, K. G. (2003). HIPAA's latest privacy rule. *Policy, Politics & Nursing Practice, 4*(1), 75–78. https://doi.org/10.1177/1527154402239459

Denecke, K., Bamidis, P., Bond, C., Gabarron, E., Househ, M., Lau, A. Y., Mayer, M. A., Merolli, M & Hansen, M. (2015). Ethical issues of social media usage in healthcare. *Yearbook of Medical Informatics, 10*(1), 137–147. https://doi.org/10.15265/IY-2015-001

Department of Justice. (2015). *Citizen's guide to U.S. law on obscenity.* https://www.justice.gov/criminal-ceos/citizens-guide-us-federal-law-obscenity

Feringa, M. M., DeSwardt, H. C., & Havenga, Y. (2018). Registered nurses' knowledge, attitude, practice and regulation regarding their scope of practice: A literature review. *International Journal of Africa Nursing Sciences, 8*(4), 87–97. https://doi.org/10.4102/hsag.v25i0.1415

Finnel, D. S., Thomas, E. L., Nehring, W. M., McLoughlin, K. A., & Bickford, C. J. (2015). Best practices for developing professional standards and scope of practice. *The Online Journal of Issues in Nursing, 20*(2). http://ojin.nursingworld.org/MainMenuCategories/ANAMarketplace/ANAPeriodicals/OJIN/TableofContents/Vol-20-2015/No2-May-2015/Best-Practices-for-Developing-Specialty-Scope-and-Standards.html

Garner, B. A. (2014). *Black's law dictionary* (10th ed.). West Publishers.

Geraghty, S., Hari, R., & Oliver, K. (2021). Using social media in contemporary nursing: risks and benefits. British journal of nursing (Mark Allen Publishing), *30*(18), 1078–1082. https://doi.org/10.12968/bjon.2021.30.18.107

Grant, S. C. (2021). Informed consent: We can and should do better. *Journal of the American Medical Association Network Open, 4*(4), e2110848. https://doi.org/10.1001/jamanetworkopen.2021.10848

Grant v. Pacific Medical Center, Inc. (2014). Supreme Court No. 90429-4 Court of Appeals No. 69643-2-I. https://www.courts.wa.gov/content/petitions/90429-4%20Answer%20to%20Petition%20for%20Review%20Pacific%20Medical%20Center%20et%20al.pdf

Guglielmo, W. J. (2013). Nurse reveals STD patient to girlfriend, patient sues and more. *Medscape Nurses.* https://www.medscape.com/viewarticle/803758

Gupta, U. C. (2013). Informed consent in clinical research: Revisiting few concepts and areas. *Perspectives in Clinical Research, 4*(1), 26–32. https://doi.org/10.4103/2229-3485.106373

Hall, D. E., Prochazka, A. V., & Fink, A. S. (2012). Informed consent for clinical treatment. *CMAJ : Canadian Medical Association Journal, 184*(5), 533–540. https://doi.org/10.1503/cmaj.112120

Hartung, K. (2018). *Lawsuits allege dancing doctor was negligent.* CNN. https://www.cnn.com/2018/05/25/health/dancing-doctor-malpractice-suits/index.html

Hayes, S. A., Zive, D., Ferrell, B., & Tolle, S. W. (2017). The role of advanced practice registered nurses in the completion of physician orders for life-sustaining treatment. *Journal of Palliative Medicine, 20*(4), 415–419. https://doi.org/10.1089/jpm.2016.0228

H.R. 5067 — 101st Congress. (1995). *Patient Self Determination Act of 1990.* https://www.govtrack.us/congress/bills/101/hr5067

Jacoby, S. R., & Scruth, E. A. (2017). Negligence and the nurse: The value of the Code of Ethics for Nurses. *Clinical Nurse Specialist, 31*(4), 183–185. https://doi.org/10.1097/NUR.0000000000000301

Kelman, B. (2022a). In nurse's trial, investigator says hospital bears "heavy" responsibility for patient death. *Kaiser Health News (KHN)*, March 24, 2022. https://khn.org/news/article/radonda-vaught-fatal-drug-error-vanderbilt-hospital-responsibility/

Kelman, B. (2022b) Tennessee nurse convicted in lethal drug error sentenced to three years probation. Retrieved from https://www.npr.org/sections/health-shots/2022/05/13/1098867553/nurse-sentenced-probation

LaMance, K. (2018). *What is tort law?* https://www.legalmatch.com/law-library/article/what-is-tort-law.html

MacMillan, C. (2013). Social media revolution and blurring of professional boundaries. *Imprint, 60*(3), 44–46.

Maloney, P., & Harper, M. G. (2016). Nursing professional development: Standards of professional practice. *Journal for Nurses in Professional Development, 32*(6), 327–330. https://doi.org/10.1097/NND.0000000000000300

McConnell v. Williams. (1949). https://casetext.com/case/mcconnell-v-williams

Moffett, P. M., & Moore, G. P. (2011). The standard of care: Legal history and definitions: The bad and good news. *Western Journal of Emergency Medicine, 12*(1), 109–112.

Moore, G. P., Moffet, P. M., Fider, C., & Moore, M. J. (2014). What emergency physicians should know about informed consent. *Academic Emergency Medicine, 21*(8), 922–927. https://doi.org/10.1111/acem.12429

Peck, J. L. (2014). Social media in nursing education: Responsible integration for meaningful use. *Journal of Nursing Education, 53*(3), 164–169. https://doi.org/10.3928/01484834-20140219-03

Pohlman, K. J. (2015). Why you need your own malpractice insurance. *American Nurse Today, 10*(11). https://www.americannursetoday.com/need-malpractice-insurance/

Reagan, W. (1998). Doctor orders nurses not to "code" patient: Case in point *Wendland v. Sparks. The Reagan Report on Nursing Law, 38*(11), 2. https://case-law.findlaw.com/ia-supreme-court/1267103.html

Riches, S., & Allen, V. (2013). *Keenan and Riches business law* (11th ed.). Pearson Co.

Rose, L., Yu, L., Casey, J., Cook, A., Metaxa, V., Pattison, N., Rafferty, A. M., Ramsay, P., Saha, S., Xyrichis, A., & Meyer, J. (2021). Communication and virtual visiting for families of patients in intensive care during the COVID-19 pandemic: A UK national survey. *Annals of the American Thoracic Society, 18*(10), 1685–1692. https://doi.org/10.1513/AnnalsATS.202012-1500OC

Sabatino, C. (2007). *Advance directives and advance care planning: Legal and policy issues.* https://aspe.hhs.gov/system/files/pdf/75366/adacplpi.pdf

Sabatino, C. P. (2010). The evolution of health care advance planning law and policy. *The Milbank Quarterly, 88*(2), 211–239. https://doi.org/10.1111/j.1468-0009.2010.00596.x

Sanbar, S. S. (2007). *Legal medicine* (7th ed.). Mosby-Elsevier.

Schloendorff v. Society of New York Hospital. 105 N.E. 92 (N.Y. 1914).

Shea, N., & Bayne, T. (2010). The vegetative state and the science of consciousness. *The British Journal for the Philosophy of Science, 61*(3), 459–484. https://doi.org/10.1093/bjps/axp046

Sohn, D. H. (2013). Negligence, genuine error, and litigation. *International Journal of General Medicine, 6*, 49–56. https://doi.org/10.2147/IJGM.S24256

Springer, G. (2015). When and how to use restraints. *American Nurse Today, 10*(1). https://www.americannursetoday.com/use-restraints/

Stern, H. (1949). *McConnell v. Williams*, Supreme Court of Pennsylvania Mar. 24, 1949 361 Pa. 355 (Pa. 1949). https://casetext.com/case/mcconnell-v-williams

The Joint Commission on Healthcare. (2016). Informed consent: More than getting a signature. *Quick Safety, 21*(2). jointcommission.org/resources/news-and-multimedia/newsletters/newsletters/quick-safety/quick-safety-issue-21-informed-consent-more-than-getting-a-signature/informed-consent-more-than-getting-a-signature/#.Y8WbEOzMLh8

Thornton, R. G. (2010). Responsibility for the acts of others. *Proceedings (Baylor University. Medical Center), 23*(3), 313–315. https://doi.org/10.1080/08998280.2010.11928641

Timms, M. (2022). Former Vanderbilt nurse RaDonda Vaught found guilty on 2 charges in 2017 death of patient. *USA Today*, March 25, 2022. https://www.usatoday.com/story/news/nation/2022/03/25/radonda-vaught-verdict-vanderbilt-nurse-guilty/7169480001/

Tovar v. Methodist Healthcare. (2005). S.W. 3d WI 3079074 (Texas App., 2005). https://caselaw.findlaw.com/tx-court-of-appeals/1158723.html

Ventola, C. L. (2014). Social media and health care professionals: Benefits, risks, and best practices. *Pharmacy and Therapeutics, 39*(7), 491–520.

Viglucci, A., & Staletovich, J. (2017). *FIU bridge collapse: Here is what we know so far.* http://www.miamiherald.com/news/local/community/miami-dade/west-miami-dade/article207358659.html

Wade, A. R. (2015). The BON's authority to interpret regulations, negligence, and nurse practice acts standards. *Journal of Nursing Regulation, 6*(3), 25–28. https://doi.org/10.1016/S2155-8256(15)30781-X

West, J. C. (2016). Vicarious liability: Is it an issue for your organization? *Journal of Healthcare Risk Management, 36*(1), 25–34. https://doi.org/10.1002/jhrm.21232

Worth, T. (2017). Lawsuits for information breaches may be on the rise. *Renal & Urology News.* https://www.renalandurologynews.com/hipaa-compliance/hipaa-noncompliance-information-breach-lawsuits-rising/article/706860/

Zhong, E. H., McCarthy, C., & Alexander, M. (2016). A review of criminal convictions among nurses 2012–2013. *Journal of Nursing Regulation, 7*(1), 27–33. https://doi.org/10.1016/S2155-8256(16)31038-9

Chapter 4 References

American Nurses Association. (2015). Code of Ethics for Nurses. *MEDSURG Nursing, 24*(4), 268–271.

Anderson, B. J., Manno, M., O'Connor, P., & Gallagher, E. (2010). Listening to nursing leaders. *Journal of Nursing Administration, 40*(4), 182–187. https://doi.org/10.1097/NNA.0b013e3181d40f65https://doi.org/10.1097/NNA.0b013e3181d40f65

Baggett, M. M., & Baggett, F. B. (2005). Move from management to high-level leadership. *Nursing Management, 36*(7), 12. https://doi.org/10.1097/00006247-200507000-00003

Barker, A. M. (1992). *Transformational nursing leadership: A vision for the future.* National League for Nursing Press.

Bass, B. M., & Avolio, B. J. (1993). Transformational leadership: A response to critiques. In M. M. Chemers & R. Ayman (Eds.), *Leadership theory and research: Perspectives and direction* (pp. 49–80). Academic Press.

Bastardoz, N., & Van Vugt, M. (2019). The nature of followership: Evolutionary analysis and review. *The Leadership Quarterly, 30*(1), 81–95. https://doi.org/10.1016/j.leaqua.2018.09.004

Bennis, W. (1984, August). The four competencies of leadership. *Training and Development Journal, 38*(8) 15–19.

Bennis, W., Spreitzer, G. M., & Cummings, T. G. (2001). *The future of leadership.* Jossey-Bass.

Bing, S. (2010). *Stanley Bing's top 10 strategies for managing up.* CBS News. http://www.cbsnews.com

Bjarnason, D., & LaSala, C. A. (2011, March). Moral leadership in nursing. *Journal of Radiology Nursing, 30*(1), 18–24. https://doi.org/10.1016/j.jradnu.2011.01.002

Blake, R. R., Mouton, J. S., & Tapper, M. (1981). *Grid approaches for managerial leadership in nursing.* C.V. Mosby.

Blanchard, K., & Miller, M. (2007, September 11). The higher plane of leadership. *Leader to Leader Journal, 46*, 25–30. https://doi.org/10.1002/ltl.253

Blanchard, K., & Miller, M. (2014). *The secret: What great leaders know and do.* Berrett-Koehler Publishers.

Buchanan, L. (2011, June). Care values. *INC Magazine*, 60–61.

Buchanan, L. (2012a). The world needs big ideas. *INC Magazine, 34*(9), 57–58.

Buchanan, L. (2012b, June). 13 ways of looking at a leader. *INC Magazine, 34*(5), 74–76.

Buchanan, L. (2013, June). Between Venus and Mars: 7 traits of true leaders. *INC Magazine, 35*(5), 64. http://www.inc.com/magazine/201306/leigh-buchanan/traits-of-true-leaders.html

Chrispeels, J. H. (2004). *Learning to lead together.* Sage Publications.

Code of Ethics for Nurses. (2001). *Nursing world.* http://www.nursingworld.org/MainMenuCategories/EthicsStandards/CodeofEthicsforNurses

Cummings, T. G., & Cummings, C. (2020). The Relevance Challenge in Management and Organization Studies: Bringing Organization Development Back In. *The Journal of Applied Behavioral Science, 56*(4), 521–546. https://doi.org/10.1177/0021886320961855

Deutschman, A. (2005). Is your boss a psychopath? Making change. *Fast Company, 96*, 43–51.

Disch, J. (2013). President's message: Professional generosity. *Nursing Outlook, 61*, 196–204. https://doi.org/10.1016/j.outlook.2013.05.006

Dorn, M. (2011). *Characteristics of caring leadership.* http://www.thecareguys.com

Feldman, D. A. (2002). *Critical thinking: Strategies for decision making.* Crisp Publications.

Goleman, D., Boyatzes, R., & McKee, A. (2002). *Primal leadership: Realizing the power of emotional intelligence.* Harvard Business School Press.

Greenleaf, R. K. (2008). Nine characteristics of effective, caring leaders. *Greenleaf Center for Servant Leadership.* http://www.greenleaf.org

Grossman, S., & Valiga, T. M. (2000). *The new leadership challenge: Creating the future of nursing.* F.A. Davis.

Hersey, P., & Campbell, R. (2004). *Leadership: A behavioral science approach.* Leadership Studies Publishing.

Herzberg, F. (1966). *Work and the nature of man.* World Publishing.

Herzberg, F., Mausner, B., & Snyderman, B. (1959). *The motivation to work* (2nd ed.). John Wiley & Sons.

Holman, L. (1995). *Eleven lessons in self-leadership: Insights for personal and professional success.* A Lesson in Leadership Book.

Ibarra, H. (2015). *Act like a leader, think like a leader.* Harvard Business Review Press.

Jackson, M., Ignatavicius, D., & Case, B. (Eds.). (2004). *Conversations in critical thinking and clinical judgement.* Pohl.

Kerfott, K. (2000). Leadership: Creating a shared destiny. *Dermatological Nursing, 12*(5), 363–364.

Kethledge, R. M., & Erwin, M. S. (2017). *Lead yourself.* Bloomsbury Publishing.

Korn, M. (2004). Toxic cleanup: How to deal with a dangerous leader. *Fast Company, 88,* 17.

Lawson, D., & Fleshman, J. W. (2020). Informal Leadership in Health Care. *Clinics in colon and rectal surgery, 33*(4), 225–227. https://doi.org/10.1055/s-0040-1709439

Leach, L. S. (2005). Nurse executive transformational leadership and organizational commitment. *Journal of Nursing Administration, 35*(5), 228–237. https://doi.org/10.1097/00005110-200505000-00006

Leclerc, L., Kennedy, K., & Campis, S. (2020). Human-Centered Leadership in Health Care: An Idea That's Time Has Come. *Nursing administration quarterly, 44*(2), 117–126. https://doi.org/10.1097/NAQ.0000000000000409Lyons, M. F. (2002, January/February). Leadership and followership. *The Physician Executive, 28(1)* 91–93.

Manning, J. (2016). The influence of nurse manager leadership style on staff nurse work engagement. *Journal of Nursing Administration, 46*(9), 438–443. https://doi.org/10.1097/NNA.0000000000000372

Maslow, A. H. (1970). *Motivation and personality* (2nd ed.). Harper & Row.

Maxwell, J. C. (1993). *Developing the leader within you.* Thomas Nelson Inc.

Maxwell, J. C. (1998). *The 21 irrefutable laws of leadership.* Thomas Nelson Inc.

Maxwell, J. C. (2018). Lessons in Leadership with Nido Qubein and John Maxwell. *Business North Carolina, 38*(1), S52, 2p.

McClelland, D. (1961). *The achieving society.* D. Van Nostrand.

McMurry. (2012). *Be a caring leader. Managing people at work.* http://www.managingpeopleatwork.com

McNichol, E. (2000). How to be a model leader. *Nursing Standard, 14*(45), 24.

Owen, J. (2015). *How to lead* (4th ed.). Pearson Education Limited.

Pavitt, C. (1999). Theorizing about the group communication-leadership relationship. In L. R. Frey (Ed.), *The handbook of group communication theory and research* (pp. 313–334). Sage Publications.

Porter-O'Grady, T. (2003). A different age for leadership, Part II. *Journal of Nursing Administration, 33*(2), 105–110. https://doi.org/10.1097/00005110-200303000-00009

Powell, C. (2012, May 21). The general's orders (Features) (Excerpts). It worked for me: In life and leadership. *Newsweek, 159*(21), 40–44.

Prufeta, P. (2017). Emotional intelligence of nurse managers: An exploratory study. *Journal of Nursing Administration, 47*(3), 134–139. https://doi.org/10.1097/NNA.0000000000000455

Public Broadcasting Service. (2021). Side by Side With Nido Qubein: John Maxwell, Author & Leadership Expert. PBS. https://www.pbs.org/video/john-maxwell-author-leadership-expert-3rbmkb/

Rhodes, M. K., Morris, A. H., & Lazenby, R. B. (2011). Nursing at its best: Competent and caring. *Online Journal of Issues in Nursing, 16*(2), 10.

Riggio, R. E. (2020). Why Followership? In New Directions for Student Leadership (Vol. 2020, Issue 167,

pp. 15–22). Wiley. https://doi.org/10.1002/yd.20395

Schick-Makaroff, K., & Storch, J. L. (2019). Guidance for Ethical Leadership in Nursing Codes of Ethics: An Integrative Review. *Nursing leadership (Toronto, Ont.), 32*(1), 60–73. https://doi.org/10.12927/cjnl.2019.25848

Scott, E., & Miles, J. (2013). Advancing leadership capacity in nursing. *Nursing Administration Quarterly, 37*(1), 77–82. https://doi.org/10.1097/NAQ.0b013e3182751998

Spears, L. C. (2010). Character and servant leadership: Ten characteristics of effective, caring leaders. *Journal of Virtues & Leadership, 1*(1), 25–30.

Spears, L. C., & Lawrence, M. (2004). *Practicing servant-leadership.* Jossey-Bass.

Spreitzer, G. M., & Quinn, R. E. (2001). *A company of leaders: Five disciplines for unleashing the power in your workforce.* Jossey-Bass.

Stewart, L., Holmes, C., & Usher, K. (2012). Reclaiming caring in nursing leadership: A deconstruction of leadership using a Habermasian lens. *Collegian, 19,* 223–229. https://doi.org/10.1016/j.colegn.2012.04.007

Tappen, R. M. (2001). *Nursing leadership and management: Concepts and practice.* F.A. Davis.

Trofino, J. (1995). Transformational leadership in health care. *Nursing Management, 26*(8), 42–47.

Turk, W. (2007, March/April). The art of managing up. *Defense AT&L,36(2)* 21–23.

White, R. K., & Lippitt, R. (1960). *Autocracy and democracy: An experimental inquiry.* Harper & Row.

Wiseman, L., & McKeown, G. (2010, May). Managing yourself: Bringing out the best in your people. *Harvard Business Review, 88*(5), 117-121. http://hbr.org/2010/05/managing-yourself-bringing-out-the-best-in-your-people/ar/1

Chapter 5 References

Clark-Burg, K., & Alliex, S. (2017). A study of styles: How do nurse managers make decisions? *Nursing Management, 48*(7), 44–49. https://doi.org/10.1097/01.NUMA.0000520721.78549.ad

Cox, S. (2017). Tips for the novice manager. *Nursing Management, 48*(7), 56.

Dantley, M. E. (2005). Moral leadership: Shifting the management paradigm. In F. W. English (Ed.), *The Sage handbook of educational leadership* (pp. 34–46). Sage Publications.

Dowless, R. M. (2007). Your guide to costing methods and terminology. *Nursing Management, 38*(4), 52–57.

Dunham-Taylor, J. (1995). Identifying the best in nurse executive leadership. *Journal of Nursing Administration, 25*(7/8), 24–31. https://doi.org/10.1097/00005110-199507000-00011

Fennimore, L., & Wolf, G. (2011). Nurse manager leadership development. *Journal of Nursing Administration, 41*(5), 204–210. https://doi.org/10.1097/NNA.0b013e3182171aff

Greenleaf, R. K. (2004). Who is the servant-leader? In L. C. Spears & M. Lawrence (Eds.), *Practicing servant-leadership* (pp. 287–293). Jossey-Bass.

Halcomb, E., Fernandez, R., Mursa, R., Stephen, C., Calma, K., Ashley, C., McInnes, S., Desborough, J., James, S., & Williams, A. (2022). Mental health, safety and support during COVID-19: A cross-sectional study of primary health care nurses. *Journal of nursing*

management, *30*(2), 393–402. https://doi
.org/10.1111/jonm.13534

Hart, L. B., & Waisman, C. S. (2005). *The leadership
training activity book.* AMACOM.

Hunter, J. C. (2004). *The world's most powerful leadership
principle.* Crown Business.

Jones, R. A. (2010). Preparing tomorrow's leaders. *Journal
of Nursing Administration, 40*(4), 154–157. https://
doi.org/10.1097/NNA.0b013e3181d40e14

Kelly, J., & Nadler, S. (2007, March 3–4). Leading from
below. *Wall Street Journal,* R4.

Kovner, C. T., Brewer, C. S., Fairchild, S., Poornima, S.,
Kim, H., & Djukic, M. (2007). Newly licensed RNs'
characteristics, work attitudes, and intentions to work.
American Journal of Nursing, 107(9), 58–70. https://
doi.org/10.1097/01.NAJ.0000287512.31006.66

Lee, J. A. (1980). *The gold and the garbage in management theories and prescriptions.* Ohio University Press.

Locke, E. A. (1982). The ideas of Frederick Taylor: An
evaluation. *Academy of Management Review, 7*(1),
14. https://doi.org/10.2307/257244

Lombardi, D. N. (2001). *Handbook for the new health
care manager.* Jossey-Bass/AHA Press.

Longmore, M. (2017). Nursing leadership being eroded.
Kai Tiaki Nursing New Zealand, 23(6), 28–29.

Mackoff, B. L., & Triolo, P. K. (2008). Why do nurse
managers stay? Building a model engagement. Part I:
Dimensions of engagement. *Journal of Nursing Administration, 38*(3), 118–124. https://doi.org
/10.1097/01.NNA.0000312758.14536.e0

McCauley, C. D., & Van Velson, E. (Eds.). (2004). *The
center for creative leadership handbook of leadership
development.* Jossey-Bass.

McGregor, D. (1960). *The human side of enterprise.*
McGraw-Hill.

Micklethwait, J. (2011). Foreword. In A. Wooldridge
(Ed.), *Masters of management* (pp. 11-16). Harper
Collins.

Mintzberg, H. (1989). *Mintzberg on management: Inside
our strange world of organizations.* Free Press.

Montebello, A. (1994). *Work teams that work.* Best Sellers
Publishing.

Owen, J. (2015). *How to lead.* Pearson Education Limited.

Schaffer, R. H. (2010, September). Mistakes leaders keep
making. *Harvard Business Review, 88*(9), 87–91.

Shirey, M. R. (2007). Competencies and tips for effective
leadership. *Journal of Nursing Administration, 37*(4),
167–170. https://doi.org/10.1097/01.NNA
.0000266842.54308.38

Shirey, M. R., Ebright, P. R., & McDaniel, A. M. (2008).
Sleepless in America: Nurse managers cope with stress
and complexity. *Journal of Nursing Administration,
38*(3), 125–131. https://doi.org/10.1097/01.NNA
.0000310722.35666.73

Spears, L. C., & Lawrence, M. (2004). *Practicing
servant-leadership.* Jossey-Bass.

Suddath, C. (2013, November 11–17). You get a D+ in
teamwork. *Bloomberg Businessweek (Online),4345,* 91.

Tokac, U., & Razon, S. (2021). Nursing professionals'
mental well-being and workplace impairment during
the COVID-19 crisis: A Network analysis. *Journal of
nursing management, 29*(6), 1653–1659. https://doi
.org/10.1111/jonm.13285

Trossman, S. (2011). Complex role in complex times. *The
American Nurse, 43*(4), 1, 6, 7.

Welch, J., & Welch, S. (2007, July 23). Bosses who get
it all wrong. *Bloomberg Businessweek (Online), 4043,*
88.

Welch, J., & Welch, S. (2008, July 28). Emotional mis-
management. *Bloomberg Businessweek (Online),
4093,* 84-.

Wiseman, L., & McKeown, G. (2010, May). Bringing out
the best in your people. *Harvard Business Review,* Reprint R1005k, 1–5.

Wren, D. A. (1972). *The evolution of management
thought.* Ronald Press.

Chapter 6 References

Agency for Healthcare Research and Quality. (2015).
Patient safety primers: Handoffs and signouts. http://
www.psnet.ahrq.gov/primer.aspx?primerID=9

Agency for Healthcare Research and Quality. (2021).
About AHRQ's quality & patient safety work. Agency
for Healthcare Research and Quality.https://www
.ahrq.gov/patient-safety/about/index.html

Alfaro-Lefevre, R. (2011). *Critical thinking, clinical reasoning, and clinical judgment: A practical approach*
(5th ed.). Mosby Elsevier.

Alfero-Lefevre, R. (2017). *Critical thinking, clinical reasoning, and clinical judgment: A practical approach*
(6th ed.). Elsevier.

American Association of Critical Care Nurses. (1990).
*Delegation of nursing and non-nursing activities
in critical care: A framework for decision making.*
Author.

American Association of Critical Care Nurses. (2010).
Delegation handbook. Author.

American Nurses Association. (1985). *Code for nurses.*
Author.

American Nurses Association. (1996). *Registered professional nurses and unlicensed assistive personnel.*
Author.

American Nurses Association. (2002). *Position statements
on registered nurse utilization of unlicensed assistive
personnel.* Author.

American Nurses Association. (2005). *Principles for delegation.* Author.

American Nurses Association. (2012a). *ANA's principles
for delegation: For registered nurses to unlicensed assistive personnel (UAP).* Author.

American Nurses Association. (2012b). *ANA's principles
of delegation by registered nurses to unlicensed assistive personnel (UAP).* Author.

Anthony, M. K., & Vidal, K. (2010). Mindful communication: A novel approach to improving delegation and
increasing patient safety. *The Online Journal of Issues
in Nursing, 15*(2), 1–3. https://ojin.nursingworld
.org/MainMenuCategories/ANAMarketplace
/ANAPeriodicals/OJIN/TableofContents/Vol152010
/No2May2010/Mindful-Communication-and
-Delegation.html

Association of Rehabilitation Nurses. (1995, May) *Registered Nurse Utilization of Unlicensed Assistive*

Association of Rehabilitation Nurses. (2017). *The role of
nursing assistive personnel in the rehabilitation setting.*
Position Paper. https://rehabnurse.org/about
/position-statements/nursing-assistive-personnel

Association for Women's Health, Obstetrics and Neonatal
Nurses. (2010). *Guidelines for professional nurse staffing on perinatal units.* Author.

Bakr, M. M. (2021). An exploration to the relationship between unlicensed assistive personnel role and patient
safety. *American Journal of Nursing and Health Sciences, 3*(1), 105–112.https://doi.org/10.11648/j
.ajnhs.20210204.15

Barrow, J. M., & Sharma S. (2021). Five rights of nursing delegation. In *StatPearls* [Internet]. StatPearls Publishing; 2022 Jan-. https://www.ncbi.nlm.nih.gov/books/NBK519519/

Berlin, G., LaPointd, M., & Murphy, M. (2022). Surveyed nurses consider leaving direct patient care at elevated rates. *McKinsey & Company Report*. https://www.mckinsey.com/industries/healthcare-systems-and-services/our-insights/surveyed-nurses-consider-leaving-direct-patient-care-at-elevated-rates#

Charett, M., McKenna, L. G., Deschenes, M. F., Ha, L., Meriser, S., & Lavoie, P. (2020). New graduate nurses' clinical competence: A mixed methods systematic review. *Journal of Advanced Nursing, 76*(11), 2810–2829. https://doi.org/10.1111/jan.14487

Cipriano, R. F. (2010). Overview and summary: Delegation dilemmas: Standards and skills for practice. *The Online Journal of Issues in Nursing, 15*(2), 1–3. http://www.nursingworld.org/MainMenuCategories/ANAMarketplace/ANAPeriodicals/OJIN/JournalTopics/Delegation-Dilemmas

DuBois, C. A., D'amour, D., Tchouaket, E., Clarke, S., Rivard, M., & Blais, R. (2013). Associations of patient safety outcomes with models of nursing care organization at unit level in hospitals. *International Journal for Quality in Health Care, 25*(2), 110–117. https://doi.org/10.1093/intqhc/mzt019

Fernandez, R., Johnson, M., Tran, D. T., & Miranda, C. (2012). Models of care in nursing: A systematic review. *International Journal of Evidence-Based Healthcare, 10*(4), 324–337.

Greene-Moton, E., & Minkler, M. (2020). Cultural competence or cultural humility? Moving beyond debate. *Health Promotion Practice, 20*(1), 142–145. https://doi.org/10.77/1524839919884912

Hawthorne-Spears, N., & Whitlock, A. (2016). Behind our eyes: The voice of the patient care assistant. *Journal of Nursing Education and Practice, 6*(6), 75–78. https://doi.org/10.5430/jnep.v6n6p75

Hicks v. New York State Department of Health. (1991). 570 N.Y.S. 2d 395 (A.D. 3 Dept).

Institute of Medicine. (2001). *Crossing the quality chasm: A new health system for the 21st century*. National Academies Press.

Institute of Medicine. (2010). *The future of nursing report*. National Academies Press.

Kalisch, B. J. (2011). The impact of RN-UAP relationships on quality and safety. *Nursing Management, 42*(9), 16–22.https://doi.org/10.1097/01.NUMA.0000403284.27249.a2

Kalisch, B. J., Landstrom, G. L., & Hinshaw, A. S. (2009). Missed nursing care: A concept analysis. *Journal of Advanced Nursing, 65*(7), 1509–1517. https://doi.org/10.1111/j.1365-2648.2009.05027.x

Keeney, S., Hasson, F., McKenna, H., & Gillen, P. (2005). Health care assistants: The view of managers of health care agencies on training and employment. *Journal of Nursing Management, 13*(1), 83–92.

Kendall, N. (2018). How new nursing roles affect accountability and delegation. *Nursing Times, 114*(4), 45–47.

LaCharity, L. M., Hosler, S. M., Kumagai, C., & Hansten, R. (2022). *Prioritization, delegation, and assignment: Practice exercises for the NCLEX-RN® examination*. Elsevier.

Lake, S., Moss, C., & Duke, J. (2009). Nursing prioritization of the patient need for care: A tacit knowledge embedded in the clinical decision-making literature. *International Journal of Nursing Practice, 15*(5),

376–388. https://doi.org/10.1111/j.1440-172X.2009.01778.x

Marquis, B. L., & Huston, C. J. (2021). *Leadership roles and management functions in nursing: Theory and application* (10th ed.). Wolters Kluwer.

Matthews, J. (2010). When does delegating make you a supervisor? *The Online Journal of Issues in Nursing, 15*(2). https://ojin.nursingworld.org/table-of-contents/volume-15-2010/number-2-may-2010/delegating-and-supervisors/McDaniel, V. P. (2021). Cultural humility in nursing: Building the bridge to best practices. *Virginia Nurses Today, 29*(2).

McHugh, M. D., Kelly, L. A., Smith, H. L., Wu, E. S., Vanak, J. M., & Aiken, L. H. (2013). Lower mortality in magnet hospitals. *Medical Care, 51*(5), 382–388.

McMullen, T. L., Resnick, B., Chin-Hansen, J., Geiger-Brown, J. M., Miller, N., & Rubenstein, R. (2015). Certified nurse aide scope of practice: State-by-state differences in allowable delegated activities. *Journal of the American Medical Directors Association, 16*(1), 20–24. https://doi.org/10.1016/j.jamda.2014.07.003

Miller, L. (2018). Delegation: Legal issues for clinicians. *Perinatal and Neonatal Nursing, 32*(2), 104–106. https://doi.org/10.1097/JPN.0000000000000327

Moss, E., Seifert, P. C., & O'Sullivan, A. (2016). Registered nurses as interprofessional collaborative partners: Creating value-based outcomes. *Online Journal of Issues in Nursing, 21*(3).

Mueller, C., & Vogelsmeier, A. (2013). Effective delegation: Understanding responsibility, authority and accountability. *The Journal of Nursing Regulation, 4*(3), 20–27. https://doi.org/10.1016/S2155-8256(15)30126-5

National Council of State Boards of Nursing. (1990). *Concept paper on delegation*. Author.

National Council of State Boards of Nursing. (1995, December). Delegation: Concepts and decision-making process. *Issues*, 1–2.

National Council of State Boards of Nursing. (1997). *Delegation Decision-Making Grid*. Author. http://www.health.ri.gov/publications/guides/Delegation-DecisionMakingTree.pdf

National Council of State Boards of Nursing. (2006). *Joint statement on delegation*. https://www.ncsbn.org/Delegation_joint_statement_NCSBN-ANA.pdf

National Council of State Boards of Nursing. (2007). *The five rights of delegation*. http://www.ncsbn.org

National Council of State Boards of Nursing. (2015). *Delegation*. https://www.ncsbn.org/1625.htm

National Council of State Boards of Nursing. (2016). National guidelines for nursing delegation. *Journal of Nursing Regulation, 7*(1), 5–14. https://doi.org/10.1016/S2155-8256(16)31035-3

National Labor Relations Act. (1935). https://www.nlrb.gov/guidance/key-reference-materials/national-labor-relations-act

Nightingale, F. (1859). *Notes on nursing: What it is and what it is not*. Harrison and Sons. (Reprint 1992. JB Lippincott.)

Parreira, P., Santos-Costa, P., Neri, M., Marques, A., Queirós, P., & Salgueiro-Oliveira, A. (2021). Work methods for nursing care delivery. *International Journal of Environmental Research and Public Health, 18*(4), 2088. https://doi.org/10.3390/ijerph18042088

Payne, R., & Steakley, B. (2015). Establishing a primary nursing model of care. *Nursing Management, 46*(12), 11–13. https://doi.org/10.1097/01.NUMA.0000473510.53926.99

Puskar, K., Berju, D., Shi, X., & McFadden, T. (2017). Nursing students and delegation. *Nursing Made Incredibly Easy, 15*(3), 6–8.

Siegel, Elena & Bakerjian, Deb & Bettega, K. & Sikma, Suzanne. (2017). Registered Nurse Delegation in nursing homes: The role of directors of nursing. *Innovation in Aging.* 1. 1070-1070. 10.1093/geroni/igx004 .3917.

Silvestri, L. (2008). *Saunders comprehensive review for the NCLEX-RN examination* (4th ed.). Saunders.

Silvestri, L. A., & Silvestri, A. E. (2020). Saunders comprehensive review for the NCLEX-RN examination (8th ed.). Elsevier.

Society of Gastroenterology Nurses and Associates, Inc. (2009). *Position statement: Role delineation of nursing assistive personnel in gastroenterology.* https://www.sgna.org/Portals/0/Education /PDF/Position-Statements/NAP_FINAL_9_20 _13.pdf

Spetz, J., Donaldson, N., Aydin, C., & Brown, D. S. (2008). How many nurses per patient? Measurements of nurse staffing in health services research. *Health Services Research, 43*(5), 1674–1692. https://doi.org/10.1111/j.1475-6773.2008 .00850.x

TeamSTEPPS. (2013). *Pocket guide: TeamSTEPPS: Strategies & tools to enhance performance and patient safety.* Agency for Healthcare Research and Quality. https://www.ahrq.gov/sites/default/files/wysiwyg /professionals/education/curriculum-tools /teamstepps/instructor/essentials/pocketguide.pdf

Ver Woert, D., & Hansten, R. I. (2020). Delegation and setting priorities for safe, high-quality patient care. In P. Kelly Vana, B. A. Vottero, & G. Altmiller (Eds.), *Quality and safety education for nurses: Core competencies* (3rd ed., pp. 143-172.). Springer Publishing.

Wagner, E. (2018). Improving patient care outcomes through better delegation-communication between nurses and assistive personnel. *Journal of Nursing Care Quality, 33*(2), 187–193. https://doi.org/10.1097 /NCQ.0000000000000282

Weiss, S. A., & Tappen, R. M. (2015). *Essentials of leadership and management* (6th ed.). F.A. Davis.

Weiss, S. A., Tappen, R. M., & Grimley, K. (2019). *Essentials of leadership & management in nursing* (7th ed.). F. A. Davis.

Weydt, A. (2010). Developing delegation skills. *The Online Journal of Issues in Nursing, 15*(2). http://www .nursingworld.org/MainMenuCategories /ANAMarketplace/ANAPeriodicals/OJIN /JournalTopics/Delegation-Dilemmas

Zimmerman, P. G., & Schultz, M. J. (2013). *Delegating to unlicensed assistive personnel.* Gannet Education Publishing.

Chapter 7 References

Agency for Healthcare Research and Quality. (2013). *Team STEPPS.* http://teamstepps.ahrq.gov

Ali, M. (2017). Communication skills 2: Overcoming barriers to effective communication. *Nursing Times, 114*(1), 40–42.

American Association of Colleges of Nursing. (2011). *Core competencies for interprofessional collaboration.* http://www.aacn.nche.edu/leading-initiatives /IPECReport.pdf

American Nurses Credentialing Center. (2012). *MAGNET designated hospitals demonstrate lower mortality rates.* http://www.medscape.com/viewarticle /773611

American Organization of Nurse Executives. (2012). *AONE guiding principles: AACN-AONE task force on academic-practice partnerships.* Author.

Arnold, J., & Pearson, G. (Eds.). (1992). *Computer applications in nursing education and practice.* National League for Nursing.

Brounstein, M. (2002). *Managing teams for dummies.* John Wiley & Sons.

Brown, C. G., Cantril, C., McMullen, L., Barkely, D. L., Dietz, M., Murphy, C. M., & Fabrey, L. J. (2012). Oncology nurse navigator role delineation study: An oncology nursing society report. *Clinical Journal of Oncology Nursing, 16*(6), 581–585.

Centers for Medicare and Medicaid Services. (2013a). *An introduction to the Medicare EHR incentive program for eligible professionals.* https://www.cms.gov /files/document/ehealthuintro-medicare-ehr -program-2014-10-01-remediatedpdf

Centers for Medicare and Medicaid Services. (2013b). *Meaningful use.* http://www.cms.gov/apps/media /press/release

Centers for Medicare and Medicaid Services. (2013c). *Research, statistics data and systems.* http://www .cms.gov/Research-Statistics-Data-and-Systems /Statistics-Trends-and-Reports/MedicareMedicaid- StatSupp/2010.html

Department of Health and Human Services (HHS) Office of Minority Health. (2013). *National CLAS Standards.* http://minorityhealth.hhs.gov/templates/browse .aspx?lvl=2&lvlID=11

Enlow, M., Shanks, L., Guhde, J., & Perkins, M. (2010). Incorporating interprofessional communication skills (ISBARR) into an undergraduate nursing curriculum. *Nurse Educator, 35*(4), 176–180.

Gartee, R., & Beal, S. (2012). *Electronic health records and nursing.* Pearson.

Haig, K. M., Sutton, S., & Whittingdon, J. (2006). SBAR: A shared mental model for improving communication between clinicians. *Journal on Quality and Patient Safety, 32*(3), 167–175. https://www.ahrq.gov /health-literacy/improve/index.html

Henry, J., Pylypchuk, Y., Searcy, T., & Patel, V. (2016). *EHR adoption: Adoption of electronic health record systems among U.S. non-federal acute care hospitals: 2008–2015.* ONC Data Brief 35. https://dashboard .healthit.gov/evaluations/data-briefs/non-federal -acute-care-hospital-ehr-adoption-2008 -2015.php

Institute for Healthcare Improvement. (2006). *Using SBAR to improve communication between caregivers.* http:// www.ihi.org/IHI/Programs/AudioAndWebPrograms /WebACTIONUsingSBARtoImproveCommunication .htm?TabId=7

Institute of Medicine. (2010). *The future of nursing: Leading change, advancing health.* Committee on the Robert Wood Johnson Foundation Initiative on the Future of Nursing at the Institute of Medicine. http://www.nap.edu/catalog /12956.html

Institute of Medicine. (2012). *Public health literacy.*

Issacson, M. (2014, May/June). Clarifying concepts: Cultural humility or competency. *Journal of Professional Nursing, 30*(3), 251–258.

Kalisch, B. J., & Lee, K. H. (2011). Nurse staffing levels and teamwork: A cross-sectional study of seven patient care units in acute care hospitals. *Journal of Nursing Scholarship, 43*(1), 82–88.

Keller, K. B., Eggenberger, T. L., Belkowitz, J., Sarsekeyeva, M., & Zito, A. R. (2013). Implementing successful interprofessional communication opportunities in health care education: A qualitative analysis. *International Journal of Medical Education, 4*, 253–259.

Konsel, K. (2016). *Medical errors and communication.* Institute for Health Improvement. http://healthcareexcellence.org/2016/06/14/medical-errors-communication/

Mahadevan, R. (2013). Health Literacy Fact Sheets; Fact sheet #1. Center for Health Care Strategies (CHCS). https://www.chcs.org/resource/health-literacy-fact-sheets/

Martin, J. S., Ummenhofer, W., Manser, T., & Spirig, R. (2010, May 4). Interprofessional collaboration among nurses and physicians: Making a difference in patient outcome. *Swiss Medical Weekly, 140*, 1–12. https://smw.ch/en/article/doi/smw.2010.13062/

National Council on State Boards of Nursing. (2018). *A nurse's guide to the use of social media.*

National League for Nursing. (2015). *Vision for interprofessional collaboration in education and practice.*

National Patient Safety Foundation. (2012). *Health literacy: Statistics at a glance.*

Nelson, B., & Economy, P. (2010). *Managing for dummies* (3rd ed.). John Wiley & Sons.

O'Brien, J. (2013). Interprofessional collaboration. *AMN Healthcare Education.* http://www.rn.com

O'Daniel, M., & Rosenstein, A. H. (2008). Professional communication and team collaboration. In R. G. Hughes (Ed.), *Patient safety and quality: An evidence-based handbook for nurses.* Agency for Healthcare Research and Quality.

Organization for Associate Degree Nursing. (2021). QSEN competency: Teamwork and collaboration #2, https://oadn.org/resource/qsen-competency-2-teamwork-and-collaboration/#:~:text=Definition%3A%20Function%20effectively%20within%20nursing,to%20achieve%20quality%20patient%20care.

Osborne, H. (2018). *Health literacy from A to Z: Practical ways to communicate your health message* (2nd ed.). Aviva Publishing.

Reinecke, S. (2015, June 15). *Is your EHR hurting your nurses?* https://www.healthcareitnews.com/blog/your-ehr-hurting-your-nurses

Robert Wood Johnson Foundation. (2013, January 9). *How to foster interprofessional collaboration between physicians and nurses?* https://www.rwjf.org/en/library/research/2013/01/how-to-foster-interprofessional-collaboration-between-physicians.html

Schwartz, F., Lowe, M., & Sinclair, L. (2010). Communication in health care: Consideration and strategies for successful consumer and team dialogue. *Hypothesis, 8*(1), 1–8.

Shea, V. (2000). *Netiquette.* Albion.

Staats, C., Capatosto, K., Wright, R., & Contractor, D. (2015). *State of the science: Implicit bias review 2015.* Kirwan Institute for the Study of Race and Ethnicity. http://kirwaninstitute.osu.edu/wp-content/uploads/2015/05/2015-kirwan-implicit-bias.pdf

Storck, L. (2017, February). Policy statement: Texting in health care. *Online Journal of Nursing Informatics (OJNI), 21*(1).

Tervalon, M., & Murray-Garcia, J. (1998). Cultural humility versus cultural competence: A critical distinction in defining physician training outcomes in multicultural education. *Journal of Healthcare for the Poor and Underserved, 9*(2), 117–125. http://melanietervalon.com/wp-content/uploads/2013/08/CulturalHumility_Tervalon-and-Murray-Garcia-Article.pdf

The Joint Commission. (2013). *Manual for Joint Commission national quality measures* (v2013A1). https://manual.jointcommission.org/releases/TJC2013A/

The Joint Commission. (2014). *Improving transitions of care: Hand-off communications.* The Joint Commission.

The Joint Commission. (2016, April). Implicit bias in healthcare. *Quick Safety Advisory, 23.*

The Joint Commission. (2017). *National patient safety goals effective January 1, 2017: Hospital accreditation program.*

UCLA Health. (2012). *Bedside report toolkit.* https://med-net.uclahealth.org/wp-content/uploads/sites/2/2017/04/BedsideReportToolkit.pdf

Wood, J. T. (2016). *Interpersonal communication* (8th ed.). Cengage Learning.

World Health Organization. (2010). *Framework for action on interprofessional education & collaborative practice.* http://whqlibdoc.who.int/hq/2010/WHO_HRH_HPN_10.3_eng.pdf

World Health Organization. (2011). *Being an effective team player. Patient safety curriculum guide.*

Chapter 8 References

Ackerman-Barger, K., Boatright, D., Gonzalez-Colaso, R., Orozco, R., & Latimore, D. (2020). Seeking inclusion excellence: Understanding racial microaggressions as experienced by underrepresented medical and nursing students. *Academic Medicine: Journal of the Association of American Medical Colleges, 95*(5), 758–763. https://doi.org/10.1097/ACM.0000000000003077

American Nurses Association. (2015). *Position statement on incivility, bullying and workplace violence July 22, 2015.* https://www.nursingworld.org/practice-policy/nursing-excellence/official-position-statements/id/incivility-bullying-and-workplace-violence

Browne, M. N., & Keeley, S. M. (1994). *Asking the right questions: A guide to critical thinking.* Prentice-Hall.

Budd, K., Warino, L., & Patton, M. (2004). Traditional and non-traditional collective bargaining: Strategies to improve the patient care environment. *The Online Journal of Nursing.* http://ojin.nursingworld.org/MainMenuCategories/ANAMarketplace/ANAPeriodicals/OJIN/TableofContents/Volume92004/No1Jan04/CollectiveBargainingStrategies.html

Christie, W., & Jones, S. (2013, December 9). Lateral violence in nursing and the theory of the nurse as wounded healer. *The Online Journal of Issues in Nursing, 19*(1). https://ojin.nursingworld.org/MainMenuCategories/ANAMarketplace/ANAPeriodicals/OJIN/TableofContents/Vol-19-2014/No1-Jan-2014/Articles-Previous-Topics/Lateral-Violence-and-Theory-of-Wounded-Healer.html

Drucker, P. F. (2002). They're not employees, they're people. *Harvard Business Review, 80*(2), 70–77, 128.

Embree, J., Bruner, D., & White, A. (2013). Raising the level of awareness of nurse-to-nurse lateral violence in a critical access hospital. *Nursing Research and Practice.* https://doi.org/10.1155/2013/207306

Fiumano, J. (2005). Navigate through conflict, not around it. *Nursing Management, 36*(8), 14, 18.

Forman, H., & Merrick, F. (2003). Grievances and complaints: Valuable tools for management and forstaff. *Journal of Nursing Administration, 33*(3), 136–138.

Girardi, D. (2015a). Conflict engagement: Creating connection and cultivating curiosity. *American Journal of Nursing, 115*(9), 60–65.

Girardi, D. (2015b). Conflict engagement: Workplace dynamics. *American Journal of Nursing, 115*(4), 62–65.

Greenfield, R. (2014). *Brainstorming doesn't work; Try this technique instead.* Fast Company. http://www.fastcompany.com/3033567/brainstorming-doesnt-work-try-this-technique-instead

Hall, W., Chapman, M., Lee, K., Merino, Y., Thomas, T., Payne, K., . . . Coyne-Beasley, T. (2015). Implicit racial/ethnic bias among health care professionals and its influence on health care outcomes: A systematic review. *American Journal of Public Health, 105*(12), 60–62.

Harter, J., & Adkins, A. (2015). Employees want a lot more from their managers. *Gallup Business Journal.*

Haslan, S. A. (2001). *Psychology in organizations.* Sage.

Hessels, A., Flynn, L., Cimiotti, J., Cadmus, E., & Gershon, R. (2015). The impact of the nursing practice environment on missed nursing care. *Clinical Nursing Studies, 3*(4), 60–65. https://doi.org/10.5430/cns.v3n4p60

Horton-Deutsch, S. L., & Wellman, D. S. (2002). Christman's principles for effective management. *Journal of Nursing Administration, 32*, 596–601.

Institute of Medicine. (1999). *To err is human: Building a safer health care system.* National Academies Press.

Isosaari, U. (2011). Power in health care organizations. *Journal of Health Organization and Management, 25*(4), 385–399.

Kim, S., Bochatay, N., Relyea-Chew, A., Buttrick, E., Amdahl, C., Kim, L., . . . Lee, Y. (2017). Individual, interpersonal and organizational factors of healthcare conflict: A scoping review. *Journal of Interprofessional Care, 31*(3), 282–290.

Kritek, P. B. (2011). *Conflict management in nursing leadership: A concise encyclopedia* (2nd ed.). Springer Publishing Company.

Lachman, V. D., Murray, J. S., Iseminger, K., & Ganske, K. M. (2012). Doing the right thing: Pathways to moral courage. *American Nurse Today, 7*(5), 24–29.

Laschinger, H., Wong, C., Regan, S., Young-Ritchie, C., & Bushell, P. (2013). Workplace incivility and new graduate nurses' mental health: The protective role of incivility. *The Journal of Nursing Administration, 43*(7/8), 415–421.

Lazoritz, S., & Carlson, P. J. (2008). Descriptive physician behavior. *American Nurse Today, 3*(3), 20–22.

Lytle, T. (2015). *How to resolve workplace conflicts.* Society of Human Resource Management. https://www.shrm.org/hr-today/news/hr-magazine/pages/070815-conflict-management.aspx

Markham, A. (2017). Your team is brainstorming all wrong. *Harvard Business Review.* https://hbr.org/2017/05/your-team-is-brainstorming-all-wrong

Martin, R. H. (2001, June). Ruling may limit ability to unionize. *Advance for Nurses, 1*(2), 9.

McChrystal, S. (2012). (Quoted by R. Safian). Secrets of the flux leader. *Fast Company, 170,* 105.

McDonald, D. (2008). Revisiting a theory of negotiation: The utility of Markiewicz (2005) proposed six principles. *Evaluation and Program Planning, 31*(3), 259–265.

McElhaney, R. (1996). Conflict management in nursing administration. *Nursing Management, 27*(3), 49–50.

Meier, L. L., Semmer, N. K., & Gross, S. (2014). The effect of conflict at work on well-being: Depressive symptoms as a vulnerability factor. *Work & Stress, 28*(1), 31–48. https://doi.org/10.1080/02678373.2013.876691

Merriam Webster. (2022). *Microaggression definition.* Retrieved April 2, 2022 from https://www.merriam-webster.com/dictionary/microaggression

Moeta, M. E., & Du Rand, S. M. (2019). Using scenarios to explore conflict management practices of nurse unit managers in public hospitals. *Curationis, 42*(1), e1–e11. https://doi.org/10.4102/curationis.v42i1.1943

Osterberg, C., & Lorentsson, T. (2010). *Organizational conflict and socialization processes in healthcare* (Master's thesis). University of Gothenburg.

Patterson, K., Grenny, J., McMillan, R., & Surtzler, A. (2003, March 18). Crucial conversations: Making a difference between being healed and being seriously hurt. *Vital Signs, 13*(5), 14–15.

Pittman, J. (2007). Registered nurse job satisfaction and collective bargaining unit membership status. *Journal of Nursing Administration, 37*(10), 471–476.

Porter O'Grady, T., & Malloch, K. (2016). *Leadership in nursing practice* (2nd ed.). Jones & Bartlett Learning LLC.

Prestia, A., Sherman, R., & Demezier, C. (2017). Chief nursing officers' experiences with moral distress. *Journal of Nursing Administration, 47*(2), 101–107.

Robbins, R., & Lesser, S. (2022). *Nurses under attack: Abuse in the workplace.* Medscape.com/slideshow/workplace-abuse-604937

Roch, G., Dubois, C., & Clarke, S. (2014). Organizational climate and hospital nurses' caring practices: A mixed method study. *Research in Nursing and Health, 37*(3), 229–240.

Sarkar, S. (2009). The dance of dissent: Managing conflict in healthcare organizations. *Psychoanalytic Psychotherapy, 23*(2), 121–135.

Siu, H., Laschinger, H. R. S., & Finegan, J. (2008). Nursing professional practice environments: Setting the stage for constructive conflict resolution and work effectiveness. *Journal of Nursing Administration, 38*(5), 250–257.

Sportsman, S. (2005). Build a framework for conflict assessment. *Nursing Management, 36*(4), 32–40.

Suddath, C. (2012, November–December). The art of haggling: When fighting for a new salary, it's all about the first number on the table. *Bloomberg.* http://www.businessweek.com/articles/2012-11-21/the-art-of-haggling

Sun, K. (2011). *Inter-unit conflict, conflict resolution methods, and post-merger, organizational integration in healthcare organizations* (Doctoral dissertation). University of Minnesota.

Tappen, R. M. (2001). *Nursing leadership and management: Concept and practice.* F.A. Davis.

The Joint Commission. (2018). *National patient safety goals effective 2018.*

The Joint Commission. (2022). *Hospital national patient safety goals effective January 1, 2022.* https://www.jointcommission.org/standards/national-patient-safety-goals/hospital-national-patient-safety-goals/

Thompson, L., & Fox, C. R. (2001). Negotiation within and between groups in organizations: Levels of analysis. In M. E. Turner (Ed.), *Groups at work* (pp. 221–266). Lawrence Erlbaum.

Thompson, L., & Nadler, J. (2000). Judgmental biases in conflict resolution and how to overcome them. In M. Deutsch & P. T. Coleman (Eds.), *The handbook of conflict resolution: Theory and practice* (pp. 213–235). Jossey-Bass Publishers.

Tjosvold, D., & Tjosvold, M. M. (1995). *Psychology for leaders: Using motivation, conflict, and power to manage more effectively.* John Wiley & Sons.

Van de Vliert, E., & Janssen, O. (2001). Description, explanation, and prescription of intragroup conflict behaviors. In M. E. Turner (Ed.), *Groups at work: Theory and research* (pp. 267–297). Lawrence Erlbaum and Associates.

Vivar, C. G. (2006). Putting conflict management into practice: A nursing case study. *Journal of Nursing Management, 14*, 201–206.

Walker, M. A., & Harris, G. L. (1995). *Negotiations: Six steps to success.* Prentice-Hall.

Willis, E., Taffoli, L., Henderson, J., & Walter, B. (2008). Enterprise bargaining: A case study in the de-intensification of nursing work in Australia. *Nursing Inquiry, 15*(2), 148–157.

Chapter 9 References

Agency for Healthcare Research and Quality. (2016). *Culture of safety.* https://psnet.ahrq.gov/resources/resource/5333/surveys-on-patient-safety-culture

Agency for Healthcare Research and Quality. (2019). *Culture of safety.* https://psnet.ahrq.gov/primer/culture-safety#

Aiken, L. H., Clarke, S. P., Sloane, D. M., Lake, E. T., & Cheney, T. (2008). Effects of hospital care environments on patient mortality and nurse outcomes. *Journal of Nursing Administration, 38*(5), 223–229.

Armstrong, K. J., & Laschinger, H. (2006). Structural empowerment, Magnet hospital characteristics, and patient safety culture. *Journal of Nursing Care Quality, 21*(2), 124–132.

Barraclough, R. A., & Stewart, R. A. (1992). Power and control: Social science perspectives. In V. P. Richmond & J. C. McCroskey (Eds.), *Power in the classroom: Communication, control and concern* (pp. 1–18). Lawrence Erlbaum.

Berkow, S., Workman, J., Arson, S., Stewart, J., Virkotis, K., & Kahn, M. (2012). Strengthening front-line nurse investment in organizational goals. *Journal of Nursing Administration, 42*(3), 165–169.

Bradbury-Jones, C., Sambrook, S., & Irvine, F. (2007). Power and empowerment in nursing: A fourth theoretical approach. *Journal of Advanced Nursing, 62*(2), 258–266.

Bradford, D. L., & Cohen, A. R. (1998). *Power up: Transforming organizations through shared leadership.* John Wiley & Sons.

Brody, A., Barnes, K., Ruble, C., & Sakowski, J. (2012). Evidence-based practice councils: Potential path to staff nurse empowerment and leadership growth. *Journal of Nursing Administration, 42*(1), 28–33.

Cameron, K., & Quinn, R. (2006). *Diagnosing and changing organizational culture.* Jossey-Bass.

Clancey, T. R. (2010). Technology and complexity: Trouble brewing? *Journal of Nursing Administration, 40*(6), 247–249.

Connaughton, M. J., & Hassinger, J. (2007). Leadership character: Antidote to organizational fatigue. *Journal of Nursing Administration, 37*(10), 464–470.

Currie, L., & Loftus-Hills, A. (2002). The nursing view of clinical governance. *Nursing Standard, 16*(27), 40–44.

DelBueno, D. J. (1987). An organizational checklist. *Journal of Nursing Administration, 17*(5), 30–33. https://doi.org/10.1097/00005110-198705000-00008

Etzioni, A. (1964). Modern organizations. Prentice-Hall, Englewood Cliffs, NJ. Adapted from Chapter 5.

Evans, M. (2013). Redesigning healthcare: Accountable care organization. *Modern Healthcare, 43*(12), 7.

Fitton, R. A. (1997). *Leadership: Quotations from the world's greatest motivators.* Westview Press.

Fralic, M. F. (2000). What is leadership? *Journal of Nursing Administration, 30*(7/8), 340–341.

Fredericks, S., Lapeim, J., Schwind, J., Beanlands, H., Romaniuk, D., & McCay, E. (2012). Discussion of patient-centered care in health care organizations. *Quality Management in Health Care, 21*(3), 127–134.

Frusti, D. K., Niesen, K. M., & Campion, J. K. (2003). Creating a culturally competent organization. *Journal of Nursing Administration, 33*(1), 33–38.

Etzioni, A. (1964). Modern Organizations. Prentice Hall, Englewood Cliffs, NJ adapted from Chapter 5 (pp. 50-58).

Haddad, L., Annamaraju, P., & Toney-Butler, T. (2022, February). *Nursing shortage.* In: *StatPearls* [Internet]. Statpearls Publishing Company. https://www.ncbi.nlm.nih.gov/books/NBK493175/#_NBK493175_pubdet_

Hannigan, T. A. (1998). *Managing tomorrow's high-performance unions.* Greenwood Publishing.

Haslam, S. A. (2001). *Psychology in organizations.* Sage.

Hess, R. (2017). Professional governance. Guest editorial. *Journal of Nursing Administration, 47*(1), 1–2.

Hinshaw, A. S. (2008). Navigating the perfect storm: Balancing a culture of safety with workforce. *Nursing Research, 57*(1S), S4–10.

Institute of Medicine. (2001). *Crossing the quality chasm; A new health system for the 21st century.* National Academies Press.

Isosaari, U. (2011). Power in health care organizations: Contemplations from the first-line management perspective. *Journal of Health Organization and Management, 25*(4), 385–399.

Krout, N. (2021). *Defining and experiencing good nursing leadership.* HealthStream Resources. https://www.healthstream.com/resource/blog/defining-and-experiencing-good-nursing-leadership

Kuokkanen, L., & Katajisto, J. (2003). Promoting or impeding empowerment? *Journal of Nursing Administration, 33*(4), 209–215.

Lawson, L., Miles, K., Vallish, R., & Jenkins, S. (2011). Recognizing nursing professional growth and development in a collective bargaining environment. *Journal of Nursing Administration, 41*(5), 197–200.

Mackoff, B. L., & Triolo, P. K. (2008). Why do nurses, managers stay? Building a model of engagement: Part 2: Cultures of engagement. *Journal of Nursing Administration, 38*(4), 166–171.

Manojlovich, M. (2007). Power and empowerment in nursing: Looking backward to inform the future. *New Hampshire Nursing News, 12*(1), 14–16.

Manojlovich, M., & Laschinger, H. K. (2002). The relationship of empowerment and selected personality characteristics to nursing job satisfaction. *Journal of Nursing Administration, 32*(11), 586–595.

Mondros, J. B., & Wilson, S. M. (1994). *Organizing for power and empowerment.* Columbia University Press.

Moore, S. C., & Wells, N. J. (2010). Staff nurses lead the way for improvement to shared governance structure. *Journal of Nursing Administration, 40*(11), 477–482.

Morgan, A. (1993). *Imaginization: The art of creative management.* Sage.

Morgan, A. (1997). *Images of organization.* Sage.

Nelson, W. (2013). The imperative of a moral compass-driven healthcare organization. *Frontiers of a Health Services Management, 30*(1), 39–45.

Perera, F., & Peiro, M. (2012). Strategic planning in healthcare organizations. *Revista Española de Cardiología, 65*(8), 749–754.

Perrow, C. (1969). The analysis of goals in complex organizations. In A. Etzioni (Ed.), *Readings on modern organizations.* Prentice-Hall.

Porter, C., Kolcaba, K., McNulty, S. R., & Fitzpatrick, J. J. (2010). A nursing labor management partnership model. *Journal of Nursing Administration, 40*(6), 272–276.

Porter O'Grady, T., & Malloch, K. (2016). *Leadership in nursing practice* (2nd ed.). Jones & Bartlett Learning, LLC.

Press Ganey. (2017). *Nursing special report: The influence of nurse manager leadership on patient and nurse outcomes and the mediating effects of the nurse work environment* [White paper].

Purser, R. E., & Cabana, S. (1999). *The self-managing organization.* Free Press (Simon & Schuster).

Redman, R. W. (2008). Symposium in tribute to a nursing leader: Ada Sue Hinshaw. *Nursing Research, 51*(15), S1–S3.

Roark, D. C. (2005). Managing the healthcare supply chain. *Nursing Management, 36*(2), 36–40.

Rosen, R. H. (1996). *Leading people: Transforming business from the inside out.* Viking Penguin.

Sabiston, J. A., & Laschinger, H. K. S. (1995). Staff nurse work empowerment and perceived autonomy. *Journal of Nursing Administration, 28*(9), 42–49.

Schein, E. H. (2004). *Organizational culture and leadership.* Jossey-Bass.

Scott-Findley, S., & Golden-Biddle, K. (2005). Understanding how organizational culture shapes research use. *Journal of Nursing Administration, 35*(7/8), 359–365.

Seago, J., Spetz, J., Ash, M., Herrera, C., & Keane, D. (2011). Hospital RN job satisfaction and nurse unions. *Journal of Nursing Administration, 41*(3), 109–114.

Sepasi, R., Abbaszadeh, A., Borhani, F., & Hossein, R. (2016). Nurses' perceptions of the concept of power in nursing: A qualitative study. *Journal of Clinical and Diagnostic Research, 10*(12), LC10–LC15. https://doi.org/10.7860/JCDR/2016/22526.8971

Spence, H. K., & Laschinger, J. F. (2005). Using empowerment to build trust and respect in the workplace: A strategy for addressing the nursing shortage. *Nursing Economics, 23*(1), 6–13.

Spreitzer, G. M., & Quinn, R. E. (2001). *A company of leaders.* Jossey-Bass.

Tappen, R. M. (2001). *Nursing leadership and management: Concepts and practice* (4th ed.). F.A. Davis.

Temple, A., Dobbs, D., & Andel, R. (2011). Exploring correlates of turnover among nursing assistants in the hospital nursing home survey. *Journal of Nursing Administration, 41*(7/8), S34–S44.

Trinh, H. Q., & O'Connor, S. J. (2002). Helpful or harmful? The impact of strategic change on the performance of U.S. urban hospitals. *Health Services Research, 37*(1), 145–171.

UCLA Health. (2009). *Mission, vision and philosophy; Staying true to what we believe.* https://www.uclahealth.org/nursing/mission-vision-philosophy

Vogus, T. J., & Sutcliffe, K. M. (2007). The safety organizing scale: Development and validation of a behavioral measure of safety culture in hospital nursing units. *Medical Care, 45*(1), 46–54.

Weissman, J. S., Rothschild, J. M., Bendavid, E., Sprivulis, P., Cook, E., Evans, R., … Bates, D. (2007). Hospital workload and adverse events. *Medical Care, 45*(5), 448–455.

Yourstone, S. A., & Smith, H. L. (2002). Managing system errors and failures in health care organizations: Suggestions for practice and research. *Health Care Management Review, 27*(1), 50–61.

Chapter 10 References

Albrecht, S. L., Connaughton, S., Foster, K., Furlong, S., & Yeow, C. J. L. (2020). Change engagement, change resources, and change demands: A model for positive employee orientations to organizational change. *Frontiers in psychology, 11,* 531944. https://doi.org/10.3389/fpsyg.2020.531944

Araujo Group. (n.d.). *A compilation of opinions of experts in the field of the management of change.* Unpublished report.

Berman-Rubera, S. (2008, August 10). *Leading and embracing change.* Business/Change-Management. http://ezinearticles.com/?Leading-And-Embracing-Change&id=1180585

Boyer, D. (2013). Paradigm shift: How *ICD-10* will change healthcare. *Health Management Technology, 34*(9), 24.

Braungardt, T., & Fought, S. G. (2008). Leading change during an inpatient critical care unit expansion. *Journal of Nursing Administration, 38*(11), 461–467. https://doi.org/10.1097/01.NNA.0000339476.73090.33

Cameron, K. S., & Quinn, Q. E. (2006). *Diagnosing and changing organizational culture.* Jossey-Bass.

Chreim, S., & Williams, B. E. (2012). Radical change in healthcare organization: Mapping transition between templates, enabling factors, and implementation processes. *Journal of Health Organization and Management, 26*(2), 215–236. https://doi.org/10.1108/14777261211230781

Cornell, P., Riordan, M., & Herrin-Griffith, D. (2010). Transforming nursing workflow, part 2: The impact of technology on nurse activities. *Journal of Nursing Administration, 40*(10), 432–439. https://doi.org/10.1097/NNA.0b013e3181f2eb3f

Dent, H. S. (1995). *Job shock: Four new principles transforming our work and business.* St. Martin's Press.

Deutschman, A. (2005a). Change or die. *Fast Company, 94,* 52–62.

Deutschman, A. (2005b). *What state of change are you in?* http://www.fastcompany.com/52596/which-stage-change-are-you

Englebright, J. D., & Franklin, M. (2005). Managing a new medication administrative process. *Journal of*

Nursing Administration, 35(9), 410–413. https://doi.org/10.1097/00005110-200509000-00011

Farrell, K., & Broude, C. (1987). *Winning the change game: How to implement information systems with fewer headaches and bigger paybacks.* Breakthrough Enterprises.

Fullan, M. (2001). *Leading in a culture of change.* Jossey-Bass.

Guthrie, V. A., & King, S. N. (2004). Feedback-intensive programs. In C. D. McCauley & E. Van Velson (Eds.), *The center for creative leadership handbook of leadership development* (pp. 25–57). Jossey-Bass.

Hansten, R. I., & Washburn, M. J. (1999). Individual and organizational accountability for development of critical thinking. *Journal of Nursing Administration, 29*(11), 39–45. https://doi.org/10.1097/00005110-199911000-00010

Hart, L. B., & Waisman, C. S. (2005). *The leadership training activity book.* AMACOM.

Heifetz, R. A., & Linsky, M. (2002, June). A survival guide for leaders. *Harvard Business Review, 80*(6) 65–74. https://hbr.org/2002/06/a-survival-guide-for-leaders

Heller, R. (1998). *Managing change.* DK Publishing.

Hempel, J. (2005, July 4). Why the boss really had to say goodbye. *Bloomberg Businessweek (Online), 3941.*

Hossainian, N., Slot, D. E., Afennich, F., & Van der Weijden, G. A. (2011). The effects of hydrogen peroxide mouthwashes on the prevention of plaque and gingival inflammation: A systematic review. *International Journal of Dental Hygiene, 9,* 171–181. https://doi.org/10.1111/j.1601-5037.2010.00492.x

Johnston, G. (2008, March 8). Change management—Why the high failure rate. *Business/Change-Management.* http://ezinearticles.com/?Change-Management—Why-the-High-Failure-Rate?&id=1028294

Kalisch, B. J. (2007). Don't like change? Blame it on your strategic style. *Reflections on Nursing Leadership, 33*(3), 4.

Kotter, J. P. (1999). Leading change: The eight steps to transformation. In J. A. Conger, G. M. Spreitzer, & E. E. Lawler (Eds.), *The leader's change handbook: An essential guide to setting direction and taking action* (pp. 87–99). Jossey-Bass.

Lapp, J. (2002, May). Thriving on change. *Caring Magazine,* 40–43.

Leonard, D. (2012, October 15). Obamacare is not an epithet. *Bloomberg Business Week,* 98–100.

Lewin, K. (1951). *Field theory in social science: Selected theoretical papers.* Harper & Row.

Lindberg, C., & Clancy, T. R. (2010). Positive deviance: An elegant solution to a complex problem. *Journal of Nursing Administration, 40*(4), 150–153. https://doi.org/10.1097/NNA.0b013e3181d40e39

MacDavitt, K. (2011). Implementing small tests of change to improve patient satisfaction. *The Journal of Nursing Administration, 41*(1), 5–9. https://doi.org/10.1097/NNA.0b013e318200285b

Maslow, A. H. (1970). *Motivation and personality.* Harper & Row.

Maurer, R. (2008, August 13). The 4 reasons why people resist change. *Business/Change-Management.* http://ezinearticles.com/?The-7-Reasons-Why-People-Resist-Change&id=1053595

Murrar, S., & Brauer, M. (2019). Overcoming resistance to change: Using narratives to create more positive intergroup attitudes. *Current Directions in Psychological Science, 28*(2), 164–169. https://doi.org/10.1177/0963721418818552

Parker, M., & Gadbois, S. (2000). Building community in healthcare workplace. Part 3: Belonging and satisfaction at work. *Journal of Nursing Administration, 30,* 466–473. https://doi.org/10.1097/00005110-200010000-00004

Pearcey, P., & Draper, P. (1996). Using the diffusion of innovation model to influence practice: A case study. *Journal of advanced nursing, 23*(4), 714–721. https://doi.org/10.1111/j.1365-2648.1996.tb00042.x

Porter-O'Grady, T. (1996). The seven basic rules for successful redesign. *Journal of Nursing Administration, 26*(1), 46–53.

Porter-O'Grady, T., & Malloch, K. (2016). *Leadership in nursing practice* (2nd ed.). Jones & Bartlett Learning.

Rieley, J. B. (2015). What to Do When Employees Are Gaming the System: Overcoming Resistance to Change. In Global Business and Organizational Excellence, *35*(2), 31–37. Wiley. https://doi.org/10.1002/joe.21653

Rodts, M. F. (2011). Technology changes healthcare. *Orthopedic Nursing, 30*(5), 292. https://doi.org/10.1097/NOR.0b013e3182352a14

"How to Overcome Resistance to Organizational Change." SafeStart, 9 June 2020, https://safestart.com/news/how-to-overcome-resistance-to-organizational-change/. Accessed 29 Mar. 2022.

Safian, R. (2012, November). Secrets of the flux leader. *Fast Company, 170,* 96–106, 136.

Schein, E. H. (2004). Kurt Lewin's change theory in the field and in the classroom: Notes toward a model of managed learning. *Reflections, 1*(1), 59–74.

Shirey, M. R. (2011). Establishing a sense of urgency for leading transformational change. *Journal of Nursing Administration, 41*(4), 145–148. https://doi.org/10.1097/NNA.0b013e3182118550

Shirey, M. R. (2012). Stakeholder analysis and mapping as targeted communication strategy. *Journal of Nursing Administration, 42*(9), 399–403. https://doi.org/10.1097/NNA.0b013e3182668149

Staren, E. D., Braun, D. P., & Denny, D. S. (2010, March–April). Optimizing innovation in health care organization. *Physicians Executive Journal, 36*(2), 54–62.

Suddath, C. (2012, December 3–9). Business by the bard. *Bloomberg Business Week,* 83–85.

Tappen, R. M. (2001). *Nursing leadership and management: Concepts and practice.* F.A. Davis.

Tombes, M. B., & Gallucci, B. (1993). The effects of hydrogen peroxide rinses on the normal oral mucosa. *Nursing Research, 42,* 332–337.

Webb, J. A. K., & Marshall, D. R. (2010). Healthcare reform and nursing. *Journal of Nursing Administration, 49*(9), 345–349. https://doi.org/10.1097/NNA.0b013e3181ee42d4

Chapter 11 References

Agency for Healthcare Research and Quality. (2013, May). *Module 4. Approaches to quality improvement.* Author. https://www.ahrq.gov/ncepcr/tools/pf-handbook/mod4.html

Agency for Healthcare Research and Quality. (2016a). *PSI 90 fact sheet. AHRQ quality indicators.* http://www.qualityindicators.ahrq.gov/downloads/modules/psi/v31/psi_guide_v31.pdf

Agency for Healthcare Research and Quality. (2016b, December). *Strategic plan.* Author. http://www.ahrq .gov/cpi/about/mission/strategic-plan/strategic-plan .html

Agency for Healthcare Research and Quality. (2017a). *Never events.* Author. https://psnet.ahrq.gov/primers /primer/3/never-events

Agency for Healthcare Research and Quality. (2017b, August). *Health information technology division's 2016 annual report.* (Prepared by John Snow, Inc. Under Contract No. HHSN316201200068W.) AHRQ Publication No. 17-0040-EF. Author.

Agency for Healthcare Research and Quality. (2018). *AHRQ strategic plan.* Author. https://www.ahrq .gov/cpi/about/profile/index.html

Agency for Healthcare Research and Quality. (2019a). *High reliability.* PSNet, September 7, 2019. Retrieved on April 6, 2022 from https://psnet.ahrq.gov/primer /high-reliability

Agency for Healthcare Research and Quality. (2019b). *Medication errors and adverse drug events.* PSNet, September 7, 2019. Retrieved on April 3, 2022 from https://psnet.ahrq.gov/primer/ medication-errors-and-adverse-drug-events.

Aiken, L. H., Sermeus, W., Van den Heede, K., Sloan, D. M., Russe, R., McKee, M., . . . Moreno-Casbas, M. T. (2012). Patient safety, satisfaction, and quality of hospital care: Cross sectional surveys of nurses and patients in 12 countries in Europe and the United States. *British Medical Journal, 344,* e1717. https://doi.org/10.1136/bmj.e1717

Anderson, J., & Abrahamson, K. (2017). Your health care may kill you: Medical errors. *Studies in Health Technology and Informatics, 234,* 13–17. https:// pubmed.ncbi.nlm.nih.gov/28186008/

Austin, M., & Derk, J. (2016). Lives lost, lives saved: A comparative analysis of avoidable deaths at hospitals graded by the Leapfrog Group. *Armstrong Institute for Patient Safety and Quality Johns Hopkins Medicine.* https://psnet.ahrq.gov/ primers/primer/34/adverse-events-near-misses -and-errors

Benner, P., Sutphen, M., Leonard, V., & Day, L. (2010). *Educating nurses: A call for radical transformation.* Jossey-Bass.

Benson-Flynn, J. (2001). Incident reporting: Clarifying occurrences, incidents, and sentinel events. *Home Healthcare Nurse, 19,* 701–706.

Brook, R. H., Davis, A. R., & Kamberg, C. (1980). Selected reflections on quality of medical care evaluations in the 1980s. *Nursing Research, 29*(2), 127.

Brown, C., Hofer, T., Johal, A., Thomson, R., Nicoll, J., Franklin, B. D., & Lilford, R. J. (2008). An epistemology of patient safety research: A framework for study design and interpretation. Part 4. One size does not fit all. *Quality and Safety in Health Care, 17,* 178–181.

Brown, T. W., McCarthy, M. L., Kelen, G. D., & Lew, F. (2010). An epidemiologic study of closed emergency department malpractice claims in a national database of physician malpractice insurers. *Academic Emergency Medicine, 17*(5), 553–560.

Burke, J., Downey, C., & Almoudaris, A. (2022). Failure to rescue deteriorating patients: A systematic review of root causes and improvement strategies. *Journal of Patient Safety, 18*(1), e140–e155. https://pubmed. ncbi.nlm.nih.gov/32453105/

Centers for Disease Control and Prevention. (2020). *2020 National and state healthcare-associated infections progress report.* https://www.cdc.gov/hai/data /portal/progress-report.html

Centers for Medicare & Medicaid Services. (2021). *Quality measurement and quality improvement.* https:// www.cms.gov/Medicare/Quality-Initiatives-Patient -Assessment-Instruments/MMS/Quality-Measure -and-Quality-Improvement-#:~:text=Quality%20im-provement%20seeks%20to%20standardize,%2C %20healthcare%20systems%2C%20and%20 organizations

Cole, L., & Houston, S. (1999). Linking outcomes management and practice improvement structured care methodologies: Evolution and use in patient care delivery. *Outcomes Management for Nursing Practice, 3*(2), 53.

Delamont, A. (2016). How to avoid the top seven nursing errors. *Nursing Made Incredibly Easy, 11*(2), 8–10.

Donabedian, A. (1969). A guide to medical care administration. In *Medical care appraisal: Quality and utilization* (Vol. II, pp. 13–45). American Public Health Association.

Donabedian, A. (1977). Evaluating the quality of medical care. *Milbank Memorial Fund Quarterly, 44*(part 2), 166.

Donabedian, A. (1987). Some basic issues in evaluating the quality of health care. In L. T. Rinke (Ed.), *Outcome measures in home care.* National League of Nursing.

Donaldson, M. S. (Ed.). (1998). *Statement on quality of care.* National Academies Press. http://www.nap .edu/

Drewniak, R. (2014). *White paper: 7 steps to healthcare strategic planning.* Hayes Management Consulting. https://www.hayesmanagement.com /wp-content/uploads/2014/06/Whitepaper-Hayes -White-Paper_7-Steps-to-Healthcare-Strategic -Planning.pdf

Dubois, C. A., D'Amour, D., Pomey, M. P., Girard, F., & Brault, I. (2013). Conceptualizing performance of nursing care as a prerequisite for better measurement: A systematic and interpretive review. *Biomed Central Nursing, 12*(7). https://doi.org/10.1186 /1472-6955-12-7

Galvin, R. S., Delbanco, S., Milstein, A., & Belden, G. (2005, January/February). Has the Leapfrog Group had an impact on the health care market? *Health Affairs, 24*(1), 228–233.

Haines, T. P., Hill, A. M., & Hill, K. D. (2011). Patient education to prevent falls among older hospital inpatients: A randomized controlled trial. *Archives of Internal Medicine, 171*(6), 516–524.

Hansten, R., & Washburn, M. (2001). Outcomes-based care delivery. *American Journal of Nursing, 101*(2), 24A–D.

Health Resources and Services Administration. (2011). *Developing and implementing a QI plan.* U.S. Department of Health and Human Services.

Hostetter, M., & Klein, S. (2012). Using patient-reported outcomes to improve health care quality. *Quality Matters. The Commonwealth Fund.* http://www .commonwealthfund.org/publications/newsletters /quality-matters/2011/december-january-2012/ in-focus

Institute of Medicine. (2000). Why do accidents happen? In L. T. Kohn, J. M. Corrigan, & M. S. Donaldson

(Eds.), *To err is human: Building a safer health system.* National Academies Press.

Institute of Medicine. (2001). *Crossing the quality chasm: A new health system for the 21st century.* National Academies Press.

Institute of Medicine. (2003). *Core competencies for health professionals.* National Academies Press.

Institute of Medicine. (2011). *The future of nursing: Leading change, advancing health.* National Academies Press.

Irvine, D. (1998). Finding value in nursing care: A framework for quality improvement and clinical evaluation. *Nursing Economics, 16*(3), 110–118.

Johns Hopkins Medicine. (2013, April 23). Diagnostic errors more common, costly and harmful than treatment mistakes. *Johns Hopkins News and Publications.* https://www.hopkinsmedicine.org/news/media/releases/diagnostic_errors_more_common_costly_and_harmful_than_treatment_mistakes

Jones, T. (2016). Outcomes measurement in nursing: Imperatives, ideals, history and challenges. *OJIN Online Journal of Issues in Nursing, 21*(2).

Kaiser Family Foundation. (2018). *The U.S. government and global health.* https://www.kff.org/search/?s=health+policy+and+research

Kalisch, B., Landstrom, G., & Williams, R. A. (2009). Missed nursing care: Errors of omission. *Nursing Outlook, 57*(1), 3–9.

Leape, L. L., Bates, D. W., & Petrycki, S. (1993). Incidence and preventability of adverse drug events in hospitalized adults. *Journal of Internal Medicine, 8,* 289–294.

Leape, L. L., Lawthers, A. G., Brennan, T. A., & Johnson, W. (1993). Preventing medical injury. *Quality Review Bulletin, 19*(5), 144–149.

Leapfrog Group. (2011). *About us.* http://www.leapfroggroup.org/about

Lichtig, L. K., Knauf, R. A., & Milholland, D. K. (1999). Some impacts of nursing on acute care hospital outcomes. *Journal of Nursing Administration, 29*(2), 25–33.

Mardon, R. E., Khanna, K., Sorra, J., Dyer, N., & Famolaro, T. (2010). Exploring relationships between hospital patient safety culture and adverse event. *Journal of Patient Safety, 6*(4), 226–232.

McLaughlin, C., & Kaluzny, A. (2006). *Continuous quality improvement in health care: Theory, implementations, and applications* (3rd ed.). Jones & Bartlett Learning.

Mitchell, P. (2008). Defining patient safety and quality. In R. G. Hughes (Ed.), *An evidence-based handbook for nurses* (Chapter 1, p. 2). Agency for Healthcare Research and Quality. https://archive.ahrq.gov/professionals/clinicians-providers/resources/nursing/resources/nurseshdbk/index.html

National Academies of Sciences, Engineering, and Medicine; National Academy of Medicine; Committee on the Future of Nursing 2020–2030; Flaubert J. L., Le Menestrel, S., Williams, D. R., et al. (Eds.). (2021, May 11). *The future of nursing 2020–2030: Charting a path to achieve health equity.* National Academies Press.

Nightingale, F., & Barnum, B. S. (1992). *Notes on nursing: What it is, and what it is not* (commemorative ed.). Lippincott-Raven.

Oliver, D., Healey, F., & Haines, T. P. (2010). Preventing falls and fall-related injuries in hospitals. *Clinical Geriatric Medicine, 26*(4), 645–692.

Oz, M. (2009). *Dennis Quaid's medical nightmare.* http://www.oprah.com/health/how-a-medical-mistake-almost-killed-dennis-quaids-twins

Patient-Centered Outcomes Research Institute. (2012). *Improving health care systems.* http://www.pcori.org/assets/PFA-Improving-Healthcare-Systems-05222012.pdf

Pham, J. C., Aswani, M. S., Rosen, M., Lee, H. W., Huddle, M., Weeks, K., & Pronovost, P. J. (2012). Reducing medical errors and adverse events. *Annual Review of Medicine, 63,* 447–463. http://www.annualreviews.org

Quisenberry, E. (2021). *How does standard work lead to better patient safety?* Virginia Mason Institute. https://www.virginiamasoninstitute.org/how-does-standard-work-lead-to-better-patient-safety/

Raduma-Tomas, M. A., Flin, R., Yule, S. J., & Close, S. (2012). The importance of preparation for doctors' handovers in an acute medical assessment unit: A hierarchal task analysis. *Quality and Safety in Health Care, 21,* 211–217.

Raduma-Tomas, M. A., Flin, R., Yule, S. J., & Williams, D. (2011). Doctors' handovers in hospitals: A literature review. *Quality and Safety in Health Care, 20,* 128–133.

Robert Wood Johnson Foundation. (2011). *Nurses are key to improving patient safety.* http://www.rwjf.org/en/about-rwjf/newsroom/newsroom-content/2011/04/nurses-are-key-to-improving-patient-safety.html

Robert Wood Johnson Foundation. (2017). *Our focus areas.* https://www.rwjf.org/en/our-focus-areas.html

Rogers, A. E., Hwang, W., Scott, L. D., Aiken, L. H., & Dinge, D. (2004). The working hours of hospital staff nurses and patient safety: Both errors and near errors are more likely to occur when hospital staff nurses work twelve or more hours at a stretch. *Health Affairs, 23*(4), 202–212.

Sternberg, S. (2016). Medical errors are third leading cause of death in the U.S. *US News and World Report.* https://www.usnews.com/news/articles/2016-05-03/medical-errors-are-third-leading-cause-of-death-in-the-us

Sutcliffe, K. (2011). High reliability organizations (HROs). *Best Practice & Research Clinical Anaesthesiology, 25*(2), 133–144.

Swansburg, R., & Swansburg, R. (2002). *Introduction to management and leadership for nurse managers* (3rd ed.). Jones & Bartlett Learning.

Taylor, M., McNicholas, C., Nicolay, C., Darzi, A., Bell, D., & Reed, J. (2013). Systematic review of the application of the plan-do-study-act method to improve quality in healthcare. *BMJ Quality and Safety.* https://doi.org/10.1136/bmjqs-2013-001862

Taylor, M. J., McNicholas, C., Nicolay, C., Darzi, A., Bell, D., & Reed, J. E. (2014). Systematic review of the application of the plan-do-study-act method to improve quality in healthcare. *BMJ Quality & Safety, 23*(4), 290–298. https://doi.org/10.1136/bmjqs-2013-001862

The Joint Commission. (2009).

The Joint Commission. (2017a). *History of The Joint Commission.* https://www.jointcommission.org/about_us/history.aspx

The Joint Commission. (2017b, June 29). *Sentinel event policy and procedures.* https://www.jointcommission.org/sentinel_event_policy_and_procedures/

U.S. Department of Health and Human Services. (2018). *Introduction about HHS.* https://www.hhs.gov/about /strategic-plan/index.html

World Health Organization. (2021). *Patient safety EURO.* https://www.who.int/europe/health-topics/patient -safety#tab=tab_1

Chapter 12 References

Agency for Healthcare Research and Quality. (2005). *Keeping patients safe: Transforming the work environment of nurses.* PSNet, May 11, 2005. Retrieved June20, 2022 from https://psnet.ahrq.gov/issue /keeping-patients-safe-transforming-the-work-environment -nurses#

Agency for Healthcare Research and Quality. (2019). *Primers culture of safety in PSNet,* September 7, 2019. https://psnet.ahrq.gov/primer/culture-safety

Agency for Healthcare Research and Quality. (2021). *Nurse and patient safety.* PSNet, April 21, 2021. https://psnet.ahrq.gov/primer /nursing-and-patient-safety

Aiken, L. H., Clarke, S. P., Sloane, D. M., Sochalski, J., & Silber, J. H. (2002). Hospital nurse staffing and patient mortality, nurse burnout, and job dissatisfaction. *Journal of the American Medical Association, 288*(16), 1987–1993.

Alexander, A., Tellner, C., & Van Embden, T. (2022, May 17). *Navigating the hazard of rising violence in health care facilities.* Reuters. https://www.reuters.com /legal/litigation/navigating-hazard-rising-violence -health-care-facilities-2022-05-17/

Altman, G. (2002). Bioterrorism's invisible threats. *Nursing Management, 33*(1), 43, 45–47.

American College of Healthcare Executives. (2017). *The culture of safety imperative in leading a culture of safety: A blueprint for success.* Author. https://www .ache.org/about-ache/our-story/our-commitments /leading-for-safety/blueprint#download

American Nurses Association. (1993). *HIV, hepatitis-B, hepatitis-C: Blood-borne diseases.* Author.

American Nurses Association. (1994). *Guidelines on reporting incompetent, unethical, or illegal practices.* Author.

American Nurses Association. (2006, December 8). *Assuring patient safety: Registered nurses' responsibility in all roles and settings to guard against working when fatigued.* Author.

American Nurses Association. (2007). *ANA's principles of environmental health for nursing practice with implementation strategies.* Author.

American Nurses Association. (2010). *Safe needles save lives fact sheet.* https://www.nursingworld.org /~48de3c/globalassets/docs/ana/snsl-fact-sheet _final110110.pdf

American Nurses Association (2011). 2011 ANA Health and Safety Survey. https://www.nursingworld.org /practice-policy/work-environment/health-safety /health-safety-survey/

American Nurses Association. (2015a). *The code for nurses.* www.nursingworld.org/practice-policy /nursing-excellence/ethics/code-of-ethics-for-nurses/

American Nurses Association (2015b). Position Statement: "Incivility, bullying, and workplace violence." https:// www.nursingworld.org/~49d6e3/globalassets/prac- ticeandpolicy/nursing-excellence/incivility -bullying-and-workplace-violence–ana-position -statement.pdf

American Nurses Association. (2018). *Work environment health and safety, hazardous chemicals.* www. nursingworld.org/practice-policy/work -environment/

American Nurses Association. (2022a). Work environment health and safety; disaster preparedness. https:// www.nursingworld.org/practice-policy/work -environment/health-safety/disaster -preparedness/

American Nurses Association. (2022b). Advocating for safe staffing. https://www.nursingworld.org /practice-policy/nurse-staffing/nurse-staffing -advocacy/

Arnetz, J. E., Hamblin, L., Ager, J., Luborsky, M., Upfal, M. J., Russell, J., & Essenmacher, L. (2015). Underreporting of workplace violence: Comparison of self-report and actual documentation of hospital incidents. *Workplace Health & Safety, 63*(5), 200–210. https://doi.org/10.1177 /2165079915574684

Association of Women's Health, Obstetric and Neonatal Nurses. (2001). *AWHONN takes action against bioterrorism.*

Bauer, X., Ammon, J., Chen, Z., Beckmann, U., & Czuppon, A. B. (1993). Health risk in hospitals through airborne allergens for patients pre-sensitized to latex. *Lancet, 342,* 1148–1149.

Beyea, S. (2004). A critical partnership-safety for nurses and patients. *AORN, 79*(6), 1299–1302.

Brooke, P. (2001). The legal realities of HIV exposure. *RN, 64*(12), 71–73.

Bureau of Labor Statistics. (2020). *Fact sheet | Workplace violence in healthcare, 2018.* https://www.bls.gov /iif/oshwc/cfoi/workplace-violence-healthcare-2018 .htm

Caruso, C. C., Geiger-Brown, J., Takahashi, M., Trinkoff, A., & Nakata, A. (2015). *NIOSH training for nurses on shift work and long work hours.* U.S. Department of Health and Human Services, Centers for Disease Control and Prevention, National Institute for Occupational Safety and Health. (Revised 10/2021). https://doi.org/10.26616/NIOSHPUB2015115revi- sed102021external icon

Centers for Disease Control and Prevention. (1998). *NIOSH alert: Preventing allergic reactions to natural rubber latex in the workplace.* DHHS (NIOSH) Publication No. 97-135. https://www.cdc.gov/niosh /docs/97-135/

Centers for Disease Control and Prevention. (2019). *COVID-19. What's new and updated?* https://www .cdc.gov/coronavirus/2019-ncov/whats-new-all .html#print

Centers for Disease Control and Prevention. (2022). *Post exposure prophylaxis sheet.* https://www.cdc .gov/hiv/risk/pep/index.html#:~:tex- t=1%2D888%2D448%2D4911&text=For%20 more%20information%20on%20the,the%20 National%20Clinicians%20Consultation%20 Center%20

Cleveland Clinic. (2021, February 25). *Shift work sleep disorder.* https://my.clevelandclinic.org/health /diseases/12146-shift-work-sleep-disorder#:~: text =Shift%20work%20sleep%20disorder%20 (SWSD)%20is%20a%20sleep%20disorder%20 that,body%20clocks%20or%20circadian %20rhythms

Daley, K. A. (2012, September). Editorial: Moving the sharps agenda forward. *American Nurse Today, 7,* 1.

Dempsey, C., & Reilly, B. (2016, January 31). Nurse engagement: What are the contributing factors for success? *OJIN: The Online Journal of Issues in Nursing, 21*(1), 2. https://doi.org/10.3912/OJIN.Vol21No01Man02

Dugdale, D. (2021, October 24). *Handling sharps and needles.* Medline Plus. https://medlineplus.gov/ency/patientinstructions/000444.htm

Edlich, R., Woodard, C., & Haines, M. (2001). Disabling back injuries in nursing personnel. *Journal of Emergency Nursing, 27*(2), 150–155.

Edwards, R. (1999). Prevention of workplace violence. *Aspen's Advisor for Nurse Executives, 14*(8), 8–12.

Equal Employment Opportunity Commission. (2018). *Reasonable accommodation policy tips.* https://www.eeoc.gov/employers/smallbusiness/checklists/reasonable_accommodation_policy_tips.cfm

Feiler, J. L., & Stichler, J. F. (2011). Ergonomics in healthcare facility design: Part 2. *Journal of Nursing Administration, 41*(3), 97–99.

Foley, M. (2012, September). Essential elements of a comprehensive sharps injury-prevention program. *American Nurse Today, 7*, 2–4.

Francis, R., & Dawson, J. M. (2016). Special report: Preventing patient-handling injuries in nurses. *American Nurse Today, 11*(5), 37–38.

General Industry Regulations Book. (2018). Subpart Z occupational safety and health standards. Title 29. *Code of Federal Regulations,* Part 1910.

Gilmore-Hall, A. (2001). Violence in the workplace. *Issues Update, American Nurses Association, 7*, 55–56. http://www.nursingcenter.com

Go Local Worcester News Team. (2017, June 16). *MA nurses call for action following Harrington Hospital stabbing.* http://www.golocalworcester.com/news/ma-nurses-call-for-action-following-harrington-hospital-stabbing

Guglielmi, C., & Ogg, M. J. (2012, September). Practical strategies to prevent surgical sharps injuries. *American Nurse Today, 7*, 8–10.

Hagen, P., Montgomery, J., & O'Reilly, J. (Eds.). (2015). *Accident prevention manual for business and industry: Administration and programs* (14th ed.). National Safety Council.

Hamilton, R., Brown, R., Veltri, M., Feroli, R., Primeau, M. N., Schauble, J. F., & Adkinson, N. F., Jr. (2005). Administering pharmaceuticals to latex allergy patients from vials containing natural rubber latex closures. *American Journal Health Systems Pharmacy, 62*, 1822–1827.

Handelman, E., Perry, J. L., & Parker, G. (2012, September). Reducing sharps injuries in non-hospital settings. *American Nurse Today, 7*, 5–7.

Hausman, M., Grimley, K., Wallace, T., & Busch, M. (2022, May 26). *Solving for healing; to achieve effective nurse staffing, you need CFO-CNO alignment.* HFMA. https://www.hfma.org/topics/cost-effectiveness-of-health/article/to-achieve-effective-nurse-staffing-you-need-cfo-cno-alignment.html

Herring, L. H. (1994). *Infection control.* National League for Nursing.

Hodge, J. G., & Nelson, K. (2014). Active shooters in health care settings: Prevention and response through law and policy. *Journal of Law, Medicine & Ethics, 42*(2), 268–271. https://doi.org/10.1111/jlme.12141

Iennaco, J. D., Dixon, J., Whittemore, R., & Bowers, L. (2013). Measurement and monitoring of health care worker aggression exposure. *Online Journal of Issues in Nursing, 18*(1), 3.

Kansas State Nurses Association (corporate author). (1996). Violence assessment in hospitals provides basis for action. *The Kansas Nurse, 71*(3), 18–20.

Kinkle, S. (1993). Violence in the ED: How to stop it before it starts. *American Journal of Nursing, 93*(7), 22–24.

Krucoff, M. (2001). How to prevent repetitive stress injury in the workplace. *American Fitness, 19*(1), 31.

Lanza, M. L., & Carifio, J. (1991). Blaming the victim: Complex (nonlinear) patterns of causal attribution by nurses in response to vignettes of a patient assaulting a nurse. *Journal of Emergency Nursing, 17*(5), 299–309.

Lilly Ledbetter Fair Pay Act of 2009, S.181, 123 Stat. 5.

Lindberg, P., & Vingård, E. (2012). Indicators of healthy work environments—a systematic review. *Work: A Journal of Prevention, Assessment and Rehabilitation, 41*(Suppl. 1), 3032–3038.

Magnavita, N., & Heponiemi, T. (2011). Workplace violence against nursing students and nurses: An Italian experience. *Journal of Nursing Scholarship, 43*(2), 203–210.

Mahoney, B. (1991). The extent, nature, and response to victimization of emergency nurses in Pennsylvania. *Journal of Emergency Nursing, 17*, 282–292.

McElwee, C. (2019, September 19). Emergency in the emergency room. *City Journal.* https://www.city-journal.org/violence-in-americas-emergency-rooms

McPhaul, K., & Lipscomb, J. (2004, September 30). Workplace violence in health care: Recognized but not regulated. *Online Journal of Issues in Nursing, 9*(3), 6. www.nursingworld.org

Nadwairski, J. A. (1992). Inner-city safety for home care providers. *Journal of Nursing Administration, 22*(9), 42–47.

National Institute for Occupational Safety and Health. (2002). *Violence occupational hazards in hospitals.* DHHS (NIOSH) Publication Number 2002–101. https://www.cdc.gov/niosh/docs/2002-101/

NPR online or Associated Press. (2022, June 5). *Police ID a suspect in the attacks on a doctor and 2 nurses at an L.A. hospital.* https://www.npr.org/2022/06/04/1103070911/attack-doctor-nurses-southern-california-hospital

Occupational Safety and Health Administration. (2003). *Back facts: A training workbook to prevent back injuries in nursing homes.* https://www.osha.gov/SLTC/healthcarefacilities/training/index.html

Occupational Safety and Health Administration. (2009). *Ergonomics for the prevention of musculoskeletal disorders.* http://www.osha.gov/ergonomics/guidelines/nursinghome/index.html

Occupational Safety and Health Administration. (2018a). *Healthcare wide hazards: Hazardous chemicals.* https://www.osha.gov/SLTC/etools/hospital/hazards/hazchem/haz.html

Occupational Safety and Health Administration, U.S. Department of Labor. (2018b). *Needlestick frequently asked questions.*

Occupational Safety and Health Administration, U.S. Department of Labor (2018c). *Safe patient handling.* https://www.osha.gov/SLTC/healthcarefacilities/safepatienthandling.html

Occupational Safety and Health Administration. (2020). *All about OSHA.* U.S. Department of Labor.

https://www.osha.gov/sites/default/files/publications/all_about_OSHA.pdf

O'Malley, P. (2011). Staying awake and asleep: The challenge of working nights and rotating shifts. *Clinical Nurse Specialist, 25*(1), 15–17.

Praug, W., & Jelsness-Jorgensen, L. P. (2014). Should I report? A qualitative study of barriers to incident reporting among nurses working in nursing homes. *Geriatric Nursing, 35*(6), 441–447.

Public Services Health & Safety Association. (2018). Intelligent safety; Annual Report 2017-2018. www.pshsa.ca https://terraform-20180423174453746800000001.s3.amazonaws.com/attachments/cjs3jez4n01vuoikk-ci4xp5l0-pshsa-2017-2018-annual-report-intelligent-safety.pdf

Roche, E. (1993, February 23). Nurses' risks and their rights. *Vital Signs, 3*.

Rogers, A. E., Hwang, W., Scott, L. D., Aiken, L. H., & Dinges, D. F. (2004). The working hours of hospital staff nurses and patient safety: Both errors and near errors are more likely to occur when hospital staff nurses work twelve or more hours at a stretch. *Health Affairs, 23*(4), 202–212.

Romjue, A. (2020, April 1). How healthcare facilities can go green in 2020. *Healthcare Facilities Today.* https://www.healthcarefacilitiestoday.com/posts/How-healthcare-facilities-can-go-green-in-2020-23988

Rosen, A., Isaacson, D., Brady, M., & Corey J. P. (1993). Hypersensitivity to latex in healthcare. *Otolaryngology Head and Neck Surgery, 109*, 731–734.

Shandor, A. (2012, May). *The health impacts of nursing shift work* (MSN thesis). Minnesota State University.

Sherman, R., & Blum, C. (2019). Finding joy in the workplace. *American Journal of Nursing, 19*(4), 66–69.

Simonowitz, J. (1994). Violence in the workplace: You're entitled to protection. *Registered Nurse, 57*(11), 61–63.

Slattery, M. (1998, September/October). Caring for ourselves to care for our patients. *The American Nurse,* 12–13.

Spector, J., & Reul, N. (2017). Promoting early, safe return to work in injured employees: A randomized trial of a supervisor training intervention in a healthcare setting. *Journal of Occupational Rehabilitation, 27*(1), 70–81. https://doi.org/10.1007/s10926-016-9633-6

Strader, M. K., & Decker, P. J. (1995). *Role transition to patient care management.* Appleton & Lange.

Trossman, S. (1999, May/June). When workplace threats become a reality. *The American Nurse, 1*, 12.

Trossman, S. (2011, May/June). Texas Nurses Association promoting enhanced nurse protection. *The American Nurse, 43*(3), 11.

U.S. Department of Labor. (1995). *Employee workplace rights and responsibilities.* OSHA.

Vahey, D., Aiken, L., Sloane, D., Clarke, S., & Vargas, D. (2004). Nurse burnout and patient satisfaction. *Medical Care, 42*(2), II-57–II-66.

Watson, C. L., & O'Connor, T. (2017). Legislating for advocacy: The case of whistleblowing. *Nursing Ethics, 24*(3), 305–312.

Wey, S. A. (2016). Healthcare and social service settings in OSHA's crosshairs. *The Florida Bar Journal, 90*(5), 42–45.

Wilkes, L. M., Peters, K., Weaver, R., & Jackson, D. (2011). Nurses involved in whistleblowing incidents:

Sequelae for their families. *Collegian, 18,* 101–106. https://doi.org/10.1016/j.colegn.2011.05.001

Chapter 13 References

Africa, L., & Trepanier, S. (2021). The role of the nurse leader in reversing the new graduate nurse Intent to leave. *Nurse Leader, 19*(3), 239–245. https://doi.org/10.1016/j.mnl.2021.02.013

Amendolair, D. (2012). Caring behaviors and job satisfaction. *Journal of Nursing Administration, 42*(1), 34–39.

American Association of University Women. (2018). *Know your rights at work: Sexual harassment, employee's guide: Sexually harassed—What should I do next?* https://www.aauw.org/what-we-do/legal-resources/know-your-rights-at-work/workplace-sexual-harassment/employees-guide

American Hospital Association, 2022. https://www.aha.org/fact-sheets/2022-06-07-fact-sheet-workplace-violence-anda-intimidation-and-need-federal-legislative

American Nurses Association. (2011). *2011 ANA health and safety survey.* https://www.nursingworld.org/practice-policy/work-environment/health-safety/health-safety-survey/

American Nurses Association. (2015). *Code of ethics for nurses with interpretive statements.* nursebooks.org

American Nurses Association. (2017). *Healthy nurses, healthy nation.* https://www.healthynursehealthynation.org/about/about-hnhn/

American Nurses Foundation (2022). *COVID-19 Two year impact assessment.* https://www.nursingworld.org/~4a2260/contentassets/872ebb13c63f44f-6b11a1bd0c74907c9/covid-19-two-year-impact-assessment-written-report-final.pdf

American Psychological Association. (2019, October). Discrimination: What it is and how to cope. https://www.apa.org/topics/racism-bias-discrimination/types-stress

ANA Ethics Advisory Board. (2019, June 7). ANA position statement: The nurse's role in addressing discrimination: Protecting and promoting inclusive strategies in practice settings, policy, and advocacy. *OJIN: The Online Journal of Issues in Nursing, 24*(3).

Annie E. Casey Foundation. (2021, April 14). *Equity vs. equality and other racial justice definitions.* https://www.aecf.org/blog/racial-justice-definitions

Baclig, J. (2015). *Compassion fatigue: Tips for coping.* Rn.com. https://www.rn.com/compassion-fatigue-tips-for-coping/

Beck, M. (2012, June 19). Anxiety can bring out the best. *Wall Street Journal,* D1.

Birks, M., Cant, R. P., Budden, L. M., Russell-Westhead, M., Sinem Üzar Özçetin, Y., & Tee, S. (2017). Original research: Uncovering degrees of workplace bullying: A comparison of baccalaureate nursing students' experiences during clinical placement in Australia and the UK. *Nurse Education in Practice, 25,* 14–21. https://doi.org/10.1016/j.nepr.2017.04.011

Blake, N. (2012). Practical steps for implementing healthy work environments. *Creating a Healthy Workplace, 23*(1), 14–17.

Boston-Fleischhauer,C. (2022). Confronting the workforce tsunami: Nonnegotiable tactics to reverse the exodus of RNs. *Journal of Nursing Administration,*

52(1), 1–3. https://doi.org/10.1097/NNA.0000000000001093

Bowers, R. (1993). Stress and your health. *National Women's Health Report, 15*(3), 6.

Burke, R. J., Ng, E. S., & Wolpin, J. (2011). Nursing staff work experiences, work outcomes and psychological well-being in difficult times: Implications for improving nursing staff quality of work life and hospital. *ISGUC: The Journal of Industrial Relations & Human Resources, 13*(2), 9–22. https://doi.org/10.4026/1303-2860.2010.0170.x

Campinha-Bacote, J. (2002). The process of cultural competence in the delivery of healthcare services: A model of care. *Journal of Transcultural Nursing, 13*(3), 181–184.

Carter, K., Crewe, S., Joyner, M., McClain, A., Sheperis, C., & Townsell, S. (2020). *Educating health professions educators to address the "isms." NAM Perspectives.* Commentary, National Academy of Medicine. https://doi.org/10.31478/202008e

Cogin, J., & Fish, A. (2009). Sexual harassment—a touchy subject for nurses. *Journal of Health Organization and Management, 23*(4), 442–462. https://doi.org/10.1108/14777260910979326

Crawford, S. (1993). Job stress and occupational health nursing. *American Association of Occupational Health Nurses Journal, 41*, 522–529.

Davidhizar, R., Dowd, S., & Giger, J. (1999). Managing diversity in the healthcare workplace. *Health Care Supervisor, 17*(3), 51–62.

Davidson, J. (1999). *Managing stress* (2nd ed.). Pearson.

Davis, M., Eshelman, E., & McCay, M. (2000). *The relaxation and stress reduction workbook* (5th ed.). New Harbinger Publications.

Dempsey, C., & Reilly, B. (2016, January 31). Nurse engagement: What are the contributing factors for success? *OJIN: The Online Journal of Issues in Nursing, 21*(1), 2. https://doi.org/10.3912/OJIN.Vol21No01Man02

Duckworth, A., Peterson, C., Matthews, M., & Kelly, D. (2007). Grit: Perseverance and passion for long-term goals. *Journal of Personality and Social Psychology, 92*(6), 1087–111. https://psycnet.apa.org/record/2007-07951-009?doi=1

Duquette, A., Sandhu, B., & Beaudet, L. (1994). Factors related to nursing burnout: A review of empirical knowledge. *Issues in Mental Health Nursing, 15*, 337–358.

Edgoose, J., Quiogue, M., & Sidhar, K. (2019). How to identify, understand, and unlearn implicit bias in patient care. *Family Practice Management, 26*(4), 29–33.

Ellrich, M., & Nelson, B. (2020). *Nurse turnover, part 2: What managers can do.* Workplace. https://www.gallup.com/workplace/295511/nurse-turnover-part-managers.aspx

Evans, G. W., Becker, F. D., Zahn, A., Bilotta, E., & Keesee, A. M. (2011). Capturing the ecology of workplace stress with cumulative risk assessment. *Environment and Behavior, 44*(1), 136–154.

Feeley, D., & Swensen, S. J. (2016). Restoring joy in work for the healthcare workforce. *Healthcare Executive, 31*(5), 70–71.

Gallup. (2022). Building a high-development culture through your employee engagement strategy. Gallup, Inc; Washington, D.C.

https://www.gallup.com/workplace/355082/employee-engagement-strategy-paper.aspx?utm_source=google&utm_medium=cpc&utm_campaign=new_workplace_non_branded_employee_engagement&utm_term=&gclid=CjOKCQiAyMKbBhD1ARIsANs7rEGjDRNeGXr9PwmKMzJrtXyIYRTPq5iKLtgpTKFTdpAXUQehnJlRLoAaApDxEALw_wcB&thank-you-report-form=1

Gelinas, L. (2018). Listening as a caring competency: Effective listening can make you a better nurse. *American Nurse Today, 13*(10), 4-5.

Golin, M., Buchlin, M., & Diamond, D. (1991). *Secrets of executive success.* Rodale Press.

Goliszek, A. (1992). *Sixty-six second stress management: The quickest way to relax and ease anxiety.* New Horizon.

Grant, S., Davidson. J., Manges, K., Dermenchyan, A., Wilson E., & Dowdell, E. (2020, June). Creating. healthful work environments to deliver on the quadruple aim: A call to action. *Journal of Nursing Administration. 50*(6), 314-321. https://doi.org/10.1097/NNA.0000000000000891.

Gustafsson, T., & Hemberg, J. (2022). Compassion fatigue as bruises in the soul: A qualitative study on nurses. *Nursing Ethics, 29*(1), 157–170.

Healy, S., & Tyrrell, M. (2011). Stress in emergency departments: Experiences of nurses and doctors. *Emergency Nurse, 19*(4), 31–37.

Henson, J. (2020). Burnout or compassion fatigue: A comparison of concepts. *MEDSURG Nursing, The Journal of Adult Health, 29*(2), 77–81, 95.

Hoolahan, S. E., & Greenhouse, P. K. (2012). Energy capacity model for nurses: The impact of relaxation and restoration. *Journal of Nursing Administration, 42*(2), 103–109.

Hughes, V., Delva, S., Nkimbeng, M., Spaulding, E., Turkson-Ocran, R. A., Cudjoe, J., . . . & Han, H. R. (2020). Not missing the opportunity: Strategies to promote cultural humility among future nursing faculty. *Journal of Professional Nursing, 36*(1), 28-33.

Hurst, K. L., Croker, P. A., & Bell, S. K. (1994). How about a lollipop? A peer recognition program. *Nursing Management, 25*(9), 68–73.

Johnson, L. (2011, August). Easing workplace stressors. *Healthcare Traveler, 19*(2), 28–34.

Kalisch, B. J., Lee, H., & Rochman, M. (2010). Nursing staff teamwork and job satisfaction. *Journal of Nursing Management, 18*, 938–947.

Kear, M. (2012, December). Caring and civility go hand-in-hand. *The Florida Nurse, 69*(4), 1, 3.

Lambert, C.E., & Lambert. V.A. (1987). Hardiness: Its development and relevance to nursing. *Journal of Nursing Scholarship, 19*(2), 92-95. https://doi.org/10.1111/j.1547-5069.1987.tb00600.x

Leana, C., Meuris, J., & Lamberton, C. (2018). More than a feeling: The role of empathetic care in promoting safety in health care. *ILR Review, 71*, 0019793917720432.

Leininger, M.M. (1999). What is transcultural nursing and culturally competent care? *Journal of Transcultural Nursing, 10*(1), 9. https://doi.org/10.1177/104365969901000105

Lenson, B. (2001). *Good stress—Bad stress.* Marlowe and Company.

Lewis, P. S., & Malecha, A. (2011). The impact of work-place incivility on the work environment, manager skill and productivity. *Journal of Nursing Administration, 41*(7/8), S17–S24.

Maslach, C., & Leiter, M. P. (2016). Burnout. In Stress: Concepts, cognition, emotion, and behavior, *Academic Press*, 351-357.

McClendon, S., & Farbman, R. (2018, February 1). *ANA addresses sexual harassment as part of # endnurseabuse initiative*. https://www.nursingworld .org/news/news-releases/2018/ana-addresses -sexual-harassment-as-part-of-endnurseabuse -initiative/

McGibbon, E., Peter, E., & Gallop, R. (2010). An institutional ethnography of nurses' stress. *Qualitative Health Research, 20*(11), 1353–1378.

McVicar, A. (2003). Workplace stress in nursing: A literature review. *Journal of Advanced Nursing, 44*(6), 633–642.

McVicar, A. (2016). Scoping the common antecedents of job stress and job. *Journal of Nursing Management, 24*, E112–E136. https://doi.org/10.1111/jonm .12326

Meyer, G., Shatto, B., Kuljeerung, O., Nuccio, L., Bergen,A., & Wilson, C. (2020). Exploring the relationship between resilience and grit among nursing students: A correlational research study. *Nurse Education Today, 84*, 104246. https://doi.org/10.1016/j .nedt.2019.104246

Mitchell, A. (1995). Cultural diversity: The future, the market and the rewards. *Caring, 14*(12), 44–48.

Murthy, V. (2022, May 23). *New surgeon general advisory sounds alarm on health worker burnout and resignation*. HHS.gov. https://www.hhs.gov /about/news/2022/05/23/new-surgeon-general -advisory-sounds-alarm-on-health-worker-burnout-and -resignation.html

Narayan, M. (2019). Addressing implicit bias in nursing: A review. *American Journal of Nursing, 119*(7), 36–43.

National Academy of Medicine. (2019). *National plan for health workforce well-being—draft for public input.* https://nam.edu/wp-content/uploads/2022/05 /NAM-National-Plan-for-Health-Workforce-Well-Being -DRAFT-FOR-PUBLIC-INPUT-5.20.22.pdf

National Institute for Occupational Safety and Health. (1999). *Stress at work.* Publication dissemination, EID; Cincinnati, OH, p. 6. https://www.cdc.gov/niosh /docs/99-101/default.html

National Institute for Occupational Safety and Health. (2022). *Stress at work.* Publication dissemination, EID; Cincinnati, OH, https://www.cdc.gov/niosh /docs/99-101/default.html

Nejati, A., Shepley, M., Rodiek, S., Lee, C., & Varni, J. (2016). Restorative design features for hospital staff break areas: A multi-method study. *Health Environments Research & Design Journal, 9*(2), 16–35.

Nowak, K., & Pentkowski, A. (1994). Lifestyle habits, substance use, and predictors of job burnout in professional women. *Work and Stress, 8*(1), 19–35.

Outwater, L. C. (1994). Sexual harassment issues. *Caring, 13*(5), 54–56, 58, 60.

Paine, W. S. (1984). Professional burnout: Some major costs. *Family and Community Health, 6*(4), 1–11.

Perlo, J., Balik, B., Swensen, S., Kabcenell, A., Landsman, J., & Feeley, D. (2017). *IHI framework for improving joy in work* (IHI white paper). Institute for Healthcare Improvement.

Peterson, K. (2016). Recognition: Is it just a bunch of fluff, or is it the right stuff? *Journal of Pediatric Nursing, 31*(2), 228–229. https:// www.sciencedirect.com/science/article/pii /S0882596315004066?via%3Dihub

Pines, A. (2004). Adult attachment styles and their relationship to burnout: A preliminary, cross-cultural investigation. *Work & Stress, 18*(1), 66–80.

Purcell, S. R., Keitash, M., & Cobb, S. (2011). The relationship between nurses' stress and nurse staffing factors in a hospital setting. *Journal of Nursing Management, 19*, 714–720.

Riahi, S. (2011). Role stress amongst nurses at the workplace: Concept analysis. *Journal of Nursing Management, 19*, 1721–1731.

Roach, M. S. (2022). *Caring, the human mode of being* (2nd ed.). CHA Press.

Roberts, R. K., & Grubb, P. L. (2014). The consequences of nursing stress and need for integrated solutions. *Rehabilitation Nursing: The Official Journal of the Association of Rehabilitation Nurses, 39*(2), 62–69. https://doi.org/10.1002/rnj.97

Rocker, C. (2012, September 24). Responsibility of a frontline manager regarding staff bullying. *OJIN: The Online Journal of Issues in Nursing, 18*(2).

Ross, S., Naumann, P., Hinds-Jackson, D. V., & Stokes, L. (2019, January 31). Sexual harassment in nursing: Ethical considerations and recommendations. *OJIN: The Online Journal of Issues in Nursing, 24*(1), 1.

Sabo, B. (2011). Reflecting on the concept of compassion fatigue. *The Online Journal of Issues in Nursing, 16*(1), 1.

Salmela, L., Woehrle, T., Marleau, E., & Kitch, L. (2020). Implementation of a "serenity room." *Nursing, 50*(10), 58–63.

Schmidt, B., MacWilliams, B., & Neal-Boylan, L. (2016). Becoming inclusive: A code of conduct for inclusion and diversity. *Journal of Professional Nursing, 33*(2), 102-107. https://www.sciencedirect.com/science /article/pii/S8755722316301302?casa _token=skYi71NkVYgAAAAA:hkEnHDrs1VXA e7PIW-zNiT5QNiWxXtxTdY8RHUnwJVB2iINi- bP923MSNHZi6c-O8vZoph qCM1M

Seago, J. A., Spetz, J., Ash, M., Herrera, C-N., & Keane, D. (2011). Hospital RN job satisfaction and nurse unions. *Journal of Nursing Administration, 41*(3), 109–114.

Sellers, K. F., & Millenbach, L. (2012). The degree of horizontal violence in RNs practicing in New York State. *Journal of Nursing Administration, 42*(10), 483–487.

Shellenbarger, S. (2012, October 10). To cut office stress, try butterflies and meditation? *The Wall Street Journal,* D2.

Sherman, R., & Blum, C. (2019). Finding joy in the workplace. *American Journal of Nursing, 19*(4), 66–69.

Smith, L. M., Andrusyszyn, M. A., & Spence-Laschinger, H. K. S. (2010). Effects of workplace incivility and empowerment on newly-graduated nurses' organizational commitment. *Journal of Nursing Management, 18*, 1004–1015.

Stubbe, D. E. (2020). Practicing cultural competence and cultural humility in the care of diverse patients. *Focus*

(American Psychiatric Publication), 18(1), 49-51. https://doi.org/10.1176/appi.focus.20190041.

Taylor, R. (2016). Nurses' perceptions of horizontal violence. *Global Qualitative Nursing Research, 3,* 2333393616641002. https://doi.org/10.1177/2333393616641002

Teague, J. B. (1992). The relationship between various coping styles and burnout among nurses. *Dissertation Abstracts International,* 1994.

Terry, P. E. (2018). Why health promotion needs to change. *American Journal of Health Promotion, 32*(1), 13–15. https://doi.org/10.1177/0890117117745445

The Joint Commission. (2022). R3 Report Issue 30: Workplace violence prevention standards. https://www.jointcommission.org/standards/r3-report/r3-report-issue-30-workplace-violence-prevention-standards/#.Y7sSK3bMJPa

Thobaben, M. (2007). Horizontal workplace violence. *Home Health Care Management & Practice. 20*(1), 82-83. https://doi.org/10.1177/1084822307305723

Trépanier, S., Fernet, C., Austin, S., & Boudrias, V. (2016). Review: Work environment antecedents of bullying: A review and integrative model applied to registered nurses. *International Journal of Nursing Studies, 55,* 85–97. https://doi.org/10.1016/j.ijnurstu.2015.10.001

Tucker, S. J., Weymiller, A. J., Cutshall, S. M., Rhudy, L. M., & Lohse, C. M. (2012). Stress ratings and health promotion practices among RNs. *Journal of Nursing Administration, 42*(5), 282–292.

Tully, S., & Tao, H. (2019). CE: Original research: Work-related stress and positive thinking among acute care nurses: A cross-sectional survey. *The American Journal of Nursing, 119*(5), 24-31.

u Long, K.A. (2003). The Institute of Medicine Report: Health Professions Education: A Bridge to Quality. *Policy, Politics, & Nursing Practice. 4*(4), 259-262. https://doi.org/10.1177/1527154403258304

Upton, K. (2018). An investigation into compassion fatigue and self-compassion in acute medical care hospital nurses: A mixed methods study. *Journal of Compassionate Health Care, 5*(7), 1–27. https://jcompassionatehc.biomedcentral.com/track/pdf/10.1186/s40639-018-0050-x.pdf

U.S. Census Bureau. (2020). *Quick facts.* https://www.census.gov/quickfacts/fact/table/US/PST045221

U.S. Department of Health and Human Services. (2022).

Wei, H., Sewell, K., Woody, G., & Rose, M. (2018). The state of the science of nurse work environments in the United States: A systematic review. *International Journal of Nursing Sciences, 5*(3), 287–300. https://doi.org/10.1016/j.ijnss.2018.04.010

Zwickel, K., Koppel, J., Katz, M., Virkstis, K., Rothenberger, S., & Boston-Fleischhauer, C. (2016). Providing professional meaningful recognition to enhance frontline engagement. *Journal of Nursing Administration, 46*(7/8), 355–356.

Chapter 14 References

Allnurses. (2018). *How to be SMART with goals.* https://allnurses.com/general-nursing-discussion/how-to-be-1136964.html

Anderson, J. (1992). Tips on résumé writing. *Imprint, 39*(1), 30–31.

Arvidsson, B., Skarsater, I., Oijervall, J., & Friglund, B. (2008). Process-oriented group supervision during nursing education: Nurses' conception one year after their nursing degree. *Journal of Nursing Management, 16*(7), 868–875.https://doil:10.1111/j.1365-2834.2008.00925.x

Banis, W. (1994). The art of writing job-search letters. In College Placement Council, Inc. (Ed.), *Planning job choices* (pp. 44–51). College Placement Council.

Beal, K. (2016). Mentoring new nurses. *American Journal of Nursing, 116*(10), 13. https://doi.org/10.1097/01.NAJ.0000503278.70682.ab

Beatty, R. (1989). *The perfect cover letter.* John Wiley & Sons.

Beatty, R. (1991). *Get the right job in 60 days or less.* John Wiley & Sons.

Bhasin, R. (1998). Do's and don'ts of job interviews. *Pulp & Paper, 72*(2), 37.

Bischof, J. (1993). Preparing for job interview questions. *Critical Care Nurse, 13*(4), 97–100. https://doi.org/10.4037/ccn1993.13.4.97

Borgatti, J. C. (2010). Choose a job you love and you will never have to work. *American Nurse Today, 5*(2). https://www.americannursetoday.com/plan-a-career-not-just-a-job-2/

Bureau of Labor Statistics. (2017). *Employment projections.* http://www.bls.gov/news.release/pdf/ecopro.pdf

Bureau of Labor Statistics (2022), *U.S. Department of Labor, Occupational Outlook Handbook, Registered Nurses.* https://www.bls.gov/ooh/healthcare/registered-nurses.htm

Carlson, K. (2017). *The nurses' guide to finding a job.* https://nurse.org/articles/nursing-job-search-guide/

Cazacu, A. (2010). *What are employers looking for in a candidate?* http://ezinearticles.com/?What-Are-Employers-Looking-For-in-a-Candidate?&id=4738932

Chestnut, T. (1999). Some tips on taking the fear out of résumé writing. *Phoenix Business Journal, 19*(47), 28.

Costlow, T. (1999). How not to create a good first impression. *Fairfield County Business Journal, 38*(32), 17.

Eubanks, P. (1991). Experts: Making your résumé an asset. *Hospitals, 5*(20), 74.

Evenden, I. (2022). *Best resume writing apps 2022.* https://www.toptenreviews.com/best-resume-writing-software

Gaines, K. (2020). *Nursing career paths: How to become a nurse and advance your career.* https://nurse.org/education/nursing-career-paths/

Gibson, A. (2018). Ultimate guide to nursing resumés. *Nurse.org Career Guide Series.* https://nurse.org/resources/nursing-resume/

Gray, J. (2012). Building resilience in the nursing workforce. *Nursing Standard, 26*(32), 1. https://doi.org/10.7748/ns2012.04.26.32.1.p8058

Green, A. (2016, February 29). How to prepare for a second interview. *U.S. News and World Report.* https://money.usnews.com/money/blogs/outside-voices-careers/articles/2016-02-29/how-to-prepare-for-a-second-interview

Hart, K. (2006). Student extra: The employment interview: Tips for success selecting an employer for the perfect fit. *American Journal of Nursing, 106*(4), 72AAA–72CCC.

Health Resources and Services Administration. (2017). *Supply and demand projections of the nursing workforce: 2014–2024.* U.S. Department of Health and

Human Services. https://bhw.hrsa.gov/sites/default /files/bhw/nchwa/projections/NCHWA_HRSA _Nursing_Report.pdf

Health Resources and Services Administration. (2021). *Projecting health workforce supply and demand.* https://bhw.hrsa.gov/data-research/projecting-health -workforce-supply-demand

Hu, H., Wang, C., Lan, Y., & Wu, X. (2022). Nurses' turn-over intention, hope and career identity: The mediating role of job satisfaction. *BMC Nursing, 21*(43). https:// doi.org/10.1186/s12912-022-00821-5

Impollonia, M. (2004, March). How to impress nursing recruiters to get the job you want. *Imprint.*

Indeed.com. (2020). *The six most important parts of a resume with examples.* https://www.indeed.com /career-advice/resumes-cover-letters/parts-of-a-resume

Indeed.com. (2020).

Institute of Medicine. (2001). *Crossing the quality chasm: A new health system for the 21st century.* National Academies Press.

Institute of Medicine. (2011). *The future of nursing: Leading change, advancing health.* National Academies Press.

Job Hunt. (2018). *The online job search guide.* http:// www.job-hunt.org/

Johnson, K. (1999). Interview success demands research, practice, preparation. *Houston Business Journal, 30*(23), 38.

Klein, E., & Dickenson-Hazard, N. (2000). The spirit of mentoring. *Reflections on Nursing Leadership, 26*(3), 18–22.

Korkki, P. (2010, February 27). Writing a résumé that shouts "Hire me." *New York Times.*

Krannich, C., & Krannich, R. (1993). *Interview for success.* Impact Publications.

Kuokkanen, L., Leino-Kilpi, H., Katajisto, J., Heponiemi, T., Sinervo, T., & Elovaninio, M. (2014). Does organizational justice predict empowerment? Nurses assess their work environment. *Journal of Nursing Scholarship, 46*(5), 349–356.

Marino, K. (2000). *Resumes for the health care professional.* John Wiley & Sons.

Martin, M. (2019, October 10). Find out how to analyze your career and goals with the SWOT method. *Business News Daily.* https://www.businessnewsdaily. com/5543-personal-swot-analysis.html

Mascolini, M., & Supnick, R. (1993). Preparing students for the behavioral job interview. *Journal of Business and Technical Communication, 7*(4), 482–488.

Moon, K. (2018). The ultimate guide to ace-ing your SKYPE™ interview. *TheMuse.* https://www.themuse.com/advice/ the-ultimate-guide-to-acing-your-skype-interview

Morgan, H. (2013, June 26). The 8 new rules of a career survivalist. *U.S. News and World Report.* http:// money.usnews.com/money/blogs/outside-voices -careers/2013/06/26/the-8-new-rules-of-a -career-survivalist

Narayanasamy, A., & Penney, V. (2014). Coaching to promote professional development in nursing practice. *British Journal of Nursing, 23*(11), 568–573. https:// doi.org/10.12968/bjon.2014.23.11.568

Papandrea, D. (2017). *Getting the nursing job: Resume tips for RNs.* https://nurse.org/articles/getting-the -nursing-job-resume-tips-for-rns/

Papandrea, D. (2018). *10 tips for landing your first nursing job: Even with no experience.* https://nurse.org /articles/tips-on-applying-for-your-first-nursing-job/

Parker, Y. (1989). *The damn good résumé guide.* Ten Speed Press.

Quast, L. (2013, April 15). How to conduct a personal SWOT analysis. *Forbes.* https://www.forbes.com /sites/lisaquast/2013/04/15/how-to-conduct-a -personal-s-w-o-t-analysis/#5a0afad28d8b

Rees, C. S., Heritage, B., Osseiran-Moisson, R., Chamberlain, D., Cusack, L., Anderson, J., Terry, V., Rogers, C., Hemsworth, D., Cross, W.,& Hegney, D. G. (2016). Can we predict burnout among student nurses? An exploration of the ICWR-1 model of individual psychological resilience. *Frontiers in Psychology, 7*, 1072. https://doi.org/10.3389/fpsyg .2016.01072

Shellenbarger, T., & Robb, M. (2016). Effective mentoring in the clinical setting. *American Journal of Nursing, 116*(4), 64–68. https://doi.org/10.1097/01 .NAJ.0000482149.37081.61

Sparacino, L. L. (2016). Faculty's role in assisting new graduate nurses' adjustment to practice. *Sage Open Nursing, 2*(1), 1–9. https://doi.org/10.1177 /23779608166351

Tyler, L. (1990). Watch out for "red flags" on a job interview. *Hospitals, 64*(14), 46–47.

Uzialko, A. C. (2018, March 15). The best fonts to use on your resume. *Business News Daily.* https://www .businessnewsdaily.com/5331-best-resume-fonts.html

Walsh, A. L. (2018). Nurse residency programs and the benefits for new graduate nurses. *Pediatric Nursing, 44*(6), 275–279.

Williamson, E. (2021). *Ensure you love your first nursing job: Choose wisely.* https://www.nurse.com /blog/2021/12/01/love-first-nursing-job-choose -wisely/

Yilmaz, E. B. (2017). Resilience as a strategy for struggling against challenges related to the nursing profession. *Chinese Nursing Research, 4*(1), 9–13. https:// doi.org/10.1016/j.cnre.2017.03.004

Zedlitz, R. (2003). *How to get a job in health care.* Delmar Learning.

Zhang, L. (2018). 30 behavioral interview questions you should be prepared to answer. *The Muse.* https:// www.themuse.com/advice/30-behavioral-interview -questions-you-should-be-ready-to-answer

Chapter 15 References

Accreditation Commission for Education in Nursing. (n.d.). https://www.acenursing.org/

Ana enterprise strategic plan 2020-2022. ANA. (2020, March 5). Retrieved January 24, 2023, from https:// www.nursingworld.org/ana-enterprise/about-us/anae -strategic-plan-2020–2023/

American Nursing Association. (2022). *Advocacy.* https://www.nursingworld.org/practice-policy /advocacy/

Benner, P. (2001). *From novice to expert: Excellence and power in clinical nursing practice. Commemorative Edition.* Prentice Hall.

Bureau of Labor Statistics, U.S. Department of Labor. (2022). *Occupational outlook handbook, registered nurses.* https://www.bls.gov/ooh/healthcare /registered-nurses.htm

Burr, S., Stichler, J. F., & Poeltler, D. (2011). Establishing a mentoring program. *Nursing for Women's Health, 15*(3), 214–224. https://doi.org/10.1111/j .1751-486X.2011.01636.x

Canadian Nurses Association. (2022). *CNA position statements.* https://www.cna-aiic.ca/en/policy-advocacy/policy-support-tools/position-statements

Cappel, C. A., Hoak, P. L., & Karo, P. A. (2013). Nurse residency programs: What nurses need to know. *Pennsylvania Nurse, 68*(4), 22–28.

Children's National Hospital. (2022). *Children's National Hospital - Ranked #5 in the nation and #1 for newborn care.* https://childrensnational.org/

Citron, J. M., & Smith, R. A. (2003). *The five patterns of extraordinary careers: The guide for achieving success and satisfaction.* Crown Business.

Cottingham, S., DiBartolo, M. C., Battistoni, S., & Brown, T. (2011). Partners in nursing: A mentoring initiative to enhance nurse retention. *Nursing Education Perspectives, 32*(4), 250–255.

Edwards, D., Edwards, D., Hawker, C., Carrier, J., & Rees, C. (2015). A systematic review of the effectiveness of strategies and interventions to improve the transition from student to newly qualified nurse. *International Journal of Nursing Studies, 52*(7), 1254–1268. https://doi.org/10.1016/j.ijnurstu.2015.03.007

Ellisen, K. (2011). Mentoring smart. *Nursing Management, 42*(8), 12–16. https://doi.org/10.1097/01.NUMA.0000399804.14328.bc

Goode, C., Lynn, M., Krsek, C., Bednash, G., & Jannetti, A. (2009). Nurse residency programs: An essential requirement for nursing. *Nursing Economic$, 27*(3), 142–159.

Harrington, S. (2011). Mentoring new nurse practitioners to accelerate their development as primary care providers: A literature review. *Journal of the American Association of Nurse Practitioners, 23*(4), 168–174. https://doi.org/10.1111/j.1745-7599.2011.00601.x

Home. Home - American Academy of Nursing Main Site. (n.d.). https://www.aannet.org/home

Jakubik, L. D. (2008). Jump starting your nursing career: Toolbox for success. *The Pennsylvania Nurse, 63*(1), 4–7.

Jones-Bell, L. J., Halford-Cook, C., & Parker, N. W. (2018). Transition to practice–Part 3: Implementing an ambulatory care registered nurse residency program: RN residency and transition to professional practice programs in ambulatory care–Challenges, successes, and recommendations. *Nursing Economics, 36*(1), 35–45.

Kramer, M. (1974). *Reality shock: Why nurses leave nursing.* CV Mosby.

Kramer, M., & Schmalenberg, C. (1993). Learning from success: Autonomy and empowerment. *Nursing Management, 24*(5), 58.

Professionalism and Canadian nursing. *On All Frontiers: Four Centuries of Canadian Nursing,* 197–211.

Murphy, L. J., & Janisse, L. (2017). Optimizing transition to practice through orientation: A quality improvement initiative. *Clinical Simulation in Nursing, 13*(11), 583–590.

National League for Nursing. (2022). About NLN. http://www.nln.org/about

National Student Nurses' Association. (2022). *About us.* http://www.nsna.org/about-nsna.html

U.S. Department of Health and Human Services. (n.d.). *NINR.* National Institute of Nursing Research. https://www.ninr.nih.gov/

Nurse Journal. (2018). *BSN vs. MSN degree. Which is best?* https://nursejournal.org/bsn-degree/bsn-vs-msn-degree/

NursingExplorer. (2022). *Nursing education & career resource website.* Nursing Explorer. https://www.nursingexplorer.com/

Organization for Associate Degree Nursing. (2022). *About OADN.* https://oadn.org/about/

Rush, K. L., Adamack, M., Gordon, J., & Janke, R. (2014). New graduate nurse transition programs: Relationships with bullying and access to support. *Contemporary Nurse, 48*(2), 219–228. https://doi.org/10.5172/conu.2014.48.2.219

Shirey, M. R. (2009). Building an extraordinary career in nursing: Promise, momentum, and harvest. *The Journal of Continuing Education in Nursing, 40*(9), 394–400. https://doi.org/10.3928/00220124-20090824-01

Strauss, E., Ovnat, C., Gonen, A., Lev-Ari, L., & Mizrahi, A. (2016). Student experience research paper: Do orientation programs help new graduates? *Nurse Education Today, 36,* 422–426. https://doi.org/10.1016/j.nedt.2015.09.002

Va.gov home. Veterans Affairs. (n.d.). Retrieved January 23, 2023, from https://www.va.gov/

Weng, R. H., Huang, C. Y., Tsai, W. C., Chang, L. Y., Lin, S. E., & Lee, M. Y. (2010). Exploring the impact of mentoring functions on job satisfaction and organizational commitment of new staff nurses. *BMC Health Services Research, 10*(1), 240. https://doi.org/10.1186/1472-6963-10-240

Zigmont, J. J., Wade, A., Edwards, T., Hayes, K., Mitchell, J., & Oocumma, N. (2015). Featured article: Utilization of experiential learning, and the learning outcomes model reduces RN orientation time by more than 35%. *Clinical Simulation in Nursing, 11,* 79–94. https://doi.org/10.1016/j.ecns.2014.11.001

Chapter 16 References

Adamy, J., & Radnofsky, L. (2012). Health law slow to win favor. *Wall Street Journal,* A1, A12.

Affordable Care Act. (2010). http://www.hhs.gov/healthcare/rights

Aiken, L. H., Clarke, S. P., Sloane, D. M., Sochalski, J., & Silber, J. H. (2002). Hospital nurse staffing and patient mortality, nurse burnout, and job dissatisfaction. *JAMA, 288*(16), 1987–1993. https://doi.org/10.1001/jama.288.16.1987

Alkema, G. E. (2016). Bringing the pieces together: Person-centeredness is key to transforming policy and services. *Generations, 40*(4), 94–100.

American Nurses Association. (2009, September 15). *Testimony before the Democratic Steering and Policy Committee, U.S. House of Representatives forum on the urgent need for health care reform.* www.nursingworld/news/news-releases/2017-news-releases/American-nurses-Association-urges-congress-to-work- on-bipartisan-solutions

American Nurses Association. (2013, July). *Health care reform.* https://www.nursingworld.org/practice-policy/health-policy/health-system-reform/

Anderson, L. M., Scrimshaw, S. C., Fullilove, M. T., Fielding, J. E., & Normand, J. (2003). Culturally competent healthcare systems: A systematic review. *American Journal of Preventive Medicine, 24*(3S), 68–79. https://doi.org/10.1016/s0749-3797(02)00657-8

Anonymous. (2013). Utah faces off with Obama over health care exchanges. *Huffington Post.* http://www.huffingtonpost.com/2013/01/03ut-health-care-reform_n_2403294.html

Bauchner, H. (2017). Health care in the United States: A right or a privilege. *Journal of the American Medical Association, 317*(1), 29. https://doi.org/10.1001/jama.2016.19687

Bever, L. (2018, February 2). "Wash your stinking hands!": ER nurse rants about "cesspool of funky flu." *Washington Post.* http://link.galegroup.com/apps/doc/A526098725/AONE?u=gale15691&sid=AONE&xid=6cea7b09

Bleich, M. R. (2012). Leadership responses to the future of nursing: Leading change, advancing health IOM report. *Journal of Nursing Administration, 42*(4), 108–184. https://doi.org/10.1097/NNA.0b013e31824ccc6b

Capretta, J. C. (2017). Building a broader consensus for health reform. *JAMA: Journal of the American Medical Association, 317*(22), 2273–2274. https://doi.org/10.1001/jama.2017.6689

Centers for Disease Control and Prevention. (2021, November 17). *Drug overdose deaths in the U.S. top 100,000 annually.* Centers for Disease Control and Prevention. https://www.cdc.gov/nchs/pressroom/nchs_press_releases/2021/20211117.htm

Cianelli, R., Clipper, B., Freeman, R., Goldstein, J., & Wyatt, T. H. (2016). The innovation road map: A guide for nurse leaders. *Innovation Works,* 1-35.

Close-Up Media, Inc. (2016, December 17). Canada's nurses release new survey findings. *Entertainment Close-Up.* http://link.galegroup.com/apps/doc/A474118277/ITOF?u=gale15691&sid=ITOF&xid=dcd62baa

Cohen, S. (2007). The image of nursing: How do others see us? How do we see ourselves? *American Nurse Today, 2*(5), 24–26.

Davis, S. (2015). *Be visionary, be visible, be vocal & add value.* https://drshirleydavis.com/blog/2015/08/06/be-visionary-be-visible-be-vocal-add-value/

Finkel, E. (2017). Being good neighbors. *Community College Journal, 88*(1), 26–32.

Fuchs, V. R. (2018). Is single payer the answer for the US health care system? *Journal of the American Medical Association, 319*(1), 15–16. https://doi.org/10.1001/jama.2017.18739

Hassmiller, S. B. (2011). Nursing leadership from bedside to boardroom. *Journal of Nursing Administration, 41*(7/8), 306–308. https://doi.org/10.1097/NNA.0b013e3182250a0d

Hassmiller, S. B., & Reinhard, S. C. (2015). A bold new vision for America's health care system. *Nursing Outlook, 63,* 41–47. https://doi.org/10.1016/j.outlook.2014.11.017

www.hse.ie/eng/about/who/nqpsd/qps-education/quality-improvement-toolkit.html

Healthcare.gov. (2022). Affordable Care Act (ACA) - Healthcare.gov Glossary." *HealthCare.gov,* https://www.healthcare.gov/glossary/affordable-care-act/.

Healthy People 2030. (2022) Lesbian, Gay, Bisexual, and Transgender Health Workgroup. https://health.gov/healthypeople/about/workgroups/lesbian-gay-bisexual-and-transgender-health-workgroup

Hewison, A., & Wildman, S. (2008). Looking back, looking forward: Enduring issues in nursing management. *Journal of Nursing Management, 16*(1), 1–3. https://doi.org/10.1111/j.1365-2934.2007.00839.x

Khoury, C. M., Blizzard, R., Moore, L. W., & Hassmiller, S. (2011). Nursing leadership from bedside to boardroom. *Journal of Nursing Administration, 41*(7/8), 299–305. https://doi.org/10.1097/NNA.0b013e3182250a0d

Mechanic, D. (2002). Sociocultural implications of changing organizational technologies in the provision of care. *Social Science and Medicine, 54,* 459–467. https://doi.org/10.1016/s0277-9536(01)00039-9

Motshedisi, E. C., Dirk, V. W., & Anna lie, B. (2015). Using appreciative inquiry to transform student nurses' image of nursing. *Curationis, 1,* 1. https://doi.org/10.4102/curationis.v38i1.1460

Nursingworld.org. Advocacy. *ANA* https://www.nursingworld.org/practice-policy/advocacy Gramlich, John.

Pew Research. (2022). "What the data says about gun deaths in the U.S." *Pew Research Center,* Pew Research Center.

Pogue, P. (2007). The nurse practitioner role. *Into the Future Nursing Leadership, 20*(2), 34–38. https://doi.org/10.12927/cjnl.2007.18900

Potter, P., & Mueller, J. R. (2007). How well do you know your patients? *Nursing Management, 38*(2), 40–41.

Redwanski, J. (2007). Is universal health care in our future? *Journal of Best Practices in Health Professions Diversity: Education, Research & Policy, 1*(2), 65-70.

Rosenbaum, S. (2011). The Patient Protection and Affordable Care Act: Implications for public health policy and practice. *Public Health Reports, 126,* 130–135. https://doi.org/10.1177/003335491112600118

Schoen, C., Doty, M., Robertson, R. H., & Collins, S. R. (2011). Affordable Care Act reforms could reduce the number of underinsured US adults by 70 percent. *Health Affairs, 3*(9), 1762–1771. https://doi.org/10.1377/hlthaff.2011.0335

Stein, R. (2017, December 21). *Life expectancy drops again as opioid deaths surge in U.S.* [Radio broadcast]. National Public Radio.

Summers, S., & Jacobs Summers, H. (2014). *Saving lives: Why the media's portrayal of nursing puts us all at risk.* Oxford University Press. https://doi.org/10.1093/acprof:oso/9780199337064.001.0001

Trinh, H. Q., & O'Connor, S. J. (2002). Helpful or harmful? The impact of strategic change on the performance of U.S. urban hospitals. *Health Services Research, 37*(1), 145–171. https://doi.org/10.1111/1475-6773.99208

U.S. Department of Health and Human Services. (2022). *Improving the Cybersecurity Posture of Healthcare in 2022.* https://www.hhs.gov/blog/2022/02/28

/improving-cybersecurity-posture-healthcare
-2022.html

Villeneuve, M., & MacDonald, J. (2006). *Toward
2020: Visions of nursing.* Canadian Nurses
Association.

Webb, J. A. K., & Marshall, D. R. (2010). Healthcare reform and nursing: What does it mean? *Journal of Nursing Administration, 40*(9), 345–347. https://doi
.org/10.1097/NNA.0b013e3181ee42d4

Wilson, L., Mendes, I. C., Klopper, H., Catrambone, C.,
Al-Maaitah, R., Norton, M. E., & Hill, M. (2016).
"Global health" and "global nursing": Proposed
definitions from the Global Advisory Panel on the
Future of Nursing. *Journal of Advanced Nursing,
72*(7), 1529–1540. https://doi.org/10.1111
/jan.12973

World Health Organization. (2012). *World health statistics 2012.* Author.

Index

References followed by the letter "f" are for figures, "t" are tables, and "b" are boxes.

331